Nurse's Guide to Successful Test-Taking

Nurse's guide

TO **SUCCESSFUL** TEST-TAKING

Marian B. Sides, R.N. , Ph.D.
Assistant Professor of Nursing, University of Wisconsin, Milwaukee, Wisconsin; Formerly, Associate Director of Nursing, University of Chicago Hospitals, Chicago, Illinois

Nancy Backus Cailles, R.N., M.S.N.
Assistant Professor of Nursing, Purdue University, Calumet, Hammond, Indiana

With 6 contributors

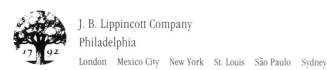

J. B. Lippincott Company
Philadelphia
London   Mexico City   New York   St. Louis   São Paulo   Sydney

Acquisitions Editor: Nancy Mullins
Coordinating Editorial Assistant: Ellen
  Campbell
Manuscript Editor: Helen Ewan
Indexer: Catherine Battaglia
Senior Design Coordinator: Anita Curry
Designer: Anne O'Donnell
Illustrations: Thomas L. Ingram

Production Manager: Carol A. Florence
Production Supervisor: Charlene Squibb
Production Coordinator: Pamela Milcos
Compositor: TAPSCO, Inc.
Printer/Binder: R. R. Donnelley and Sons
  Company

6 5 4 3

Library of Congress Cataloging in Publication Data

Sides, Marian B., [DATE]
  Nurse's guide to successful test-taking.

  Includes index.
    1. Nursing—Examinations.   2. Nursing.
  3. Nursing—Examinations, questions, etc.
  4. Reasoning (Psychology)—Problems, exercises, etc.
  I. Cailles, Nancy Backus. II. Title. [DNLM:
  1. Educational Measurement—nurses' instruction.
  2. Learning—nurses' instruction.   3. Nursing—
  examination questions.   4. Problem Solving—nurses'
  instruction. WY 18 S568n]
  RT55.S48   1989   610.73'076   88-23110
  ISBN 0-397-54689-0

Any procedure or practice described in this book should be applied by the health-care
practitioner under appropriate supervision in accordance with professional standards
of care used with regard to the unique circumstances that apply in each practice
situation. Care has been taken to confirm the accuracy of information presented and to
describe generally accepted practices. However, the authors, editors, and publisher
cannot accept any responsibility for errors or omissions or for consequences from
application of the information in this book and make no warranty, express or implied,
with respect to the contents of the book.
  Every effort has been made to ensure drug selections and dosages are in accordance
with current recommendations and practice. Because of ongoing research, changes in
government regulations, and the constant flow of information on drug therapy,
reactions, and interactions, the reader is cautioned to check the package insert for each
drug for indications, dosages, warnings, and precautions, particularly if the drug is new
or infrequently used.

To my mom, Evelyn, and my dad, Daniel,
in recognition of their constant support,
interest, and encouragement

MARIAN B. SIDES

In loving memory of Joyce A. Ellis Ed.D., R.N.,
teacher, mentor, friend

NANCY B. CAILLES

CONTRIBUTORS

Marytherese Balskus, R.N., M.S.N.
Chief Flight Nurse
University of Chicago Aeromedical
  Network
Chicago, Illinois

Diane M. Black, R.N., M.S.
Instructor, Medical Surgical Nursing
Thornton Community College
South Holland, Illinois

Ann Sheerer Filipski, R.N., M.S.N., C.S.
Assistant Professor, Psychiatric and
  Mental Health Nursing
St. Xavier College
Chicago, Illinois

Barbara Etling Murphy, R.N., M.S.N.
Perinatal Clinical Nurse Specialist
Washington Hospital
Fremont, California

Wayne Nagel, R.N., M.S.N.
Director, Harbor Home Support
  Services
Chicago, Illinois;
Lecturer, University of Wisconsin,
Milwaukee School of Nursing
Milwaukee, Wisconsin

Cynthia Smego, R.N., B.S.N.
Clinical Nurse Specialist
University of Chicago Hospitals
Chicago, Illinois

FOREWORD

The dilemmas of taking the entry examination for one's chosen profession are apparent to all who deal with individuals faced with taking this test, and to the test-takers themselves. Most adults face trepidation when they have to take tests, whether laboratory tests ordered by a family physician or those required on renewal of a driver's license. Those of us in continuing and staff development education recognize the anxiety in instructional situations when adult learners are required to take tests to assess the extent of their ability to grasp the material. Whether a pretest or post-test, or a final course examination, throughout an individual's learning experiences from childhood on, tests create uneasiness. The magnitude of a test that will permit or restrict the practice of one's professional career choice, then, becomes obvious.

What causes the apprehension, and what can be done about it? Surely, this extreme discomfort is not merely to be accepted as a rite of passage into the profession. There must be a way of easing the pain, whether or not it was assuaged for us.

In some academic situations, students are encouraged to form study groups, given sample test questions, and generally assisted with learning and applying appropriate test-taking behaviors in a specific circumstance. Unfortunately, the student's ability to transfer this experience to other academic courses often is finite. Although it worked for one course, the student frequently does not realize that the same activities will be effective in a subsequent course. If, in succeeding courses, faculty do not replicate these helpful tactics, the student's effective test-taking performance will cease.

Assistance with test-taking occurs less frequently in staff development situations, where passing a final examination after an orientation course may be required for assignment into the work area of a nurse's choice. Even success with the state board examination is not consistently transferred to test-taking occasions in the work setting.

Individuals faced with test-taking and its accompanying tension in educational and practice settings seek relief in a variety of ways. Often, there are "quick fixes" that can be applied, but these may have only a short-term, limited effect, and the results may not be generalizable beyond the specific testing situation.

Although numerous preparation courses for taking the nursing state board examination, NCLEX, are offered by continuing education providers, they tend to focus more on review of the content of the examination than on managing test-taking. Time constraints restrict the potential effectiveness of these courses. And, individual learner differences cannot be addressed. Attention to learning styles and preferences of those attending a review course is limited at best.

In this handbook, the authors provide new graduates facing state boards with a systematic, organized, efficient means to prepare themselves. But this is not an ordinary state board test review book. The focus of this review book is cognitive skill development, the underlying learning necessary for success not only in taking the state board test, but in problem-solving in general.

In Part I, patterns of learning are described. All people do not learn the same way, and the chapters in this section are sensitive to individual differences. The characteristic students and learners have in common, of course, is their attitude toward the learning situation, the content, the instructors, and the demonstration of what they have learned, in this case the state board examination. Attitude often spells success or failure. The underlying approach to success on the NCLEX examination is based on confidence and the person's view of self as successful. In addition, every reader will recognize a specific test-taking personality as similar to his or her own. But, beyond that, ways to correct or at least minimize the effects of inappropriate test-taking personalities are offered.

The concepts and ideas presented in Part I of this text will help new graduates organize their learning and their review for the exam, using a framework with which every nursing student and graduate is familiar, the nursing process. In contrast with other approaches that perpetuate memorization, this book offers a method for the reader to understand and use learning based on knowing the how and why of nursing actions. In its approach to demonstrating nursing knowledge and skill on an examination, this text replicates the cognitive behaviors that are expected of nurses and that they will use in their practice.

In Part II, readers have the opportunity to apply what they learned to 17 concepts essential for health. In each of these chapters, learning and problem-solving are based on the nursing process. Principles underlying the conceptual foundations are illustrated, and "memory jogs" are included to illustrate critical points. Sample test questions are provided to assess comprehension and application along with rationales for correct responses, thus reinforcing learning. The division of these essentials into one chapter each allows readers to focus on areas where learning needs exist, reviewing only those in which they perceive a deficiency.

Beyond the stated focus on state board test-taking, this book deals with problems facing all new graduates of nursing programs, problems of self-esteem, inadequacy, and uncertainty. These are the problems that affect retention in the profession. The methods used to prepare to take state boards are applicable throughout a career in nursing.

The same strategies and techniques can be used to problem-solve and achieve goals in a myriad of instances, such as finding a job, interviewing for a promotion, becoming certified, wherever thinking skills, learning ability, and a positive attitude are crucial—the list is endless. In providing strategies for success in state boards, the authors also have produced the ways and means for practicing nurses to prepare themselves for many professional endeavors.

In addition to contributing to the likelihood of success of individuals preparing to enter the profession, this book is a valuable asset to nurses in practice. The sage counsel in this book will prove to be a worthwhile benefit to faculty in academic settings, continuing and staff development educators in hospitals and other health care agencies, all those who work with nurses in any stage of their professional careers.

Belinda E. Puetz, Ph.D., R.N.
President
Belinda E. Puetz & Associates, Inc.;
Editor-in-Chief
Journal of Nursing Staff Development
Pensacola, Florida

PREFACE

we must not forget that
the beauty of a learned
man is
  not what he's learned
  but . . .
  that he knows how
  to learn!!

Marian B. Sides

This inspirational quotation carries a powerful message to all new professionals and practicing nurses. It stresses the importance of learning as a process rather than as a product.

The impetus for writing this book evolved from the results of research efforts that focused on determining cognitive skill patterns in students and graduate nurses. These efforts revealed that nurses performed poorly on test questions that stressed higher level thinking and problem solving and performed better on questions that emphasized memorization and recollection of facts. This was true regardless of whether the subjects graduated from BSN, ADN, or diploma schools.

Through years of work with new graduates, my colleagues and I have learned that nurses find solace and comfort in clutching to facts and value concrete information as key to their future success. The practice of nursing today calls for greater sophistication in the process of higher level thinking and problem-solving with less emphasis on memorization and regurgitation of facts. Likewise, the use of lecture as a vehicle for imparting information, traditionally the most common form of knowledge dissemination, must give way to more diverse and sophisticated forms of inquiry and intellectual exercises. Such reform, in shaping the minds of new professionals, will enable them to grasp key concepts and apply selected principles to the practice of nursing.

This book is written for anyone who wishes to refine his or her approach to teaching and learning. Part I focuses on patterns of learning and provides strategies to guide the mental skill development for lower level and higher level learning. Concepts include the nursing process as a problem solving model, strategies for test-taking, and personalities of test-takers. A positive mental attitude is stressed as a key to success. Part II presents a concise and simple model of 17 fundamental concepts that are essential for health. These concepts form the foundation for nursing practice. A special feature of Part II lies in its simplicity and the easy manner in which it portrays the core concepts that shape wellness and balance in humans. Sometimes we tend to make learning so complex that we overlook the basic principles that shape health and its deviations. These principles are presented and illustrated in health and illness patterns. Test questions in the form of reasoning exercises follow each chapter. Based on clinical situations, these exercises challenge the nurse's use of the nursing process and levels of thinking in problem-solving and managing patient care. Part III consists of a series of specifically designed comprehensive tests to provide opportunities for the practice and refinement of cognitive development and test taking skill. Part IV contains rationales for the reasoning exercises in Part III.

This book is designed to bring pleasure to learning and to help new professionals meet the challenge that lies ahead.

Marian B. Sides, Ph.D., R.N.

ACKNOWLEDGMENTS

This manuscript has been a vehicle for the bonding of professional friendships and camaraderie among the special people who have contributed to the development of its contents. Special thanks to Marytherese Balskus, Diane Black, Nancy Cailles, Ann Filipski, Barbara Murphy, Wayne Nagel, and Cynthia Smego.

I express my appreciation to my co-author, Nancy Cailles who worked diligently with me in shaping the conceptual framework for this book. Special thanks to Nancy for leading the item writing team in meeting the specifications for the comprehensive tests in Part III. I gratefully acknowledge the contributions of item writers, Ann Filipski, Barbara Murphy, and Cynthia Smego, who met faithfully to create and refine the items for this volume. I wish to acknowledge and thank Maureen Marthaler and Joan O'Connell for their contribution of test items.

I appreciate the efforts and support of 750 graduate nurses and the educational administrators of schools of nursing in the state of Illinois who participated in a statewide research project to determine cognitive skills of nurses from BSN, ADN, and diploma schools. The outcome of this work prompted the writing of this volume.

Likewise, a special recognition to all 800 graduate nurses who participated over the last five years in The Education Enterprise State Board Review, taught by the authors and contributors of this volume. Results generated from these reviews provided a focus and direction for this volume.

A special thank-you is owed to medical illustrator, Thomas L. Ingram, whose creative and skillful work adds flavor and spirit to the concepts presented herein.

I wish to acknowledge the inspiration and influence of Benjamin S. Bloom, Distinguished Service, Professor Emeritus, professor and mentor during my doctoral studies at the University of Chicago. His powerful teachings in the taxonomy of thinking and learning encouraged me to devote my time and talents to the promotion and expansion of higher level thinking and problem-solving among nurses.

I am grateful for the skillful secretarial services of Sharon Massey and Charlene Knox, for their many hours of timely dedication to the preparation of this manuscript.

I wish to extend a special appreciation to Nancy Mullins and the staff of J. B. Lippincott Company for their interest, encouragement, and support in the preparation of this volume.

Marian B. Sides, Ph.D., R.N.

INTRODUCTION

New graduates are ready and waiting for this unique book, and nurse educators in schools and in health-care agencies will welcome it as a valuable resource. A number of books currently in print assist the new graduate with the task of preparing for the R.N. licensing examination. Unique in this book are the orientation to process and to action and the personalization to the reader. Part I, Patterns of Learning, is not merely an exposition of cognitive strategies. It is a model for concept formation, effective thinking and self-assessment. More importantly for the new graduate, it is a guide to action. Even the inspirational message of Chapter 1, Forming the Psychology of Success, is offered in the format of the model for the use of ideas: concept, principle, illustration of the principle. The principles for building a successful attitude reside not only in Chapter 1, but function implicitly throughout the following chapters. The reader begins to experience control, freedom, and enhanced self-esteem through mastery of concepts and strategies. Self-awareness develops as the reader compares personal characteristics with the test-taking personality typologies presented, and later tracks errors and corrects deficiencies in response to reasoning exercises. Imagery stimuli are presented both for the test-taking situation and for nursing practice situations. The action impetus moves from general to specific, from attacking the problem of getting organized to prepare for the licensing examination, to employing alternative test-taking techniques to test items representing different levels of learning.

NCLEX-RN candidates, facing the important challenge of the licensing examination, form the principal audience for this book. Everyone who has the privilege of exposure to this energetic group of beginning practitioners knows that these individuals want to be where the action is and feel ready to begin to assert control over their professional careers. The new graduate is impatient to get out of the seat in the classroom and into the full-time practice of nursing.

This book appeals to the new graduate by addressing the need to put learning to use. Of course, the book should be read and studied in the conventional fashion (*i.e.,* sitting down), but it demonstrates consistently how to put knowledge into action. The format of the book models the process being taught; the importance of organization on the part of the reader is emphasized and then exemplified in carefully constructed tables throughout the book. The conversational style helps to vitalize concepts, principles, and the nursing process. The language is appropriate to this time of transition from the academic setting to the world of nursing practice. The reader benefits from plenty of practice and diagnostic feedback through reasoning exercises imbedded in the text, as well as those assembled as practice tests in a separate section. The nursing curriculum has primed the new graduate to receive the information presented about synthesizing knowledge for action and applying test-taking techniques based on levels of learning. This book builds on student experiences in synthesizing and applying knowledge and in taking examinations to formulate strategies for state board success. The authors' experience in teaching nursing and test-taking to this audience is evident in the personalized approach they have taken, showing respect for the reader as an individual who brings knowledge and experience to the task of NCLEX preparation and providing a readable text, complete with winning thoughts, memory jogs, and characterizations of test-taking personalities.

The nurse educator, whether primarily responsible for the education of basic students or for the professional development and continuing education of practicing nurses will find this book to be an important resource. The keystones for building a successful attitude (Chapter 1) are relevant to many educational and career goals toward which nurse educators assist students and nurses, and are not at all limited to success with the licensing examination. The strategies and techniques for test-taking are useful throughout the nursing curriculum to help students sharpen their thinking and discriminating skills as well as to improve their performance on multiple choice tests. The patterns of learning information contained in Part I is valuable in preparing students for examinations and in analyzing and interpreting examination results with students, including discussion of particular test items. Nurse educators who develop and present review sessions for certification examinations will find use not only for the test-taking strategies suggested, but also for the approach modeled in the text. The book is satisfying reading for the nurse educator because of the emphasis on levels of learning, development of concepts, and application of knowledge. The usefulness of the sophisticated analysis of errant responses, diagnosis, and remediation for learning errors is not limited to the test-taking situation, but can be employed effectively in individual or group conferences in which nursing actions selected in clinical situations are discussed.

Nurse's Guide to Successful Test-Taking makes a special contribution. The NCLEX candidate can feel confident that, while success still depends on individual effort applied to preparation for the examination, an effective guide has been provided which, by organizing the task of preparation in a conceptual, yet practical, format and providing practice materials with constructive feedback, helps the new graduate identify personal priorities in preparation and focus preparation time to maximize individual performance. The nurse educator has gained a significant adjunct to resources for refining skills in goal achievement, thinking, problem solving, concept formation, and application of knowledge, as well as maximizing test performance. This book will enjoy great popularity because it offers exceptional support and assistance to new graduates in facing the challenge of the licensing examination and because it presents and models approaches that nurse educators will find helpful in facilitating accomplishment of learning outcomes.

Bette B. Case, Ph.D., R.N.

Contents

I

PATTERNS OF LEARNING

FORMING THE PSYCHOLOGY OF STATE BOARD SUCCESS

MARIAN B. SIDES

One's attitude is truly a vital human quality. For you as a new graduate, it will play an important role in determining how well you perform on state boards. Several prominent ideas serve as keystones for building a successful attitude. This chapter will set forth eight important principles that embrace these ideas. If you learn them well and modify your behavior as directed, you will feel the power, the inspiration, and the "I can" attitude necessary to achieve your goal to pass state boards.

CONCEPT: CONTROL

PRINCIPLE

WINNERS SET GOALS, ESTABLISH PLANS, AND TAKE CONTROL

Illustration of Principle

Winners do not leave the development of their potential to chance. They find out exactly what to do to succeed, and they establish a plan to achieve that success. Remember, *you* are in control. Your future is in your own hands. How important is your future? How important are you? I hope your answers to these two questions are both dynamic and invigorating. If so, you *will* take control.

Your mission in life, right now, is to become a professional nurse, and your goal is to pass state boards. In order to accomplish that goal, you must create an action plan based on clearly defined objectives and selected activities. The plan must have realistic time frames and deadlines to keep you focused and to prevent procrastination (Fig. 1-1). It should start soon after graduation and continue until the date of the scheduled exam. You may begin earlier if you desire.

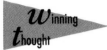

Winning thought

> An action plan gives you control over your immediate future. It provides organization, discipline, and a sense of direction. It helps reduce stress, anxiety, frustration, and unnecessary use of time and energy. If you don't have a plan, you may jeopardize your chance to succeed and increase your chance for failure.
>
> A winner has a plan!
>
> A loser has an excuse!

Your commitment to state board success may involve sacrifice. Climber Clara could effectively reduce her work stress on her journey to the top of the moun-

Preparation for State Board Success

Sample Action Plan

Mission: Become a professional nurse

Goal: Pass state board examination

Objectives	Activities	Date Accomplished

I. Organize my knowledge around basic concepts.
  A. Describe in my own words how fluids and electrolytes work in the body
  B. Identify key principles in growth and development
	1. Read Chapters 9 and 20 in review book.
	2. Form small study group and meet once a week.
	3. Take state board review course.
		June 1–4
		
		May 15–July 10
		
		June 18–25

II. Answer correctly 90% of test questions in review book and understand rationale. (Med/Surg items first)	1. Look for the key idea in test item. 2. Don't erase my answers. 3. Review test questions in review book.	Ongoing Ongoing Review 20 questions every day, except weekends, between June 1–July 1
III. Decrease my anxieties from present level	1. Establish study plan. 2. Work with someone who can help me identify and correct my weaknesses.	May 15 Once a week
IV. Establish a positive attitude about myself	1. Identify those things I do well. 2. Reward myself when I finish a task.	May 15–ongoing

Note: This plan is a model. It provides a framework that must be tailored by you to meet your specific needs.

FIGURE 1-1. SAMPLE ACTION PLAN IN PREPARATION.

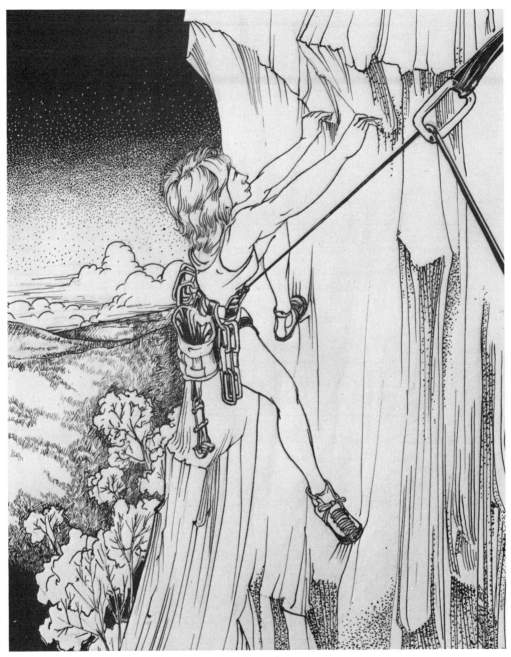

Climber Clara

tain if she unloaded her backpack and left behind those items that will not help her reach that goal. Likewise, if you are to be successful on state boards, you may need to temporarily give up some things that you enjoy, want, and even need, to provide more time to focus on your goal. If you work full time, you may need to reduce your hours. If you do not work, it might be wise to delay employment until after boards. During this time, use your support network effectively. If you have children, for example, ask a friend to watch them so you can arrange an uninterrupted study time. Ask a family member or friend to assist with laundry or to shop for groceries. You can return the favor after you pass boards. Remember, you have limited time and energy to devote to this effort. Therefore, it is important that you manage your time and yourself effectively. Everything that you do or allow to have an impact on your life should contribute in a healthy way to your goal and should not detract from it.

Balance

Remember that all work and no play reduces productivity. You need balance in your life during this important time. You must match work and study with appropriate rest, relaxation, and recreation. Set measurable goals with positive reinforcement. Reward yourself appropriately and frequently for work well done.

> There are those who travel, and there are those who are going somewhere. If a man knows not where he is going, any wind will get him there.
>
> *Great Quotations, Inc.*

The power to achieve success on state boards is within your control. "I can pass" is power. "I will pass" is control.

CONCEPT: FREEDOM

PRINCIPLE

ATTITUDE IS A FREEDOM

Illustration of Principle

As human beings, we are endowed with the freedom to choose our attitude. Victor Frankl, a distinguished psychiatrist and survivor of the Nazi concentration camp, wrote in his book *In Search of Meaning,* "The last of the human freedoms is to choose one's attitude in any given set of circumstances. Attitude is an inner quality that can keep us free, even happy, during difficult times." A healthy attitude is one that views the state board exam as an opportunity, not an obstacle. State board success is a freedom. It is not rationed. Success has no quotas—everyone can pass. Performance on boards is measured against a behavioral standard. That standard is the same for everyone. Attitude plays an important role in determining who meets that standard. Adopt a winning attitude: "I will pass!"

> In the mind's eye lies the fulfillment of a dream. No one can give it to you. No one can take it away.

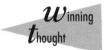

*W*inning *t*hought

CONCEPT: SELF-FULFILLING PROPHECY

PRINCIPLE

THE OUTCOME OF YOUR EFFORTS IS DIRECTLY RELATED TO YOUR SELF-EXPECTANCY AND YOUR SELF-IMAGE

Illustration of Principle

A powerful relationship exists between the mind and the body in which the mind is able to produce expected outcomes. You become what you think about most. In preparing for boards you have the choice to project your own performance in pass or fail terms. A winner's attitude is one that says, "I'm going to pass."

As normal human beings, we are driven to predict the consequences of our actions. Unfortunately, we often concentrate on the negative outcomes, those that we don't want to happen. Does this self-talk sound familiar to you?

> Gee, I know I'm not going to pass this test. What'll I do if I fail? I'll kill myself. I'll lose my job. I won't be able to face anyone at work. I won't be able to pass meds. What if I don't make it?

This self-talk is truly self-fulfilling. You can talk yourself into almost anything. So, why not talk yourself into passing? Expect the best; it will happen! Success is a self-fulfilling prophecy.

An effective technique used by many successful people in pursuit of important goals is guided imagery. This technique is demonstrated in the following exercise. I invite your participation.

Find a quiet spot somewhere in your home where you can concentrate for about 20 minutes without interruption. Guide yourself through this mental exercise.

Guided Imagery Exercise

Step 1. Commitment (5 minutes)

Think for a moment: How badly do you want this RN licensure? What does it mean to you to pass state boards? How important is it to your future? What are you willing to sacrifice to get it? How much time does this goal deserve out of your busy schedule in the next few months? Will it drive you to get up early some mornings, stay up late at night, stay at home some nights when other, more exciting things are happening?

Step 2. Self-actualization (10 minutes)

Imagine for a moment what it will feel like when you reach that dream, when you actually achieve your success on state boards. Think about how you will feel when you open that envelope from NCLEX. In large black letters, it reads **PASS.** You are a registered nurse! Think about your new name tag with the letters *RN* after your name. You have worked hard for this. Your efforts, your determination, your hopes, your dreams have brought you to a true sense of knowing who you really are!

Think of the satisfaction you feel, the pride your family has in you. Your patients are waiting, they need you. You have a new sense of importance, a new recognition, a new kind of responsibility, a new privilege. You have entered a rewarding and challenging profession. You are a professional nurse! Congratulations!

 Winning thought

> You have a choice to be your own creator. Winners make things happen. Losers let things happen!

Step 3. Mental Pole Vault (5 minutes)

In this phase of the guided imagery, you will visualize your activity. Create the details of preparing for boards in your imagination. See yourself in the process of getting there. Let's examine some related success stories where guided imagery has enhanced performance.

Winners All Our Lives is a film that portrays the use of imagery in cross-country marathon and other related activities. Positive imagery has guided elderly participants, aged 75 to 80 years, to successfully run 13 miles a day. A pianist who was imprisoned in a concentration camp mentally rehearsed his skill by playing the piano over and over every day. When he left the camp, he could immediately perform an award-winning concert.

Now, bring forth your own best capabilities and rehearse them repeatedly in your mind. As you move through this book, you will become aware of some of your own barriers to success. You will encounter them courageously, and you will mentally pole vault to heightened levels of success. For example, if you have a habit of erasing answers and entering the wrong answer (second guesser), you will practice disciplining your mind to break this habit. You will visualize yourself in a test situation in which you never use your eraser.

If you are a very slow test taker, you will visualize yourself moving more quickly through the test. Of course, you must accompany this mental activity with actual practice. Select 20 test items in a review book, for example, and allow yourself 20 minutes to answer them. Practice pacing your work, both mentally and physically. Eventually the new winning behavior will become engrained in your muscle memory, and you will be on the road to success.

A key attitude for your success is a belief in yourself, a positive self-image. You must believe that you can do it. Remember you *did* make it through nursing school. In belief you will find power. In that power is your future.

CONCEPT: SELF-ESTEEM

PRINCIPLE

THE QUALITY OF YOUR PERFORMANCE EXISTS IN DIRECT PROPORTION TO YOUR FEELING OF SELF-WORTH

Illustration of Principle

The person most likely to succeed is the one who has a deep sense of self-worth. She likes herself, has self-respect, and accepts herself. The easiest thing in the world to be is what you are. Your goal in life is to become the best you.

Do you feel you should pass state boards? Whenever I ask this question of new graduates, I get an initial pause, a hesitancy to answer, then some will say, "I think so," "I guess so," "I hope so," even, "I don't think so." If you don't think you'll pass, you probably won't.

> Those who say, I can, *will.* Those who say, I can't, *won't.*

*W*inning *t*hought

Let's ask that question again. Will you pass state boards? Your answer is, Yes, absolutely! Now, list the reasons why you should pass. Don't stop until you've listed at least five, starting with

1. I worked hard; I deserve to pass.
2.
3.

4.

5.

A sense of self-worth means that you *are* an important person. You *can* make a difference in your chosen profession. If you don't feel good about yourself, you won't win the respect and confidence of those you plan to serve.

It's always nice to get praise and recognition from others. But you should not rely on external reinforcement alone to give you a feeling of worthiness. Self-respect and self-esteem come from within.

CONCEPT: SELF-AWARENESS

PRINCIPLE

SUCCESS BEGINS WITH KNOWING THYSELF

Illustration of Principle

How well do you really know yourself? How much self-awareness do you really have? What strengths and weaknesses do you bring to this state board exam?

Somewhere in your nursing program you probably developed a favorite subject or a clinical practice area that you really enjoyed, in which you excelled. You also probably can identify an area in which you performed poorly. It is important at this time to sort out these differences because the kind and amount of attention you give to each will differ.

As you identify your strengths you can pride yourself in your skills and perhaps guide others less skilled towards a better understanding of these concepts. Few of us enjoy hearing and learning about our weaknesses. It takes courage to recognize and acknowledge imperfection. Achievement, however, relies upon an open examination of these areas.

The wise graduate will form a network of friends or a small study group of colleagues who can provide useful, objective feedback about self-performance. One should avoid defensive behavior. Accept constructive criticism and apply corrective measures when necessary. If you concentrate on strengthening these skills in a deliberate way, you will see noticeable improvement in your performance.

*W*inning *t*hought

> Take responsibility for your errors, your imperfections. The day you stop making excuses is the day you start to the top.
>
> *O. J. Simpson*

CONCEPT: COURAGE/FAILURE

PRINCIPLE

FAILURE IS A NATURAL CONSEQUENCE OF A COURAGEOUS MAN

Illustration of Principle

The only one who fails is the one who doesn't try. Most successful people fail time and time again. Have you ever failed an exam? Most of us have. How do you usually behave? How many excuses do you try to make?

> I was just getting over a fever, I wasn't feeling well. . . . Wouldn't you know, my boyfriend (girlfriend) decided to break up with me right before state boards. . . . It was a bad day. . . . I knew the material, but they didn't ask what I studied. . . . The room was just too cold, and I couldn't concentrate with all the noise.

Don't make excuses. Take full responsibility for your errors. Spend your time understanding your weaknesses and correcting deficiencies. Use the diagnostic grid in Chapter 4 to help you categorize your errors and focus on ways to correct your thinking.

If you intend to pass state boards, you must establish a healthy attitude toward failure. Between now and state boards, you are going to answer many questions incorrectly. Failing an exam is like hitting a pothole on the road to success. You have a temporary setback, maybe a little bruise. But you pick yourself up and move on. Failure is an opportunity to begin again more intelligently.

> There can be no failure to a man who has not lost his courage, character, self-respect and self-confidence. He is still a King.
>
> *Great Quotations, Inc.*

*W*inning *t*hought

You gain strength, courage, and confidence with every error you make if you confront it honestly and sensibly. If you don't err, you don't grow. Remember, it's unnecessary to correct every weakness, every error. The state board exam is a measure of minimal competency. You don't have to strive for perfection. Just do your best.

CONCEPT: PERSEVERANCE

PRINCIPLE

NO GOAL IS ACHIEVED WITHOUT PERSEVERANCE

Illustration of Principle

A powerful attribute underlying success is endurance. How many times have you thought about quitting? How often have you wished it were all over? You have recently completed a long and difficult course of study, and you probably feel physically and mentally exhausted. You still have several difficult months ahead. How will you survive?

The successful graduate recalls that the body expresses what the mind thinks. Therefore, you need to program the mind for state board success. Psychologists tell us that the average person uses less than 10% of her human potential. You realize, then, that you still have reserve energies. If you establish self-discipline and perseverance in a consistent and determined manner, you will create a positive, healthy attitude that will carry you through these next few months.

A fundamental principle to remember is that "no man is an island." The successful graduate will rely upon her support networks to help maintain perseverance and a sense of direction. The following activities will guide those efforts:

1. Work closely with one other person upon whom you can rely to lift your spirits and provide encouragement when you feel discouraged.

2. Break down your workload into manageable units of study. Completion of small, short tasks and self-made assignments will give you a sense of accomplishment and a feeling of progress. Persistence is best maintained on small tasks.

3. Openly seek feedback to give you an objective evaluation of your progress.

4. Challenge one another's thoughts and ideas. Explore options to test questions and be able to defend your answers.

Remember, focus intensely on your goal. Maintain a strong sense of commitment. Don't give up when you're at the 1-yard line.

*W*inning *t*hought

> Success is failure turned inside out. The silver tint of the clouds of doubt. And you never can tell how close you are. It may be near when it seems so far.
>
> So stick to the fight when you're hardest hit. It's when things seem worse that you must not quit.
>
> *Great Quotations, Inc.*

CONCEPT: MOTIVATION

PRINCIPLE

MOTIVATION IS THE MUSCLE BEHIND SUCCESS

Illustration of Principle

Two sources of motivation exist in relation to new graduates' preparation for state boards—fear and desire.

Fear

New graduates fear failure, the unknown, and the discovery of imperfection.

Failure

No one likes to fail, especially something as important as state boards. Therefore, each new graduate is motivated to harness this fear by establishing a well-designed plan to succeed.

Unknowns

A correlation exists between anxiety and the unknowns. An increase in unknown factors causes a corresponding increase in anxiety. Your goal, therefore, is to reduce fear and anxiety to a level of comfort, one that will circulate enough adrenalin to keep you alert and on your toes. What are some common unknowns? You don't know how many questions are in the exam. You don't know how the test is organized. You don't know how to pick the right option on the test question when you've narrowed it down to two answers. You don't understand the question. You don't know how to pace yourself. You don't have all the knowledge you'd like to have. You don't know the questions on the test, and many, many more. In the past five years, through state board reviews and test-taking clinics, *The Education Enterprise* has identified common unknowns from student nurses and new graduates across the country. Throughout this review book, strategies are offered to help you reduce the number of these unknowns.

Discovery of Imperfection

The best way to deal with the fear of imperfection is to acknowledge that you aren't perfect and then see how close to perfect you can become. The first step is to learn your imperfect ways. You may have developed some bad learning habits over the years. Glance for a moment at the caricatures in Chapter 5. Do you recognize yourself anywhere? Do you read into questions? Do you cram for tests? Are you a slow test taker? Your efforts should be directed at correcting those behaviors that will hinder your pursuit toward perfection. These efforts, designed to improve yourself to avoid failure, are the intrinsic motivators that will enhance your journey to success.

Desire

Desire is a second source of motivation. It is derived from your ambition to reap the rewards of your hard work. Rewards come in many forms. They include your licensure as an RN, the personal satisfaction of achievement, your first paycheck, power, prestige and status, the power to help people in ways that no one but a professional nurse can. These rewards that automatically accompany success are powerful motivators.

Additional personal rewards provide inspiration and incentive to spur your efforts towards your goal. Nurses often think that the more they study, the smarter they will become. To the contrary: working harder is not always better. Your life during the next few months must have balance between work and play. You should treat yourself to rewards, such as a good TV show, a movie, a night out to dinner, or a favorite dessert. Something as trite as a coffee break from a grueling itinerary can be stimulating and pleasurable. Your productivity will improve substantially with a healthy balance between study and relaxation. Anticipation of these built-in rewards is an effective motivator and should be used generously.

If you apply the eight principles discussed in this chapter in a consistent and wise manner, you will find yourself in the Winner's Circle!

*W*inning *t*hought

When you have done your best, wait for the results in peace.
J. Lubbock

Reference

Davis W: The Best of Success. Lombard, Great Quotations, Inc., 1984

Developing Thinking Skills 2

Marian B. Sides

Your success on state boards is highly influenced by how effectively you think. What are thinking skills and how do you learn them?

Through years of formal and informal learning you established your own techniques and patterns of thinking. How effective are they—how well do they work for you? Effective thinking begins with an awareness of your own thinking. Unless you are consciously aware of your own thought processes, you cannot take control of what goes on in your own mind. This chapter will offer some simple and basic guidelines to improve your learning and thinking in preparation for state boards. Attention will be focused on the common problems that new graduates face in developing higher level problem-solving skills.

The taxonomy of thinking consists of six levels. The first two are memory and comprehension. They form lower level thinking. The next four levels—application, analysis, synthesis, and evaluation—form higher level or problem-solving behaviors.

The test plan for the state board examination includes test items at the first four levels, which will therefore be the focus of this chapter. Although most of the items are written for application and analysis skills, you must have a good understanding of the basics before you attempt to master the higher level processes.

Memorization

Most new graduates, upon completion of their nursing program, have more than enough knowledge needed to pass state boards. Unfortunately, a substantial amount of that information is learned through memorization and has not been systematically incorporated into higher forms of learning that can be readily used to solve problems or to answer complex test questions. Such infor-

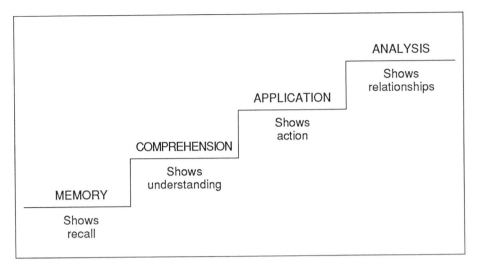

FIGURE 2-1. THE TAXONOMY OF THINKING.

mation exists as isolated, disjointed, and disconnected facts that simply clog and confuse the mind.

Did you ever feel overwhelmed at the amount of information you tried to learn and wonder how you would be able to retain it long enough for the test? New graduates are often compelled to memorize everything. Consequently, they often store in memory useless data and forget the important information. Remember, you don't need to memorize a lot of detail. For example, you will never need to recite every skill a child can perform for each year of growth. Instead, you should learn key developmental behaviors for specific age categories, such as the age at which a typical child learns to walk. Remember to establish frameworks and categories of information rather than memorize details and isolated facts. Other examples include drug classifications, stages of labor, common lab tests and ranges, and the basic principles of body processes for circulation, respiration, and movement.

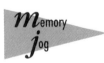

> Know *what* to learn. Don't find security in quantity. "The more you learn, the better you'll do" assumption is false. Effective learning is selective and useful memorization.

A second problem that new graduates face is that they often choose short-term memory strategies like rehearsing words or repeating phrases over and over. Information learned by simple repetition usually fades as soon as the test is over or even before the test is taken.

An effective way to improve memory performance is to invent memory techniques for situations that cause memory difficulties.

Acronyms

The use of acronyms is a helpful technique often used to retrieve information from memory. The following scenario may be a *déjà vu* for you:

> Oh, I know the answer to that. . . . I learned it yesterday. I can just see it . . . it's on page 37 . . . on the top right hand corner . . . give me a minute, I know it'll come. . . .

For important information, you want to be prepared with a retrieval tool that will trigger recall. You've learned acronyms like TLC, COPD, and PEARL that have been widely used as mental crutches to facilitate recall. Effective learners will create their own jargon or gimmicks to assist them in retrieving information.

Acrostics

This mental tool is an arrangement of words into a familiar phrase that triggers the recall of other information to be learned. An example is the familiar phrase "On Old Olympus Towering Tops a Sin in German Viewed Some Hop." The first letter or each word is also the first letter of one of the 12 cranial nerves—the mind has a tendency to recall unique and creative jingles or phrases more easily than straightforward content.

ABCs

Another strategy commonly used to facilitate retrieval is the formation of words from the ABCs. The words are intended to trigger key signs that form a vivid portrait of a classical patient problem.

CLINICAL PORTRAIT: EMPHYSEMA

Apprehension
   Barrel chest
      Cyanosis
         Dyspnea
            Engorged neck veins
               Frown on forehead

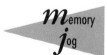

Memory Jog

Image-Name Technique

Another effective retrieval strategy is the linkage of a name to a clinical problem that clinically portrays the patient. For example, the names *pinkpuffer* or *blue bloater* are used to depict patients with specific chronic obstructive pulmonary disorders.

The amount of information you should actually memorize and store is a very small percentage of information that is actually available. The key to success in the first level of learning is to create and use strategies that will trigger retrieval of relevant information rather than to recall isolated data. Your goals in preparing for state boards at the first level of learning are to improve memory and to reduce forgetting.

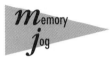

> Treat your mind like a palace with a golden gate and reserved seating. Don't let information into the gate if it doesn't belong there and if you don't have room. Ask yourself, "Do I really need to memorize this?" If you memorize without discrimination or cram carelessly, valuable information may be lost or pushed aside.

Comprehension

Effective memorization is a prerequisite to understanding. However, effective understanding requires more than simple recall or recognition. Comprehension puts memorized information into a context that gives it meaning. It bridges the gap between simply parroting information and really knowing what you're talking about.

Effective comprehension is the ability to translate information from one form to another. This can be done by paraphrasing, summarizing, explaining, or demonstrating your understanding. For example, Mrs. Jones has a potassium level of 2.8 today. You once learned that serum potassium normally ranges from 3.5 to 5.5 mEq/L. So far you have demonstrated retrieval of memorized data. Now, interpret the meaning of the 2.8 potassium level. What is the implication of this lab value for nursing practice? The mental activity in which you are now engaged is comprehension.

In preparing for state boards you must be highly sensitive to your level of understanding and your ability to discuss relationships among important facts. Unfortunately, students and graduates often slight this level of learning, moving impulsively to the action or solution without a clear notion of how the information fits together. It's like the baker who rushes to put the cake into the oven without paying attention to whether all the proper ingredients are present or whether they are mixed together effectively.

Several comprehension strategies have been effectively used by new graduates and are recommended in preparing for boards.

Small Group Work

Comprehension is most effectively accomplished by working in small groups or with at least one other person. It provides a forum for verbalizing your thought processes and critiquing each other's thinking. One way to expand your comprehension is to listen to someone else's viewpoint on selected topics of interest and to challenge customary patterns of thinking. Debate and disagreement usually provoke a deeper, richer, and more meaningful understanding of material being learned. Often a colleague will detect flaws in your thinking and can assist you in taking corrective measures to fine tune your cognitive skills. You cannot get this kind of healthy exchange and feedback when you work alone. Therefore, small group work should be used for the comprehension level of learning.

Creative Use of Questions

The use of questions in classroom teaching and testing is not a new concept. Traditionally, questions have been a useful mechanism for determining the end result of learning and for determining course grades. As you prepare to take state boards, a more creative use of questions is encouraged to enhance learning at the comprehension level.

Somewhere in your nursing program you probably encountered the question, "What is the most critical sign of distress displayed by your patient who has emphysema?" You probably answered, "He's dyspneic." Now, build on this scenario by generating questions that start with the answer and work backward. List as many relevant questions as you can.

Answer: The patient is dyspneic.

Questions: Why is he dyspneic?
What specifically triggered this episode of dyspnea?
If he's dyspneic now, what could happen next?
Can I explain the relationship between dyspnea and the pathophysiology of emphysema?
What signs of improvement should I be looking for?

Use these questions in your small discussion groups. Ask for clarification, build on the original answer, ask deeper questions until you feel you can comfortably discuss this clinical problem and all ramifications intelligently. Then you have mastered the second level of thinking, comprehension.

Relevance of Facts

An awareness of the differences between memory strategies and comprehension strategies should help you to progress from one to the other. Memory learners digest facts. They learn, for example, that arteries are elastic. Comprehension learners try to understand the relevance of these facts. They probe more deeply into a further interpretation of the facts. For example, "Why are arteries elastic? Will they always be elastic? If not, what will cause them to lose elasticity? How will circulation occur if arteries lose elasticity? What can we do to maintain the integrity of artery elasticity?" Discussion of these questions will draw a more vivid understanding of the basic principles of circulation, a valuable and productive experience.

Imagery

A final strategic technique to bring comprehension skills to brilliance is the use of visual imagery or the creation of mental pictures about your patients or the patients whom others have described to you. Fix these images in your memory. Retrieve them during test-taking to aid you in answering questions correctly.

Memorization and comprehension form the lower mental processes in the taxonomy of learning. If you have mastered these skills for important concepts that frame health and its disorders, you are ready to move on to higher level problem-solving skills, application and analysis.

Reasoning Exercises for Lower Mental Process Items (Knowledge–Comprehension)

1. During normal ventilation, the volume of air that does not participate in gas exchange is called
   *A. Residual
   B. Expiratory
   C. Tidal
   D. Total lung

2. A disturbance or loss of ability to use words or to understand them is
   A. Apraxia
   *B. Aphasia
   C. Dysphagia
   D. Dyskinesia

3. Mrs. James is in labor with a vertex fetal presentation. Appearance of meconium-stained fluid may indicate
   A. Abrupto placenta
   B. Normalcy
   *C. Fetal distress
   D. Premature rupture of membranes

4. Mr. Grady has emphysema. Which alteration in lung volume and capacity would you expect?
   A. Increase in tidal volume
   B. Decrease in residual volume
   *C. Decrease in vital capacity
   D. Increase in total volume

5. Sara is 18 months old. Which of the following behaviors is most typical for this stage of developmental growth?

   A. Building a tower with blocks

   B. Turning on TV by pulling the knob

   *C. Placing toys in a box

   D. Pulling a toy with a rope

6. If Mrs. Moss is given an intermediate-acting insulin at 8:00 AM, the most likely time for a hypoglycemic reaction would be

   A. 10:00 AM

   B. 12:00 PM

   *C. 6:00 PM

   D. 10:00 PM

Application

Application is the process of using information in the practice of nursing to maintain, promote, or restore health. A vital step in the application process is knowing *why* you are going to do what you plan to do. It involves the awareness and use of previously learned principles to justify your intended actions. Application *is* the implementation phase of the nursing process and is at the heart of nursing practice.

The foundation of nursing practice is built on a set of principles that explain health and its deviations. These principles are drawn from nursing and related disciplines. For our use, a principle is defined in the following way:

> *Principle:* A basic fact or truth that can be applied in practical situations; a specific guideline that can be used to explain and support actions.

If you cannot identify the principle or provide a rationale for your nursing actions, you should not perform them.

> The less you know about why, the more you know about error.

The following model test item will illustrate the properties of application items and the strategies to be used in selecting the correct answer.

Application Test Item

Mrs. Miller—Depression

Mrs. Miller was admitted to the hospital with a recent history of depression. She has eaten very little since her admission. Which response to Mrs. Miller, during breakfast, would be most appropriate initially?

A. Please start eating, Mrs. Miller; I'll be back in 10 minutes to see how you're doing.

B. If you don't eat, Mrs. Miller, we'll have to start IVs on you or give you injections.

C. You'll be hungry in a few hours, Mrs. Miller, if you don't eat.

D. Let's eat just a little of everything, Mrs. Miller. I'll help fix your tray.

Properties of Application Items

Application items usually provide a brief scenario or description of the context within which the situation is based. The description is usually followed by a stem or question that leads to the four completion options or answer choices.

Selection Strategies

Before you choose an answer to this question, you must form a logical rationale based on principle to support your choice of action. Your thinking should flow something like this:

A is incorrect because I cannot assume that a depressed patient will initiate appropriate behavior upon request.

Principle: Depressed patients are not self-directed and require a guided and assertive approach.

B is incorrect because it can be perceived as threatening and may increase anxiety.

Principle: Nursing actions should convey respect for the dignity of the patient; nursing action should effectively reduce anxiety.

C is incorrect because it appeals to rational thinking.

Principle: Nursing intervention for depressed patients should be concrete, direct, and should not seek response that relies on sound cognitive processes.

D is correct.

Principle: Nursing action should show the therapeutic use of self in the form of a caring presence. Depressed patients need guidance and direction in conducting basic activities. Depressed patients consume food more effectively when served in small portions.

This item should serve as a model to guide your thinking through application questions. Repeat this mental process with each question to strengthen and refine your problem-solving skills. In a short time it will become a habit in your thinking.

Analysis

The skills involved in analysis occur at a more complex and difficult level of thought than do the skills of comprehension and application. Because analysis appears above memory, comprehension, and application in the taxonomy, their skills are a prerequisite to one's ability to analyze. Analysis itself can be divided into various levels of abstract thought, characterized by increasing difficulty. These skills are frequently exercised by scientists, scholars, detectives, and others whose jobs engage them in complex problem-solving and application of logical thinking.

It is not the intent of this discussion to make an instant scientist out of you. Nor is it necessary that you be able to masterfully distinguish between the levels of comprehension and analysis. It is important, however, that you recognize that differences exist and that you know how to approach intellectually the test questions and clinical situations that require such thinking.

For purposes of the board review, this discussion will focus on the structure of the analysis question in its most simple and basic form so that you can begin to tailor your thinking and develop efficiency in this form of thought.

No clear distinction exists between levels of learning. Their boundaries are blurred, and the processes blend and overlap. To illustrate this phenomenon, let's examine the item about Mrs. Miller, the depressed patient, and the levels of learning upon which this item was built. This item encompasses all four of the levels that you have learned in this chapter. For example, you must be able to retrieve basic knowledge about depression (Level 1) as a state of the mind. Secondly, you must comprehend and understand the meaning of the condition, depression, and the meaning of the communication chosen. It requires your interpretation of depression as it relates to eating and includes your ability to explain the relationship between depression and patterns of eating (Level 2).

So far the information needed to perform the lower level skills, memory and comprehension, is provided for you in the scenario or test question. In the next two levels, you must show your ability to draw upon appropriate abstract and logical forms of thought (not provided in the text) that will lead you to correct answers or conclusions. Application, for example, involves the selection of appropriate rationale or principles to justify your nursing action as illustrated in the discussion following the test item on Mrs. Miller. These principles were not provided. You were required to supply this substance in the form of thinking.

Analysis is the ability to think at a level beyond comprehension and application. You may be able to comprehend the meaning of the communication used with Mrs. Miller, but you may not be able to analyze it effectively.

Analysis emphasizes the breakdown of material into its parts and detection of the relationships of the parts to the whole.

Bloom 1956

Analysis is an aid to fuller comprehension. It requires the ability to distinguish the cause-and-effect relationships among depression, reduced appetite, and response to different forms of communication. Can you recognize and analyze the technique used to get Mrs. Miller to eat? Can you trace the traits of thought and the relationships that you must draw to accurately answer the question? Skill development in analytic thought requires much practice.

Errors in Analysis

New graduates face some common problems in answering analysis questions that result in error.

Problem 1. Incomplete Analysis

Graduates often miss important elements in the content or a communication that must be considered in the analysis. For example, selecting a nursing response for a pregnant woman may be very different from the response for a pregnant *diabetic* woman. That response may differ from the one selected for the pregnant diabetic who is experiencing a high level of stress. The following test question illustrates this concept:

> What effect will an unusual amount of *stress* have on the insulin requirement of an *overweight diabetic* who becomes *pregnant?*

You may be essentially on the right track in answering this question, but you may miss one of the important elements, relationships, or principles. If that occurs, you will answer the question incorrectly.

Problem 2. Overanalysis

The "philosopher" nurse goes too far in analyzing situations (see Chap. 5). This person breaks the situation up into more elements than necessary or sometimes adds information that is not provided or is irrelevant. This graduate often misses important relationships and does not see the forest for the trees.

Problem 3. Quality Error

Analytic test questions often provide options that have differing degrees of accuracy or completeness. The distinction is not between right and wrong but is a matter of the best response or the one that offers the highest quality.

Effective strategies for developing analytic skills are a combination of the methods offered in this chapter. Group work is high on the list. Working with others will enhance and deepen your familiarity with all important elements and relationships that exist in test questions.

Practice reviewing test questions and analyzing your thinking patterns. Practice with purpose; experience is the best teacher.

Reasoning Exercises for Higher Mental Process Items (Application–Analysis)

1. A meconium-stained vaginal discharge is noted in Mrs. Gregory during the early stage of labor. Your first action is to

    A. Determine fetal presentation

    B. Notify the doctor

    *C. Assess fetal heart tone and rate

    D. Provide information to the patient

2. Brian has been hospitalized with an acute asthmatic attack. He is receiving 2000 cc of 5% D/W with 20 mEq of KCl per day. The drop factor is 60 drops per milliliter. How many drops per minute should you administer?

    A. 48

    B. 68

    C. 76

    *D. 83

3. Mrs. Hurley continues to see "bugs" everywhere. The most appropriate response of the nurse to Mrs. Hurley's experience is

    A. "Believe me, Mrs. Hurley, there really are no bugs in your room."

    B. "I'll get rid of all the bugs so you won't see them again, Mrs. Hurley."

    *C. "I'm right here next to you, Mrs. Hurley. What you're experiencing will soon pass."

    D. "I'm going to give you some medication so you'll feel better, Mrs. Hurley."

4. Mr. Brown was admitted to the emergency room with multiple injuries suffered in an automobile accident. He has a crushed chest, abdominal trauma, probable head injury, and multiple fractures. Which of the following emergency care interventions are most appropriate and in proper order?

    A. Assess vital signs, obtain a history, arrange for emergency x-ray films

    *B. Assess breathing, control accessible bleeding, determine presence of critical injuries

    C. Conduct physical assessment, control bleeding, cover open wounds

    D. Start an IV, get blood for typing and cross-matching, assess vital signs

5. Mr. Roberts had a colon resection for removal of a malignant tumor. The day after surgery, he went into hypovolemic shock. What is an observable effect of Mr. Robert's compensatory efforts?

    A. Level of consciousness maintained because of adequate blood flow to myocardium

    B. Cold, clammy skin as a result of peripheral vasodilation

    *C. Reduced urinary output as a result of decreased blood flow to kidneys

    D. Increased pulse rate caused by further reduction in cardiac output

Reference

Bloom BS et al: Taxonomy of Educational Objectives: The Classification of Educational Goals, Handbook 1. New York, David McKay, 1956

THE NURSING PROCESS: A PROBLEM-SOLVING MODEL

MARIAN B. SIDES

The framework for the state board exam is based on the nursing process and client needs. You will do well on state boards and subsequently in your professional practice if you can effectively use the nursing process to meet the needs of clients with commonly occurring health problems.

This chapter describes and illustrates each phase of the nursing process and provides test questions to measure your skills. The blueprint for the NCLEX test plan is incorporated into the discussion.

The nursing process is a diagnostic and management tool that guides the practice of nursing. It uses a scientific problem-solving approach to gather data, determine client problems, select appropriate interventions, and measure outcomes.

Client needs are grouped into four categories. The weightings given to each category are illustrated in Figure 3-2. They are based on the results of a job analysis on entry level performance of registered nurses (Kane, 1986). A description of client needs is included at the end of this chapter. The state board exam uses the five-phase nursing process model, which includes assessment, analysis, planning, implementation, and evaluation. Each phase is given equal emphasis on the exam and will therefore be treated accordingly in this chapter's discussion.

Assessment

The first step in the nursing process is the collection of information about the client. The purpose of this assessment is to bring into focus the relevant data about your client's health status to enable you to make an intelligent and valid problem statement or nursing diagnosis.

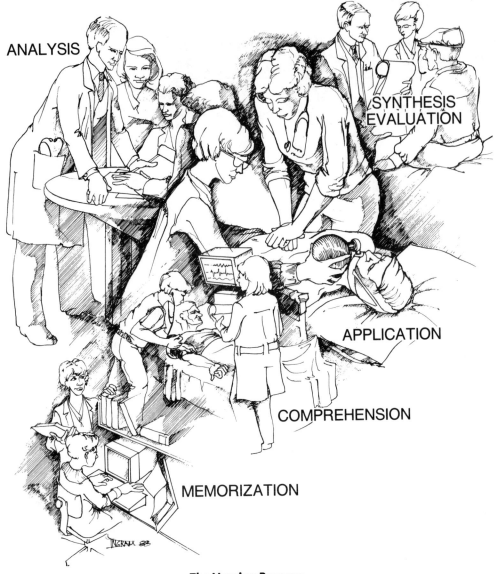

ANALYSIS

SYNTHESIS
EVALUATION

APPLICATION

COMPREHENSION

MEMORIZATION

The Nursing Process

Assessment data are characterized as subjective and objective. Subjective data are obtained from the client either through a planned interview or through incidental sharing of information by the patient. Subjective information includes symptoms such as dizziness, palpitations, pain, anger, fear, and others that also clearly express the patient's experience.

Objective data are obtained about the client by yourself, the patient's family, or others who might have useful information. Data are gathered through direct observation and by use of the senses of vision, hearing, touching, and

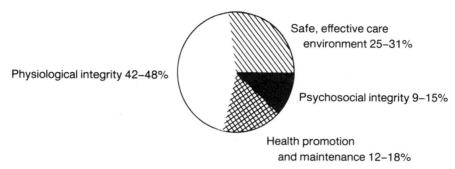

FIGURE 3-2. WEIGHTING ASSIGNED TO EACH CATEGORY OF CLIENT NEED ON THE STATE BOARD EXAM.

smelling. They include signs such as facial grimacing, crying, unsteady gait, vital signs, clammy skin, or bloody urine.

Data collection is done purposefully and selectively. You should seek objective information that verifies the subjective complaints or symptoms reported by the patient. These data should relate to the knowledge you have about nursing theory or about the other basic sciences. As information is gathered it should begin to form a pattern and take on meaning. The goal of data gathering is to provide a basis for interpretation and problem definition.

Assessment: Establishing a data base

A. Gather objective and subjective information relative to the client:
1. Collect verbal and nonverbal information from the client, significant others, health team members, records, and other pertinent resources.
2. Review standard data sources for information.
3. Recognize symptoms and significant findings.
4. Determine client's ability to assume care of daily health needs.
5. Determine health team member's ability to provide care.
6. Assess environment of client.
7. Identify own or staff reactions to client, significant others, and health team.

B. Verify data:
1. Confirm observation or perception by obtaining additional information.
2. Question orders and decisions by other health team members when indicated.
3. Check condition of client personally instead of relying upon equipment.

C. Communicate information gained in assessment.

(National Council, 1987)

Reasoning Exercises: Assessment

Mrs. Jones, a 20-year-old patient with a history of Hodgkin's disease, was admitted through the emergency room to a medical unit. You observe Mrs. Jones returning from the bathroom in a slightly unsteady gait.

1. Which of the following measures by the nurse would be most appropriate first?

   A. Question Mrs. Jones to be sure that she feels all right.

   B. Consult the medical record for the latest vital signs and blood count.

   C. Recheck Mrs. Jones' blood pressure and pulse.

   D. Put Mrs. Jones back to bed to protect her from falling.

In this question you are involved in the assessment or data collection phase of the nursing process. You know that Mrs. Jones has Hodgkin's disease. You have observed Mrs. Jones' unsteady gait. This observation suggests a possible deviation from the body's normal health state of balance or homostasis. Additional information should be sought to verify the presence or absence of a problem. Having analyzed the item scenario, you are now ready to look at the options. Option **D** is an implementation measure. Since you cannot determine the presence or extent of a problem from the information provided, you do not have a logical scientific rationale for option **D**. Therefore, you must withhold judgment until your data are more complete.

Each of the first three responses are forms of assessment or data gathering. The first response (**A**) provides the most direct lead to information about Mrs. Jones' unsteady gait. Subjective data that validate your assumptions are best provided by the client himself and can give accurate direction for your nursing actions.

A common problem in answering assessment questions or conducting the assessment process is the inability to accurately prioritize nursing responses. Eager to take action, nurses often jump to conclusions before having the necessary information. Perhaps in choosing option **A** you will learn that Mrs. Jones was having difficulty seeing without her glasses, and your action would logically be to get her glasses rather than put her to bed.

Memory jog

> When in doubt about the presence or nature of a problem, seek more information if time permits and if the patient's safety is not in jeopardy. Seek the most current, valid, and reliable information first, to rule out life threats and to expedite problem definition.

Johnny was admitted to the emergency room with complaints of a headache and nausea. Two weeks ago he had fallen from a bicycle and struck his head on the cement pavement.

1. What is your first nursing action?

   A. Obtain an order for pain medication.

   B. Conduct a neurological evaluation on Johnny.

   C. Ask Johnny's mother to describe what led to this episode.

   D. Ask Johnny if he was unconscious after he fell.

In this item, option **A** is an action response and must be withheld until a problem definition is made. The last three options are assessment responses. The appropriate response is the one that seeks the most direct, relevant, and up-to-date information about Johnny (option **B**). It is the only response that provides useful information about his current health status, which could be life-threatening.

Analysis

When all available data have been obtained or when all data that time permits have been obtained, the significance of that data must be determined. The process of interpretation of the data to form a definition or statement of the problem is called analysis. Defining the presence of a problem and determining its characteristics are the most difficult and critical aspects of problem solving. If you err here, the rest of the process is invalid and off course.

    One activity that is useful in the analysis of data is to discuss the assessment information with someone. Ask questions, communicate your understanding of the data, and put the facts into your own words. What are the possible needs and problems that could evolve from a sudden blow to the head? What are the problems that a nurse can identify? What conditions can the nurse plan to care for and treat?

Analysis: Identifying actual or potential health care needs and problems based on assessment

A. Interpret data:
    1. Validate data.
    2. Organize related data.

B. Collect additional data as indicated.

C. Identify and communicate client's nursing diagnosis.

D. Determine congruency between client's needs and problems and health team member's ability to meet client's needs.

(National Council, 1987)

Reasoning Exercises: Analysis

Mrs. Brown had an uneventful delivery of a normal, healthy baby boy 3 days ago. When the nurse entered her room that afternoon she found Mrs. Brown sitting up in bed, crying softly.

1. How would you interpret Mrs. Brown's behavior?
    A. This is a beginning psychosis following a stressful event.
    *B. Patient is experiencing postpartum blues related to hormone changes following delivery.
    C. Patient feels sadness over termination of pregnancy.
    D. This is a normal emotional response caused by exhaustion and episiotomy discomfort.

Mental activity required to answer this question involves an understanding of the normal physiological changes following childbirth. Consider the information provided about Mrs. Brown in the question and make an assumption about her behavior. Option **A** is incorrect because it suggests a medical diagnosis. Although the other three opinions are stated within the parameters of nursing knowledge, option **B** is the most logical and accurate interpretation of her situation.

Steven, an athletic 20-year-old college student, suffered a fractured shoulder and sprained wrist in a fall at a ski resort.

1. In developing Steven's care plan following surgery, which of the following typical problems would you anticipate?
    A. He will undergo an alteration in self-concept.
    B. He will experience anxiety as a result of flashbacks about the skiing accident.
    *C. He will have impaired mobility caused by immobilization of upper extremity.
    D. There will be abnormal tissue perfusion caused by swelling.

If you use both the information provided and your understanding of surgical needs following reduction of a fracture, the only problem that would normally occur is impaired mobility. In analyzing data you would first attempt to recall and understand typical scenarios or patterns of needs that commonly occur. Validate your problem definition by incorporating specialized data or individualized signs and symptoms presented by your client. These specialized data should be accompanied by a statement of cause. For example, if you note that Steven's fingertips are cold and pitting edema is forming on the back of the hand, your analytic statement might be option **D**, abnormal tissue perfusion caused by swelling. An accurate analysis of data provides a valid and useful framework for planning patient care.

Planning

The planning process begins with setting goals for client care and determining strategies to meet these goals. Client goals are an expression of outcomes that are realistic, measurable, and achievable and will be accomplished within a designated time frame. For example, an activity goal for a patient following surgery is to ambulate with assistance the full length of the room by evening of the first day after surgery.

Planning is a complex process because it involves many variables that are interrelated. These variables include the following:

1. Locus of decision making: Who should be involved in this plan of care and to what extent should the clients themselves, family, and others participate in this plan of care?
2. Return to normalcy: What limitations are placed on the client's ability to return to the original state of health? What impact has this illness or intervention had on the client's potential to return to normalcy?
3. Availability of resources: Are the necessary social, community, or institutional resources available to achieve the goals you plan to set?
4. Prognosis or potential for resolution of problems: What impact do the pathological, physiological, and psychological changes make on your client's potential for recovery? How great is the need for acceptance of limitations and the need to adapt to alternate states of health and balance?
5. Collaboration with health team members: Are the right people involved to provide the most comprehensive and highest quality plan for this client's care?
6. Additional data: Are more data needed to complete the plan of care, and are avenues available to obtain that data?
7. Diagnoses: Does the plan of care accurately address both medical and nursing diagnoses?
8. Intervention outcomes: Can you predict and provide reasonable assurance that the plan of care, when implemented, will lead to the expected outcomes? Are the strategies realistic and valid, and will they guide nursing actions?

Planning: Setting goals for meeting client's needs and designing strategies to achieve these goals

A. Determine goals of care:
   1. Involve client, significant others, and health team members in setting goals.
   2. Establish priorities among goals.
   3. Anticipate needs and problems on basis of established priorities.

B. Develop and modify plan:
   1. Involve the client, significant others, and health team members in designing strategies.
   2. Include all information needed for managing the client's care, such as age, sex, culture, ethnicity, and religion.
   3. Plan for client's comfort and maintenance of optimal functioning.
   4. Select nursing measures for delivery of client's care.

C. Collaborate with other health team members for delivery of client's care:
   1. Identify health or social resources available to the client and significant others.
   2. Coordinate care for benefit of client.
   3. Delegate actions.

D. Formulate expected outcomes of nursing interventions.

(National Council, 1987)

Reasoning Exercises: Planning

Mr. Hathaway expresses his dislike of the hospital and his feelings of insecurity about being there.

1. The nursing staff's plan to make him feel more secure should include:
   A. Allowing him to do as he pleases
   B. Providing for all of his needs
   C. Assigning specific tasks for him
   D. Being consistent in their approach to him

2. To prevent Mr. Hathaway from reacting defensively, what types of nursing actions should the nursing staff plan?
   *A. They should be nonjudgmental and accepting of his responses.
   B. They should be nondefensive and provide a good role model.
   C. They ought to have a matter-of-fact attitude when he has problems.
   D. They should make him aware of the goals to be accomplished.

Both questions above have a key word that provides a focus for your thinking in answering the question. The word *insecurity* in the first and the word *defensively* in the second are key to the intent of the questions. A common characteristic of planning items is that they provide or refer to basic principles that should guide your nursing actions.

In question 1, the lack of security generally comes from the presence of "unknowns" in the environment. Security comes from being able to predict the unknown and set reasonable expectations for what is going to happen. The best way for a nurse to help a patient accomplish this sense of security, then, is to be consistent in one's approach to the client. Appropriate interventions include anything that shows consistency.

The same form of thinking applies to the second question. Discuss this question, and exercise your thinking about planning times by using the items in the sample tests in Part III.

Implementation

Once the planning phase is complete, you are ready to implement the strategies you designed to achieve the goals of care. Nursing actions span a wide range of activities, including directly providing care, teaching the client, and recording information. Implementation is simply putting your plan into action.

When you answer an action-oriented item you must first identify the rationale or principle that supports your actions. Always ask yourself the question, "Why am I going to do this? Why should I take this action?" If you cannot answer this question with a logical and convincing argument, you should not choose the response or take the action option. In action items the principle and rationale are not provided. You must figure out the appropriate principle.

Implementation: Initiating and completing actions necessary to accomplish the defined goals

A. Organize and manage client's care.

B. Perform or assist in performing activities of daily living:
   1. Institute measures for client's comfort.
   2. Assist client to maintain optimal functioning.

C. Counsel and teach client, significant others, and health team members:
   1. Assist client, significant others, and health team members to recognize and manage stress.
   2. Facilitate client relationships with significant others and health team members.
   3. Teach correct principles, procedures, and techniques for maintenance and promotion of health.
   4. Provide client with health status information.
   5. Refer client, significant others, and health team members to appropriate resources.

D. Provide care to achieve established client goals:
   1. Use correct techniques in administering client care.
   2. Use precautionary and preventive measures in providing care to client.
   3. Prepare client for surgery, delivery, or other procedures.
   4. Institute action to compensate for adverse responses.
   5. Initiate necessary life-saving measures for emergency situations.

E. Provide care to optimize achievement of the client's health care goals:
   1. Provide an environment conducive to attainment of client's health care goals.
   2. Adjust care in accord with client's expressed or implied needs or problems.
   3. Stimulate and motivate client to achieve self-care and independence.
   4. Encourage client to follow a treatment regimen.
   5. Adapt approaches to compensate for own and health team member's reactions to factors influencing therapeutic relationships with client.

F. Supervise, coordinate, and evaluate the delivery of client's care provided by nursing staff.

G. Record and exchange information:
    1. Provide complete, accurate reports on assigned client to other health team members.
    2. Record actual client responses, nursing actions, and other information relevant to implementation of care. (National Council, 1987)

Reasoning Exercises: Implementation

Mr. Brown has recently been told by his doctor that he has high blood pressure and should be eating a low-sodium, low-salt diet.

1. Which of the following food selections provides the least amount of these substances?
    A. Hotdog with cole slaw and french fries
    B. Bologna sandwich with hard boiled egg
    *C. Tuna salad and fruit cup
    D. Bread with split pea soup and ham

2. Mr. Brown asks the nurse for a late tray since he missed the dinner meal. Which of the following food preparations would you bring him?
    A. Hotdog with cole slaw and french fries
    B. Bologna sandwich with hard boiled egg
    *C. Tuna and fruit cup
    D. Bread with split pea soup and ham

What is the difference in the cognitive level of these two questions? The first item is a lower level question. It challenges the nurse's knowledge about the relative salt and sodium content in selected foods. It does not engage the nurse in nursing action, teaching, or patient care. The second item demands a selective knowledge and understanding of hypertension and the effects of sodium on the hemodynamics of the human body. The nurse assists the patient in decision making by recommending the selection foods that are lowest in sodium and salt. The principles that support this item rationale come from the biological and physical sciences. Both on state boards and in clinical practice you will be expected to know the relationship between sodium and salt intake, blood pressure changes and fluid volume precautions. You will be expected to take appropriate action in diverse situations. Therefore, it is important to challenge your own understanding of common health problems and to question the implications they have for patient care.

Reasoning Exercises: Implementation

Brian, aged 4 years, is sitting in the pediatric day room with Michael, another patient. He suddenly realizes that he has wet his pants and runs to the nurse, crying.

1. The most appropriate initial response by the nurse is:

    A. Why, Brian, what happened? Why did you wet your pants?

    B. You know better than this, Brian; next time you'll get a good spanking.

    *C. Let's take off those wet pants, Brian, and put on something dry so you'll be more comfortable.

    D. Wait until I tell Michael what you did. Aren't you ashamed of yourself?

Several relevant principles come into play in this item in selecting the correct answer. A very basic principle is, "The nurse shows *respect* for the individual in treating human responses to actual or potential health problems." In other words, focus on treating the patient with respect first, and then attempt to modify wrong behavior. This principle shows an acceptable standard of nursing action.

The following principles show behavior that supports unexceptable standards:

1. A rational approach to solving an emotional, psychological, or even a physiological health care problem is seldom effective (option **A**).
2. Punitive behavior creates anxiety and is not therapeutic (option **B**).
3. Imposing shame and ridicule increases anxiety and is not therapeutic (option **D**).

Review other implementation items in Part III. After reading the stem, before looking at the options, practice identifying the principles and rationale to support your action choices. Then read the options and select the answer that best matches your rationale.

Evaluation

The last phase of the nursing process is evaluation. It focuses on the outcomes of patient care, a process that is often neglected. How effectively do *you* evaluate patient care? Let's complete the exercise in Figure 3-3 and find out how well you actually do.

The evaluation phase of the nursing process is an excellent monitor of the effectiveness of your care. It provides guidance and direction in continuing the

Directions for use: Answer each question by checking the numbered column that corresponds best to your performance in the particular care aspect described. After completion of the exercise, total your points and compare it to the effectiveness scale key.

	Strongly Agree				Strongly Disagree
	5	4	3	2	1

1. I give pain medication to my patients and always follow up to see how effective the medication was.

2. After meals I always observe what and how well my patient ate.

3. I always compare my patient's health progress with the needs and problems stated on admission.

4. I can state precisely my patient's care goals and can describe how well the goals are being achieved.

5. I know how well my patient is complying with physician and nursing orders.

6. I can describe change in my patient's status by citing the patient record and progress notes.

7. I can specifically describe the cause and effect between my patient's health status and my nursing intervention.

8. I modify the nursing care plan based on my patient's response.

Evaluation Effectiveness Rating Scale

Total Points	Effectiveness
40–37	Excellent
36–29	Good
28–21	Average
20–13	Poor
12–8	Unsafe

FIGURE 3-3. EVALUATION TOOL FOR PATIENT CARE EFFECTIVENESS.

nursing process. It validates your actions, ensures patient safety, and promotes compliance with your legal responsibilities to your patient.

Evaluation: Determining the extent to which goals have been achieved

A. Compare actual outcomes with expected outcomes of therapy:
    1. Evaluate responses (expected and unexpected) in order to determine the degree of success of nursing interventions.
    2. Determine need for change in the goals, environment, equipment, procedures, or therapy.

B. Evaluate compliance with prescribed or proscribed therapy:
    1. Determine impact of actions on client, significant others, and health team members.
    2. Verify that tests or measurements are performed correctly.
    3. Ascertain client's, significant other's, and health team member's understanding of information given.

C. Record and describe client's response to therapy and or care.

D. Modify plan as indicated; reorder priorities.

(National Council, 1987)

Reasoning Exercises: Evaluation

The nursing staff recognizes that Mrs. Jones is the primary support person for her husband. Mrs. Jones has identified her problem as role conflict between being a mother to teenage children, a wife of a hospitalized husband, and a person with rights of her own.

1. Which action by Mrs. Jones would indicate that she has analyzed her problem?
    A. She takes the children to visit her husband daily.
    *B. She gives the children some of the home responsibilities.
    C. She describes the roles of each member of the family.
    D. She talks to Mr. Jones about his physical limitations.

2. The nurse approaches Mrs. Jones and states, "I see you are not staying at night with your husband anymore. Is there a problem?" What answer would indicate that Mrs. Jones is coping realistically?
    *A. "I feel so angry at times. I need time to think."
    B. "The children said that they needed me at home."
    C. "My husband asked that I not stay anymore."
    D. "The staff does everything for my husband."

Several additional evaluation item stems are presented below:

3. Which of the following comments indicate that Mrs. Turner has *accepted* her *illness?*

4. The following progress note indicates that *hemodialysis* was effective:

5. Which of the following behaviors are signs that Mrs. Brown feels *confident* in *taking care* of her 3-day-old baby girl, Melissa?

In the questions above, the italicized words are actually goals being measured. In these items as well as in your clinical practice you should be looking for evidence that these goals are being met.

The nursing process is a valuable and powerful problem-solving tool. If you use it well, it will guide you successfully through state boards and will serve as a vehicle to your success as a professional nurse.

Client Needs*

I. Safe, Effective Care Environment

The nurse meets client needs for a safe and effective environment by providing and directing nursing care that promotes achievement of the following client needs:

1. Coordinated care
2. Quality assurance
3. Goal-oriented care
4. Environmental safety
5. Preparation for treatments and procedures
6. Safe and effective treatments and procedures

Knowledge, Skills, and Abilities. In order to meet client needs for a safe, effective environment, the nurse should possess knowledge, skills, and abilities in areas that include but are not limited to the following examples: knowledge of bio/psycho/social principles; teaching/learning principles of group dynamics and interpersonal communication; expected outcomes of various treatment modalities; general and specific protective measures; environmental and personal safety; client rights; confidentiality; cultural and religious influences on health; continuity of care; and spread control of infectious agents.

II. Physiological Integrity

The nurse meets the physiological integrity needs of clients with potentially life-threatening or chronically recurring physiological conditions, and of clients at risk for the development of complications or untoward effects of treat-

---

* National Council of State Boards of Nursing: Test plan for the national council licensure examination for registered nurses. Chicago, 1987. Reprinted with permission.

ments or management modalities by providing and directing nursing care that promotes achievement of the following client needs:

1. Physiological adaptation
2. Reduction of risk potential
3. Mobility
4. Comfort
5. Provision of basic care

Knowledge, Skills, and Abilities. In order to meet client needs for physiological integrity, the nurse should possess knowledge, skills, and abilities in areas that include but are not limited to the following examples: normal body structure and function; pathophysiology; drug administration and pharmacologic actions; intrusive procedures; routing nursing measures; documentation; nutritional therapies; managing emergencies; expected and unexpected response to therapies; body mechanics; effects of immobility; activities of daily living; comfort measures; and use of special equipment.

III. Psychosocial Integrity

The nurse meets client needs for psychosocial integrity in stress- and crisis-related situations throughout the life cycle by providing and directing nursing care that promotes achievement of the following client needs:

1. Psychosocial adaption
2. Coping and adaption

Knowledge, Skills, and Abilities. In order to meet client needs for psychosocial integrity, the nurse should possess knowledge, skills, and abilities in areas that include but are not limited to the following examples: communication skills, mental health concepts; behavioral norms; psychodynamics of behavior; psychopathology; treatment modalities; psychopharmacology; documentation; accountability; principles of teaching and learning; and appropriate community resources.

IV. Health Promotion/Maintenance

The nurse meets client needs for health promotion and maintenance throughout the life cycle by providing and directing nursing care that promotes achievement, within clients and their significant others, of the following needs:

1. Continued growth and development
2. Self-care
3. Integrity of support systems
4. Prevention and early treatment of disease

Knowledge, Skills, and Abilities. In order to meet client needs for health promotion and maintenance, the nurse should possess knowledge, skills, and abilities in areas that include but are not limited to the following examples: communication skills, principles of teaching and learning; documentation; community resources; family systems; concepts of wellness; adaptation to altered health states; reproduction and human sexuality; birthing and parenting; growth and development including dying and death; pathophysiology; body structure and function; and principles of immunity.

References

National Council of State Boards of Nursing, Inc: NCLEX-RN Test Plan For the National Council Licensure Examination for registered nurses. Chicago, 1987

Kane M, Kingsbury C, Colton D, Estes C: A Study of Nursing Practice and Role Delineation and Job Analysis of Entry-Level Performance of Registered Nurses. Chicago, National Council of State Boards of Nursing, Inc., 1986

STRATEGIES FOR EFFECTIVE TEST-TAKING

MARIAN B. SIDES

An important objective in preparing for state boards is to develop and refine your test-taking skills. Competence in test taking requires mastery of both content and process skills. As a new graduate you may have a good knowledge base for the practice of nursing, but if you can't take a test, you won't be able to demonstrate what you really know.

The purpose of this chapter is to examine your strengths and weaknesses in test taking. Common problems and errors in performance will be presented. You will evaluate your own intellectual practices to determine patterns or trends in your thinking that may lead you to the correct or incorrect answers. This is an exercise to get to know yourself better so you can develop and refine your skills.

The first step in developing test-taking wisdom is to learn as much about the examination and the condition of testing as possible. Familiarity breeds comfort and contentment. In Chapter 3 you learned about the test plan that provides a framework for your thinking and learning. This chapter will focus on the development of specific strategies for effective test taking.

The state board examination consists of four separate integrated tests. Each book consists of 90 questions. Each item is usually preceded by a brief vignette or patient situation that provides the framework for the question. Approximately four to six items accompany each situation.

Basic Rules for Test-Taking Success

In the following paragraphs, ten basic rules for test taking will be presented. These rules provide solutions to the most common problems faced by over 500 graduate nurses who took the NCLEX-RN exam during 1984–1987.

Rule 1. Know the Parts of a Test Question and how to Read Them

A multiple choice test question consists of three main parts: a background statement, a stem, and a list of options. The background statement is a brief scenario that provides information that is necessary or useful in answering the question.

The stem is the element that contains the specific problem or intent of the item. It can be presented in the form of a question or an incomplete statement, formed by a subject and a verb. These components are shown in the following chart.

Stem Forms of a Test Question

Mrs. Green arrived at the hospital in early labor.	Background statement
Which of the following signs is the best indicator that labor is progressing?	Stem in question form
The best indicator that labor is progressing is	Stem in incomplete statement

The background statement does not always provide information essential to answering the question. It may be included to provide a framework for the stem or to flavor the test with interest and personality. It may be included to determine how effectively you can sort through data and select pertinent information. The chart above, for example, provides a background statement that is not necessary in answering the question. The background statement in the chart below, however, is critical to answering the question correctly. In developing test-taking skill, you will learn how to discriminate essential from nonessential information in the background statement and the stem.

Mrs. Green, aged 41, at term and a diabetic, arrived at the labor and delivery suite in early labor.	Background statement
Which of the following assessment data should the nurse obtain upon admission?	Stem in question form
The assessment data that the nurse should gather includes	Stem in incomplete statement form

The options are a list of possible answers to the question or solutions to the problem. The correct answer is called the *keyed response* and the other options are called *distractors*. The words, option, distractors, response, and answer are used interchangeably in this text. A question is usually followed by four single-option choices. The state board exam does not include multiple choice answers.

In answering the test question you will select the option that best completes the question or solves the problem. In the chapters to follow you will have many opportunities to work with options and develop your skill in selecting the correct one.

Rule 2. Read the Question Carefully Before Looking at the Options;
Identify Key Words in Stem

The stem is the heart of the item. It provides the focus and directs your thinking. Your key words will be found in the stem. Read it carefully and grasp the complete thought before looking at the options. Then, read each option and select the one that best solves the problem or answers the question. If you don't read the entire stem, and you if gloss over words or misread them, you will misinterpret the question. A common error is to miss the word *except,* as shown in the following question:

1. All of the following behaviors are typical of a 3 year old except
   A. Putting on make-up and playing grown up
   *B. Reciting her address and telephone number
   C. Throwing a ball about 5 feet
   D. Identifying animals from a picture book

The word *except* in the stem directs you to look for the response that is not typical of a 3-year-old child. If you miss the word you will select the wrong answer.

> Haste makes waste! Read each word in the stem carefully before looking at the options. Look for key words such as first, primary, initial, early, most important, except.

Michael, aged 3 years, was admitted to the emergency room after being rescued from a fire in his home. He is having difficulty breathing.

2. An early sign of respiratory distress that you might observe in Michael is
   *A. Increased pulse rate
   B. Cyanosis
   C. Decreased pulse rate
   D. Clammy skin

If you missed the word *early* in the stem you may have chosen cyanosis as the answer. Although cyanosis is a sign of respiratory distress, it's a late sign rather than an early sign.

Other key words commonly used in test stems are: primary, initial, best, except, and most. These words will not be highlighted or emphasized in any way on the test. You must be alert and read each word carefully to extract the true meaning of the stem.

Rule 3. Identify the Theme of the Item, and Base It on Information Provided in the Stem; Don't Assume Information that is not Given

Each test question is designed to measure a specific unit of knowledge or process skill. When you read the stem you need to identify the precise idea it intends to convey. Confine your thinking to the information provided and don't add to it. A common error is to choose a response that might have been appropriate for a patient you previously cared for or a response that worked in another situation. Remember, each person is different; what's appropriate in one instance may not apply for the patient in your test question.

Mrs. Brown's husband was admitted to the emergency room in delirium tremens (DTs). This admission is his third visit in 2 weeks. While waiting to see her husband, Mrs. Brown said to the nurse, "What in the world can I do to help Joe get over this drinking problem?"

1. The best initial response for the nurse is
   A. Don't feel guilty, Mrs. Brown; I know this must be difficult for you.
   B. Let's go into the lounge, so we can talk more about your concern, Mrs. Brown.
   C. You need to convince Joe to seek professional help, Mrs. Brown.
   D. How long has your husband been drinking, Mrs. Brown?

If you chose Option A, you are reading into the question and adding a factor that was not provided—that Mrs. Brown is feeling guilty. Perhaps you know of someone who did feel guilty in a situation like this, or perhaps you thought she should feel guilty. Because this background statement does not tell you how Mrs. Brown feels, you can't make this assumption (option **A**).

Option **C** is incorrect because you don't have enough information about the situation to offer this advice. You should be in the assessment or data collection phase of the nursing process. Option **D** is not the best choice because it focuses on Mr. Brown's problem and channels the interaction specifically, rather than encouraging Mrs. Brown to express her concerns. Since Mrs. Brown is concerned about what *she* can do to help her husband, the correct response is one that first encourages her to verbalize how she is feeling (option **B**).

Rule 4. Answer Difficult Questions by Eliminating the Obviously Incorrect Responses First; then Select the Best of the Remaining Options

If you can reduce your options on a difficult question to two choices, you can sharpen your focus, and the task will seem more manageable. Eliminate the obviously wrong distractors, then reread the stem. Identify rationale for each of the remaining answers, and select the strongest option. This process can take several minutes at first, but you will develop speed as you gain skill through practice.

If you cannot eliminate any of the options, skip the question and return to it later, or take a wild guess and select any answer. You are not penalized for guessing, and you will have a 25% chance of getting it right.

Rule 5. Select Responses that are Therapeutic, Show Respect, and Communicate Acceptance; Eliminate Responses that are Bizarre, Inappropriate, and Punitive

Your actions should always be guided by the basic principles of interpersonal relationships. The intent to respect others should underlie every interaction. In school you were taught to "accept the patient as he is." Therefore, you can automatically eliminate distractors that violate these principles because they are always inappropriate. The use of basic principles to guide your thinking can help you select the correct response even if you don't understand or recognize the item idea or condition described in the stem. The following question illustrates this concept.

Mrs. Durham is recovering from a colon resection for removal of a malignant mass in the large bowel. Following breakfast one morning she told the nurse, "I'm tired of waiting, I want my bath now. You're never here when I need you."

    1. Which of the following responses by the nurse is most appropriate?

        A. What do you mean, I'm never here? I spent all 3 hours with you yesterday, Mrs. Durham.

        B. I'm sorry you've been waiting Mrs. Durham. Let's get you comfortable now, and I'll be back in 20 minutes to give you a bath.

        C. I'm doing my best, Mrs. Durham. You know I have three other patients to take care of today, besides you.

        D. I must see Mrs. Jones right now Mrs. Durham. She's really sick today. I'll be back as soon as I can.

The only appropriate response is option B. Acknowledge her feelings and give her a clear, factual response to her concern. Never challenge a patient's statements and don't be defensive (option A). Do not reprimand the patient unnecessarily or talk about the needs of the other patients (options C and D). In this case you did not need to know a lot about colon resections to answer this question. You did need to have skill in basic communication and human interaction.

Rule 6. Know the Basic Principles that Guide the Practice of Nursing

The best preparation for test-taking success is to know your professional discipline, nursing. Know your subject matter. Part II presents the basic principles that underlie the practice of nursing. Focus on learning principles and broad concepts for client problems that are prevalent in our society. Recognize and learn common needs and aspects of care of high-volume patient populations. You may become skilled in recognizing familiar illness portraits even if you don't recognize the medical disorder described in the item. Consider the following two items:

Mrs. Joan Andrews, aged 48 years, was brought to the Sunny Manor Nursing Home in a debilitating state with Helsink's disease. Mr. Andrews, her husband, says that she has become very unstable on her feet; her motor skills have become very spastic. She is becoming increasingly irritable and is having difficulty eating by herself. Mr. and Mrs. Andrews appear very depressed.

1. Following the initial assessment, the best action for the nurse is to
   A. Give the Andrews a few hours of privacy so they can gather their composure
   B. Introduce them to other clients in the day room so they won't feel so isolated
   C. Get Mrs. Andrews settled in her room; give her and Mr. Andrews a basic orientation to their immediate surroundings
   D. Assist Mrs. Andrews to ambulate in the corridor to regain her strength

2. Activities that would be appropriate for Mrs. Andrews are those that would allow her to
   A. Compete with others
   B. Succeed at a task
   C. Promote social interaction
   D. Tax her thinking skills

The answer to question 1 is option **C.** The answer to question 2 is option **B.** Did you answer these questions correctly? Did you recognize the disease, Helsink's? If not, did you proceed to answer the questions anyway, or did you panic and wonder what you should do because you never learned this disorder, or at least you don't remember learning it?

The purpose of this demonstration item is to expose you to an exercise with a fictitious disorder (*Helsink's disease*) and to see if you could answer the question correctly by interpreting the information provided and recognizing the familiar clinical portrait described. Whether you know Helsink's disease or not you probably did recognize these behavior patterns.

Mrs. Andrew's complaints and symptoms are typical of a degenerative neurological condition. Persons with this type of problem sense a loss of independence and control. The important implication for nursing is to assist the client to gain control over the environment and to achieve a sense of autonomy and independence whenever possible. These individuals are not ready to socialize or spend time in day rooms with other people. They are focused on their own personal needs. These problems and care needs are very fundamental, regardless of whether the client has Huntington's chorea, Parkinson's disease, CVA, or Helsink's disease.

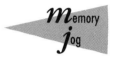

> When you confront strange or unfamiliar background statements or vignettes, don't panic. Proceed with the question. Look for behavior patterns or clinical portraits that will provide clues for nursing action.

Rule 7. Look for Patterns in Your Performance and Flaws in Your Thinking.
Analyze Your Test-taking Behaviors, then Establish Strategies to Correct these Problems

Typically students and new graduates learn by trial and error. Seldom is learning well designed and led by a systematic plan. Even more seldom do students evaluate their performances and analyze their learning strengths and weaknesses.

The test-taking grid diagrammed in Figure 4-2 is a tool that will assist you to track your patterns of thinking and identify flaws in your practices. It will help you establish a mental mechanism for higher level thinking and problem solving. Guidelines for use are provided (see Fig. 4-1). This tool can be used in answering test questions in Part III of this book.

Rule 8. Manage Your Time Effectively During Test Taking

Each test booklet on the exam contains 90 questions. You are allowed 90 minutes for each test, so that you have approximately 1 minute per item. Pace yourself accordingly so you can complete the exam during this time allowance.

When you feel you have mastered the content for a particular aspect of nursing, start timing yourself in the practice tests. If you are a slow test taker, practice reading at a faster pace. Pay attention to your comprehension. If you are making more errors when you pick up speed, perhaps your knowledge base is weak for the content you are reviewing. Familiarity and mastery of the material will certainly enhance your speed in test taking.

The quality of concentration during test taking can also affect your pacing and your speed. Try to block sound and motion interference during test taking. Don't be distracted by candidates coming to or going from the test site. You shouldn't care what others are doing, how soon they finish, how far they are, or whether you're the last one done. You are not competing with them. Concentrate on your own test, your time, and yourself.

Directions for Use

of

Diagnostic Grid for Recording Test-Taking Errors

The purpose of this grid is to display your errors in test taking. The form consists of a column for each of the four tests included in this book. An extra column is included for adult health and one for an integrated exam. These columns can be used in reviewing items from other sources. Categories of test-taking errors are listed in the left margin.

When you miss an item, place a mark in the square that you think best describes errors in thinking. Make sure you place the mark in the appropriate test column.

Once you have listed all your errors, look for patterns in your thinking. Begin to analyze the thoughts that led to the wrong answers. Do you frequently miss key words? Do you read into the question something that isn't stated? Make appropriate corrections in your thinking by applying the principles and ideas presented in this book.

Continue to practice test taking. Your weaknesses should gradually decline, and you should see fewer errors.

FIGURE 4-1. DIRECTIONS FOR USE OF DIAGNOSTIC GRID FOR RECORDING TEST-TAKING ERRORS.

Don't spend too much time on one item. If you cannot eliminate any distractors, skip the question and return to it later, if time permits. If you can eliminate two options, but can't decide on the answer, take a guess. You may not have time to return to the question.

If you progress in a timely fashion, you will feel confident about your performance, and you will maintain control and composure in the testing situation.

Keep in mind that separate answer sheets are no longer used in the state board exam. You will record your answers directly in the test booklet. This system reduces the possibility of error in matching test items with the corresponding answer sheet and should help you pick up speed in test taking.

Try not to leave stray marks on your test booklet. You must erase them, or they may be interpreted as your intended answers. Clearing up stray marks takes time, detracts from your thinking, and affects your progress. Notepaper is provided in the test booklet for calculations.

Rule 9. Do Not Change Answers Without Good Reason or Sound Rationale

Your first attempt at answering a test question is usually accomplished with an orderly and well-disciplined thought process. Your thinking is logical and systematic. When you decide to change an answer, usually you are acting impulsively, and you are not using a good problem-solving technique.

If you are a *second guesser* and have a habit of changing answers, you should not review your entire test. Review only those questions about which you were unsure or those you did not answer. Do not change answers you have marked unless you have a good reason and can provide a defensible rationale. If you are a *second guesser,* refer to Chapter 5 for further discussion of this test-taking personality.

ERROR CATEGORIES	PRACTICE TESTS						ITEMS WRONG PER ERROR CATEGORY
	Women's Health	Child Health	Adult Health	Adult Health	Mental Health	Integrated Exam	
1. Did not recognize or remember subject matter							
2. Did not understand subject matter							
3. Did not recognize item idea							
4. Did not recognize principle or rationale for correct answer							
5. Missed key word							
6. Did not read all distractors carefully							
7. Did not understand question							
8. Read into question							
9. Used incorrect rationale for selecting response							
10. Changed the answer							
11. Other							
TOTAL ITEMS WRONG PER TEST							

FIGURE 4-2. DIAGNOSTIC GRID FOR RECORDING TEST-TAKING ERRORS.

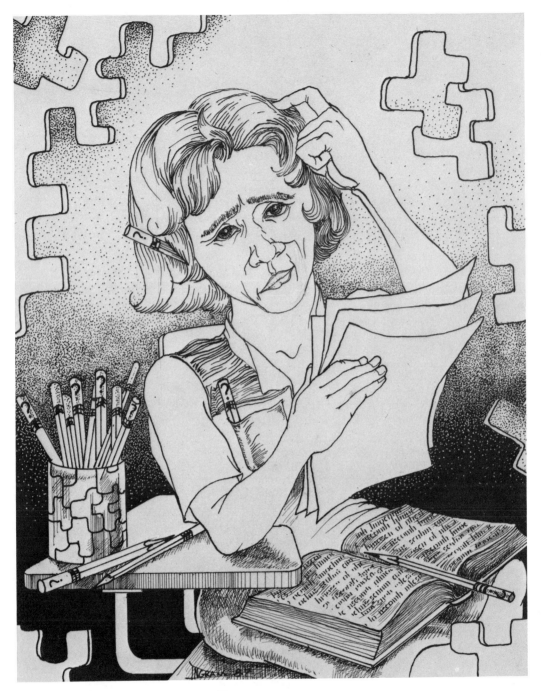

THE SECOND GUESSER

Rule 10. Choose Options that are Within the Realm of Nursing; Be Able to Differentiate the Need for Nursing Judgment from Physician Judgment

Test questions that are action-oriented are based on clinical situations that require nursing judgment. Occasionally distractors will be used that call for physician action. The nurse may inappropriately call the doctor and refer to physician judgment when the situation really calls for nursing judgment. Such behavior can result in negligence.

Mr. Ebstein, 58 years old, is recovering from a suprapubic prostatectomy. His urinary output in the past 2 days has been satisfactory; however, the nurse now notices that it is becoming increasingly bloody.

1. The initial action of the nurse should be to
    A. Irrigate the Foley catheter
    B. Notify the physician
    C. Take vital signs
    D. Empty the drainage bag

Your immediate goal is to determine if the increase in bleeding is causing a life threat to the patient and if it is threatening his stability. Taking the vital signs (option **C**) is the only action that will give you information on Mr. Epstein's physiological status. The nurse should not notify the physician until she can provide further assessment of his condition.

Mr. Parker is receiving Dilantin to stabilize his seizure condition. One morning when Mr. Parker is taking a walk in the corridor, you, his nurse, notice his gait is extremely ataxic and he complains of dizziness.

1. Which of the following nurse's notes indicates that appropriate nursing action was taken?
    A. Very unsteady gait probably owing to dilantin toxicity. Notify physician.
    B. Complaining of dizziness while walking. Gait unsteady, returned to bed, blood pressure 110/70, pulse 112, respiration 32. Physician notified.
    C. Gait very unsteady. Returned to bed. Physician notified.
    D. Gait unsteady. AM dose dilantin withheld. Blood pressure 110/70, pulse 112, respiration 32.

Options **A** and **D** are not within the realm of nursing judgment. You don't know that Dilantin is causing the unsteady gait, and you should not withhold the medication without proper assessment. Option **C** is appropriate but not sufficient. The nursing notation in option **B** provides factual information related to appropriate assessment and provides a data base for physician analysis.

Reducing Stress and Anxiety

Stress is simply the wear and tear imposed on the body by the normal or abnormal events of life. The environment in which we live surrounds us with stressors that affect our ability to maintain a sense of balance and equilibrium. The activities of walking, breathing, eating, and talking all stress the body in different ways to keep us alive and healthy.

Stress related to test taking can produce unusual demands upon the body. The key to success during this particular time lies in the ability to control and balance the stressors in your life. I refer you to Chapter 1 for guidelines and inspirational tips on managing these stresses.

Remember to create a plan that will realistically blend this additional responsibility with other stressors in your life. Adopt and use stress reduction and relaxation exercises to assist you in managing stress. Relaxation tapes are available from local book stores and can be purchased from textbook publishing companies.

Anxiety related to test taking is often a major impediment to effective test performance. Although anxiety and stress are related phenomena, anxiety differs from stress in several ways. Whereas stress is a generalized state of tension resulting from many different life events, anxiety is a specific state of uneasiness produced by a particular stressor. Anxiety related to test taking can result from lack of information, lack of skill, or the presence of unknowns surrounding the test-taking situation. Strategies to decrease anxiety should focus on these three areas, that is, gaining information, developing skill, and decreasing unknowns. A reduction in anxiety will effectively reduce stress.

Pre-Exam Preparation

Preparation for the state board examination should be systematic and well spaced to allow for the natural assimilation and digestion of information.

Application Process

Each state has its own state board application protocol. Application should be made to the state in which you wish to be licensed. Therefore, it is best to contact your State Board of Nursing directly or follow the procedures outlined by your professional school. A list of State Boards of Nursing is in the appendices.

State Board Review Course

Many new graduates benefit from state board reviews. Others do well without them.

Benefits

A well-designed state board review will assist you to

1. Organize your knowledge for the practice of nursing
2. Improve your understanding of the basic principles and concepts that form the practice of nursing
3. Strengthen problem-solving skills
4. Improve test-taking skills
5. Reduce anxiety and stress
6. Establish confidence
7. Formulate a positive attitude
8. Develop wisdom and insight into your own strengths and weaknesses

A good state board review will offer you a support network of instructors and colleagues who share a common interest. It will also share some of the decision making that you would otherwise be making independently in preparation for state boards. Many graduates gain a sense of security in this experience.

Limitations

Be aware that a state board review is not a crash course in nursing and is not intended to offer you an entire nursing curriculum in a few days. It will not perform miracles, nor will it bridge the gap between a life-long deficit in learning and success on state boards. You must enter the review with an adequate foundation in the nursing discipline. A review will help you put the finishing touches on your learning.

State Board Review Books

In addition to this review book you may want to consult another resource book with test questions for additional opportunity to practice test taking. Use the test grid (see Fig. 4-1) to track your errors. Make sure you analyze your strengths and weaknesses as you proceed.

Last-Minute Preparation

When you receive information about the location of the exam, you should familiarize yourself with the test site, the building, parking facilities, and route of travel. Make a trial run and note the mileage and travel time for the time of day you will be traveling. You may want to register at a nearby hotel during the exam period. You will avoid travel time, enjoy hotel meals, swimming, and other guest amenities. Go for it!

Make a checklist of things you should bring and do. Be sure to read the instructions you received from your State Board of Nursing and assemble all required materials.

Don't eat or drink excessively the night before the exam. Avoid unusual, different, or spicy foods that could cause disturbances in your digestive system and interfere with your test performance.

Don't study the night before the exam. Heavy concentration and cramming will reduce your effectiveness and your powers of thinking. Have a relaxing evening and go to bed at a reasonable hour. Do not take stimulants or depressants.

Wear clothes that are comfortable on the day of the exam. A layered outfit is appropriate so you can remove or add clothing in response to temperature changes in the room or to your own body temperature changes.

Bring a "warm fuzzy," such as a charm, snapshot of a special person, or a small trinket that can provide psychological warmth and a sense of security. If these articles cannot be displayed, place them in a jacket or pants pocket.

Pack a few pieces of hard candy or other quick source of energy. Chewing gum sometimes helps to dissipate anxiety.

Get up early the morning of the exam to allow enough time to get yourself ready and travel to the test site. Review your checklist to make sure you have gathered everything you need. Eat a healthful breakfast. Spend a few moments in silence; meditate, pray, or do whatever will provide the mental and spiritual uplift that you need to start the day off right. Now, you've done your best. What else could you ask of yourself?

During the Testing Period

You will complete two 90-minute test booklets on each day of the exam, one in the morning and one in the afternoon. A 2-hour break separates each exam period. After you complete the first booklet you will break for lunch. A word of caution: do not get caught in the panic circle, surrounded by anxious people. You will gain nothing by getting emotionally involved in test item review. Quietly remove yourself from the presence of this activity.

The evening of the first exam day should again be spent quietly and in a relaxed environment. You might spend an hour or so alone or with a colleague, analyzing the test as a whole, how it was structured, content focus, and how you felt during the test. Avoid any detailed, tedious review.

Once the exam is over, take a well-deserved break and await the results in peace. Then move on to the next phase in your career plan.

PERSONALITIES OF TEST TAKERS

NANCY B. CAILLES

Throughout our lives, demands to obtain and process knowledge, develop skills and insights, and synthesize solutions and strategies are placed upon us as growing individuals. As young children, we are challenged by the intricate handwork of tying a shoe lace. At school age, we are at first baffled by the complexity of long division. Approaching adulthood, we attempt to conquer the intangibles of geometry, theology, or a foreign language.

Learning that occurs in the very early years tends to occur on a continuum with maturation. If a child has difficulty learning to balance himself on a bicycle and ride independently at the age of four years, it is most likely because he has not yet achieved the developmental or maturational level required. However, after frequent falls and multiple attempts, the child at the age of five years will acquire the skill of bike riding and then maintain that skill throughout life. Learning, then, occurs over a period of time, on a continuum with the maturation and development of the growing child. There is no mandate—no time frame—limiting the learning period.

In the academic environment, such mandates—such as time frames—*do* certainly exist. Learning is often quantified for measure by means of regularly scheduled examinations, framing a set of chapters, a period of weeks, or a series of lectures. The adult student in the academic environment becomes acutely aware that tests mandate achievement and accomplishment within a set period of time. It is easy to understand, then, that students may come to fear examinations or to view them as hurdles in the learning process that must be overcome in order to continue onward through the chosen course of study.

Nursing educational systems not only mandate accomplishment of specific concepts and content within preset time frames, they require *application* of the newly acquired knowledge almost immediately. The nursing student is expected to utilize new knowledge of nursing principles and actions gathered

59

in the classroom to make decisions about patient care in the clinical setting. The transfer of practice in the laboratory to practice in the clinical setting is most often a very rapid one for the student nurse, mandating a rapid processing of newly acquired knowledge. An additional stressor is placed upon the student nurse by the realization that errors in practice could well be harmful to a human patient. The learner, then, naturally begins to identify testing in nursing as a potential barrier or as a possible threat, and test-related anxiety is a natural consequence of that perception.

Since the national licensure examination is that series of tests by which the student nurse verifies his or her achievements and abilities as a professional nurse and thereby receives licensure by which to practice in the health-care setting, the examinee must face and cope with an unyielding timeline: the few weeks between graduation from a program of nursing and the dates for the licensure examination. The purpose of this chapter is to explore some typical reactions to the stresses of testing that students might use in order to cope with test-related anxiety. Suggestions for controlling undesirable testing behaviors are identified. The reader should attempt to identify how she *personally* copes with testing by relating her own behaviors to those of the test-taking personalities discussed in this chapter. With new insight into testing behaviors developed, the reader may then practice more successful or appropriate testing behaviors, which will optimally result in better performance on the licensure examination for nursing.

"The Rusher"

The Rusher is an individual who hurries through the entire process of taking an examination in a desperate rush to complete the test before essential facts that have been studied are forgotten. The Rusher arrives at the testing room one-half hour early, waits anxiously outside, and mumbles to herself tidbits of information that are rapidly becoming confused and jumbled. "Let's see . . . if the pH goes up, the CO_2 goes down . . . or is it the other way around? Well then what does the HCO_3 do? Up? Down? Left? Right?" The anxiety that the Rusher experiences as she readies for the examination causes her body to tighten up, and she prepares to begin the test while entwining her legs around the base of her seat and taking a vicelike grip on her pencil. While most students are yet completing the first few items, the Rusher is already one third completed with the exam. She flies through each item and circles a chosen response as quickly as possible, escalated not only by her fear of forgetting information but also by the physiological forces that take hold when anxiety occurs—racing pulse, rapid respirations, neuromuscular excitement. It's a sure bet that the Rusher will be the first person to complete the exam and will hurry out of the testing room as quickly as she entered. Once away from the testing situation, the test-related anxiety decreases, and the Rusher experiences feelings of exhaustion, both physiological and mental.

The problem that the Rusher experiences while racing through the exami-

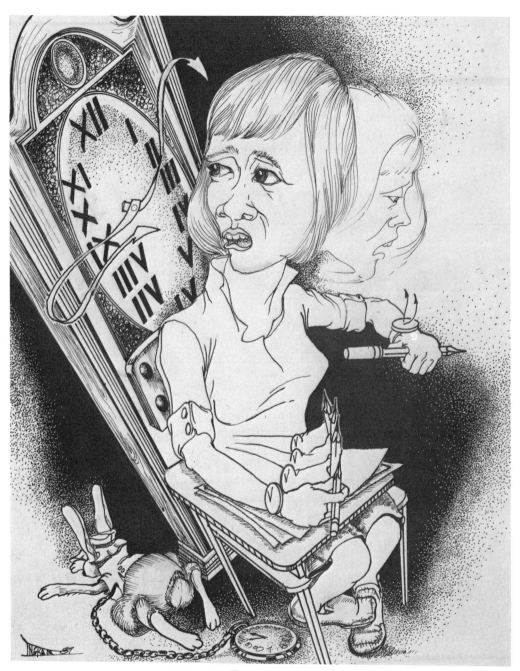

THE RUSHER

nation is that she is unable to read carefully and completely the situation and questions before her. She is at high risk for misreading, misinterpreting, and mistaking, because she focuses her attention on getting *through* the test, finishing the test, rather than accepting and *taking* the test. If the Rusher encounters a difficult item that she is not readily able to answer, her anxiety to complete the examination is heightened, and she is likely to quickly pick a guessed response to the question simply to continue moving through the exam.

The Rusher should employ two techniques to alter rushing behaviors in testing situations. First, she should practice progressive relaxation exercises while preparing for the scheduled examination, in order to reduce feelings of increasing anxiety as the test time approaches. Secondly, the Rusher should develop a plan of study prior to the examination that will allow ample time for the review of important concepts and content, thereby eliminating the need to "cram" knowledge to be learned just prior to the test, which will likewise significantly reduce testing anxiety. The Rusher may also find it helpful to practice test-taking strategies at home by taking sample test questions and attempting to slow down her pace of reading and answering.

"The Turtle"

The Turtle, in contrast to the Rusher, does nothing fast when it comes to testing. Often fearful of missing important points or necessary details in items on an examination, the Turtle moves slowly, methodically, and deliberately through each question—reading and then rereading, underlining important points, scratching out unwanted responses, and then rereading the item to check over the selected response. Although it might seem at first that this careful process would help the examinee to perform better on the test, such may well not be the case. Turtles often are the last to finish an examination, *if* in fact they are able to complete the examination at all. Typically the Turtle has far too many questions to complete in the limited time period left, and thus must hasten through a last series of items and quickly jot down an answer, any answer. Turtles, then, tend to score much better in the first section of a test than in the last, having taken undue time and caution in the first section and leaving insufficient time for the last section.

The average multiple choice examination is designed to allow 1 minute per item Simple, straightforward items will require 20 to 30 seconds, leaving a bit extra time to answer more difficult or complex items. Turtles may take up as much as 60 to 90 seconds simply reading the questions, however, with additional time needed to select the correct response. Turtles, then, tend to have great difficulty finishing the entire examination within the set time limitations, and thus their scores suffer, not from lack of knowledge or poor preparation, but from lack of time and inability to complete all of the examination items.

Turtles can best overcome their tendency to test too slowly by taking practice tests at home, focusing on the time spent on each item. With continued practice with reading and answering items, the Turtle should note an increase in speed and comprehension in reading. She would also benefit by wearing a watch with a large face and easy-to-read numbers, in order to keep aware of the passage of minutes during testing. To reduce wasted time in moving the wrist to glance at the watch, she should place the watch just in front of her on the desk. Finally, the Turtle should make a mental note of the total number of items on the examination in conjunction with the total time for the examination and mark on the test sheet approximately where in the test she should be halfway through the test period, so that there is adequate time to complete all the questions on the test in an unhurried and relaxed manner.

"The Personalizer"

The Personalizer is most often an older, more mature graduate who has gained personal knowledge and insight more through undergoing life experiences than through formal, structured education. Although experiential learning is indeed valuable and often leaves a more lasting impression than classroom or laboratory settings may provide, there is an inherent risk in relying upon what one has learned through observation and experience only. The graduate nurse preparing for the licensure examination, who attempts to understand broad concepts and applications based upon her experience with a limited population in practice, faces a great risk for developing false understandings and stereotypes about the larger populations. Personalizers can easily err in testing situations, because their personal beliefs and experiences may not, in fact, be the norm, the standard, the expected.

The national licensure examination for registration of nurses maintains set standards of nursing practice in its questions for the examinee. The focus is placed on an expected duty of care owed to selected patients, and the examinee must be able to choose appropriate measures to enact that expected duty of care. The Personalizer who relies upon personal exposures to patients and clinical situations may have significant difficulty in identifying the expected measures to meet the standard or the duty of care owed to a selected patient.

Consider the following example: An examination item requires the reader to identify an appropriate nursing intervention for the patient undergoing detoxification from alcohol toxicity. The Personalizer's thought process might be:

> When I was in my Psych rotation at County Hospital, I had a patient that was going through alcohol detox, and I remember that he became very agitated and combative, and the staff was really worried that he would become violent. They didn't want him to hurt anyone—they put him in restraints—that's the right answer, then! It's **C.** Place the patient in leather restraints.

What appears in this example as a process of deductive reasoning based upon life experiences and personal clinical exposure is in reality faulty thinking and even stereotyping. The Personalizer relied upon personal exposure to the detoxifying patient rather than on the standards for care for that type of patient. It is *not* considered standard or expected practice to place the detoxifying patient in restraints, because this may serve only to agitate the patient more. In this example, the Personalizer reflected upon an experience she had as a student. Unfortunately, the care delivered to the remembered client was incorrect and inappropriate, in violation of a standard practice for that type of patient. In selecting responses in the examination based upon personal experience and exposure, the Personalizer erred and thus selected the incorrect response.

The Personalizer can best alter this pattern of test taking by focusing on the broad principles and standards that guide and support nursing actions. The Personalizer should avoid making mental connections between patients in case situations included on an examination with single individual patients whom she may have met in practice. Even though the experience of illness is unique for each individual, many generalities occur among groups of types of patients, thus allowing health-care givers to predict patient needs and anticipate care requirements. The Personalizer should focus on the generalities about the type of patient and formulate decisions in testing situations based on standards of care established for nursing practice.

"The Squisher"

The Squisher is an individual who views examinations as a hurdle to jump, a barrier to cross, and a threat to self-esteem, rather than as a natural and expected event in a course of study. Squishers tend to be very preoccupied with grades, placing great value on personal accomplishment and fearing personal failure. Since a testing situation may result in less than desired achievement, or even worse, with failure, the Squisher attempts to avoid the responsibility and accountability associated with the testing experience, thus reducing anxiety over failure to achieve the personally determined level of achievement.

Rather than pursuing a plan of ongoing study and preparation for an examination, the Squisher faces an upcoming test with an attitude of "I'll worry about it tomorrow." The defense mechanism of suppression (placing an anxiety-causing event out of the mind and away from immediate thought) is overutilized by the Squisher, resulting in the development of "mental lists" for test study and preparation that are never fully actualized.

Typical mental lists of the Squisher personality include the following steps:

The test is in 2 weeks. I'll do the required readings this weekend.

Well, I can always read the textbook during the following week.

I'm sure I won't need to do the readings if I review my class notes very thoroughly.

I'll take a peek at the class notes this weekend before the exam, so the material will be fresh in my mind.

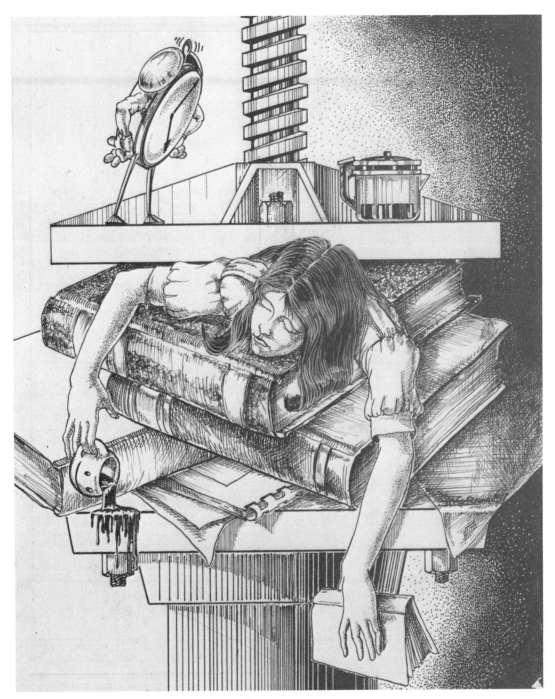

THE SQUISHER

I'll probably remember the material even better if I study the morning of the test.

Gosh, the test is in 2 hours! What should I do? I'll flip through my notebook and hope for the best!

The pattern of avoidance behavior exhibited by the Squisher in the above scenario clearly demonstrates this individual's inability to cope with the uncertainties of examinations and the associated feelings of performance anxiety. The Squisher spends excess time and psychic energy in planning avoidance *of* the examination, rather than simply preparing *for* the examination. Unfortunately, as pretest anxiety increases as the actual examination approaches, the ability of the human mind to absorb facts, organize knowledge, and correlate information markedly decreases. The Squisher thus attempts to focus or "squish" knowledge into her mind just before the examination, when the mind's ability to learn and process new knowledge is at its lowest level. The effort to avoid feelings of anxiety prior to the test are thus actually exacerbated by the increase of anxiety and guilt generated by avoidance behavior that inhibits the ability to learn, perform, and succeed.

The Squisher can best correct her inappropriate, personally hazardous behaviors by setting a plan for progressive, disciplined study. A prescription for study and test preparation should be devised, with defined time frames identified for completion of a unit of study. The Squisher then will not view the process of test preparation as an overwhelming one, but rather, as a step-by-step process that can readily be accomplished and completed. Just as an Olympic athlete must train for competition through consistent and progressive practice, so too the Squisher can "train" for the testing experience through consistent and progressive study.

"The Philosopher"

The Philosopher is typically a talented, thoughtful, intelligent student who has enjoyed a successful academic career, mainly as a result of persistent, disciplined, and well-structured study. The Philosopher places a high value on understanding or at least recognizing the complexities of a situation, but somehow never really believes that she knows *enough* about a topic or subject. Thus, when placed in a testing situation, she tends to "pore over" selected questions with great intensity and concentration, looking for an underlying, hidden meaning of the item. She studies the item with undue care and caution, searching for an unstated intent or "trick" in the question. It is quite likely that she has been told by her faculty or colleagues that she "reads into" the questions on examinations, yet she has great difficulty reading items as they are printed for the obvious content and intent of the questions.

Philosophers are easy to recognize in a testing situation, because much of the philosophic, "searching" process is evidenced in their outward behavior. They have a tendency to stroke their chins while studying the item, calling to

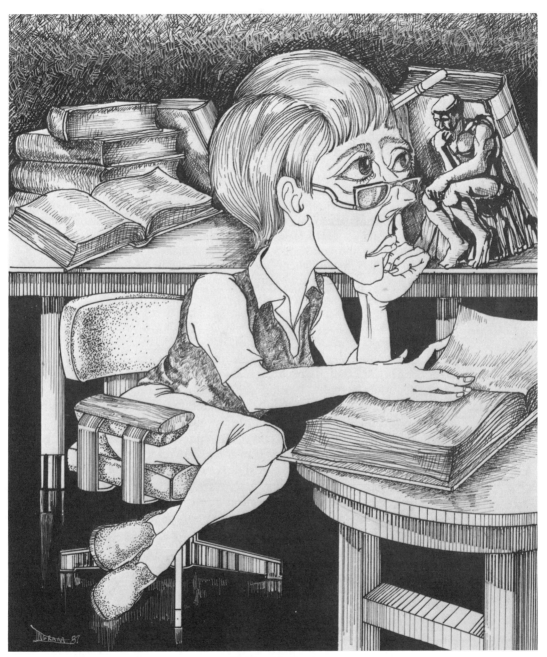

THE PHILOSOPHER

mind images of a famous statue, *The Thinker*. Often, they will look all around the test room or stare upwards toward the ceiling, deep in thought, unaware of others around them. Inevitably, they begin to lose sight of the actual intent of the item, overanalyzing even simple or straightforward questions, reading information *into* the item that does not exist. They answer the question, then, with their own additional information added rather than with what intent the original question was written.

The mental process of a Philosopher answering a question, "What pancreatic hormone does a diabetic patient lack?" would be as follows:

> Okay, well, the patient with diabetes does not manufacture insulin in his pancreas. So, it seems reasonable that the answer is insulin. But that seems so *obvious*. Maybe this is a trick question. I wonder if this question is really talking about the adult onset or Type II diabetic. Then the answer would not be insulin. Maybe they could be managed on diet alone, and they wouldn't need insulin. Of course, the pancreas also manufactures glucagon. Glucagon raises blood sugar. Does the diabetic manufacture glucagon? Well, since his pancreas does not function correctly, he probably doesn't. It *was* a trick question! The answer is *definitely* glucagon!

The obvious answer *is* insulin. The *correct* answer is insulin. The Philosopher had chosen the correct answer at first. But because she overstudied the item, she eventually chose an incorrect response. In her effort to allay her anxieties over not knowing *everything,* or not understanding completely enough, the Philosopher actually developed a misconception about the intent of the above question and will inevitably end up feeling even greater anxiety, when she discovers that her chosen response was, in fact, an incorrect one.

The Philosopher can best correct her inappropriate testing behavior by progressively developing self-esteem and self-confidence so that there will be less tendency to question initial responses to test questions. The Philosopher must learn to focus on the items *as they are written,* and avoid the tendency to read the item over and over, adding information or meanings unintended by the test authors. Continued practice with sample test items included in this book should help the graduate preparing for the State Board Examination to overcome "Philosopher" behavior.

"The Second Guesser"

The Second Guesser attempts to forestall feelings of anxiety in testing situations by playing the roles of both student and teacher, examinee and examiner. First, the Second Guesser carefully answers each question on the examination, taking the role of examinee. Then, however, she assumes the role of examiner and grades her own examination. This individual believes that a second look at each answered question will allow her to "catch" any possible error, and so she proceeds through the completed examination, changing initial responses as she goes. In that sense, she is "grading" her own test, playing the role of examiner.

Of course, the Second Guesser cannot with certainty know each answer to each question. But erasing the believed incorrect response and filling in a second, supposedly correct response gives the individual a sense of control, thus reducing her testing anxiety. Unfortunately, the examinee is far more likely to respond correctly to a question with a first answer than if she repeats the item and alters the initial response. When a human experiences anxiety, the perceptual field narrows, and the ability to think clearly, logically, and reasonably wanes. For this reason, the Second Guesser, experiencing increasing levels of anxiety as she progresses through the examination, is likely to have greater difficulty processing information and formulating correct responses as she goes through her examination the second time "correcting" it. The pencil eraser that seems her greatest ally in "fixing" her responses on a test then in fact is her biggest foe. Invariably, the Second Guesser will comment after receiving a graded examination, "Gosh! I had it right, but then I changed it to the wrong answer. I did that on about five of my questions!"

Second Guessers likewise court danger in testing by changing selected responses because they "seem" wrong—they don't fit into a pattern, or there is too much repetition of the same response. This individual becomes ill at ease when, as she rereads her examination answers, she notes that she has six **B** responses in a row, or too many *True* answers. Convinced that there must be an error to have so many answers in one pattern, she randomly changes one or two initial responses, forming a new pattern of response that she deems more acceptable.

The Second Guesser can easily alter this nonproductive behavior by rereading *only* the few items she is very unsure of and avoiding erasing or changing any initial response unless absolutely necessary. The examinee should focus on moving through the examination progressively and carefully, without setting aside the end of the examination period for rereading and "grading" behaviors.

"The Lawyer"

The hallmark characteristic of a good attorney is the ability to carefully formulate questions in order to get the most valuable and informational response. An attorney will attempt to get at the truth of a situation by following a successive series of questions that ultimately lead to the needed or desired answers. When the lawyer oversteps appropriateness in his questioning and attempts to place ideas or words into the witness' responses that the witness did not intend, the lawyer will be called upon for *leading the witness.*

It seems that communication questions, especially when placed in psychosocial settings, test the "lawyer" out in many test takers. When presented with a situation of nurse–patient or nurse–family interchange that requires selection of the most appropriate nurse response, examinees often veer away from obviously appropriate responses and select responses that place words or ideas into the patient's statements that were not really intended. The examinee who attempts to get at the truth or reality of what a patient is saying by choosing a "leading the witness" response is only *providing his own view* of the truth.

Consider the sample below:

Patient: Life has been so difficult since my husband's death. I can't seem to get involved in anything. I feel so empty and lifeless.

Nurse response: Have you thought about suicide?

In this example, the nurse, in an effort to get at the reality of the patient's feelings and thoughts, oversteps appropriateness in her questioning, placing meaning into the patient's words that may not have been intended. Simply, the nurse in this example is "leading the witness," as a *lawyer* might, rather than seeking to help the patient to express herself, as a *nurse* should. The nurse did *not* verbalize the implied, because the patient never alluded to a desire to end her own life. Rather, the *nurse provided her view* of the patient's reality.

Let's try another example:

Patient: I'm nervous about this open heart surgery tomorrow. Do you think I'll be all right?

Nurse response: You seem terribly frightened. Perhaps you should talk with your surgeon about your fears.

Wow! If the patient wasn't frightened at first, he sure is now! The patient simply states his nervousness about impending surgery and seeks reassurance from the nurse. The nurse, however, oversteps the real meaning of what the patient is saying and "leads the witness" to feelings of being "terribly frightened." Exaggerating the patient's feelings into intense fear may well cause the patient considerable emotional upset, an undesired effect of communication, especially just prior to a major surgery.

The Lawyer needs to focus on listening to the patient and hearing his thoughts and feelings, rather than on formulating responses targeted at getting certain information. Reflecting the patient's remarks is often a very effective way to encourage greater and fuller expression by the patient. Likewise, sharing observations made about the patient by the nurse can facilitate communication and ideally foster greater interaction between patient and nurse. Several helpful tips and examples of strategies that may be utilized by the examinee in answering communication questions are offered under the heading "Communication" in a later chapter of this book.

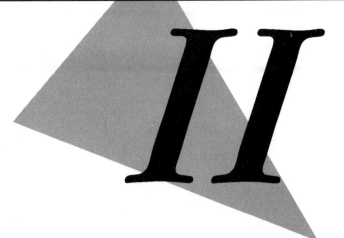

II

CONCEPTUAL FOUNDATIONS FOR NURSING PRACTICE

A CONCEPTUAL MODEL FOR LEARNING: ESSENTIALS FOR HEALTH

MARIAN B. SIDES

The framework for the organization of this nursing review is based on the conceptual foundations of nursing practice. It applies the philosophy that man, as a human being, constantly aspires to achieve an optimal state of health. This state of being requires internal harmony among all the processes that contribute to human functioning.

Health occurs along a continuum from wellness to illness. Each of us falls somewhere along this continuum. Optimal health depends upon our ability to maintain a delicate internal balance while relating to the environment around us.

This section presents 14 core concepts that frame health and common deviations from health. Chapters are organized around the model illustrated in Figure 6-1.

Each chapter focuses on a fundamental health concept such as oxygenation or acids and bases. Key principles for each concept are identified and illustrated in the text. Throughout, you will be led into thinking about how these concepts are acted out in the human body. Who is at risk for development of disease or illness? How are they manifested? What interventions are appropriate to regain balance? How do you know when the balance has occurred? This strategy for reviewing nursing will make you an active, thinking participant in the nursing process. It guards against the rote memorization of materials and encourages the understanding and application of principles to new and different situations.

This review does not include detailed description of every illness or disease. Certain broad concepts and principles are common to many disease and illness states. Once you become familiar with them, through use of this book, you will possess the skills that can be used to answer questions about most health situations.

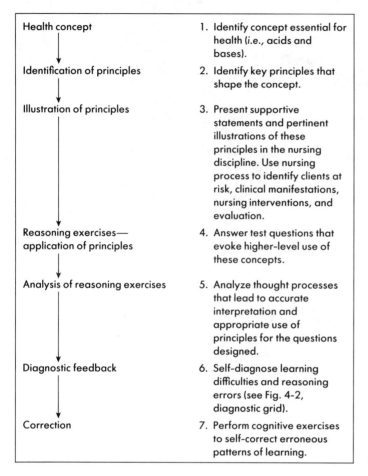

Health concept	1. Identify concept essential for health (*i.e.*, acids and bases).
Identification of principles	2. Identify key principles that shape the concept.
Illustration of principles	3. Present supportive statements and pertinent illustrations of these principles in the nursing discipline. Use nursing process to identify clients at risk, clinical manifestations, nursing interventions, and evaluation.
Reasoning exercises—application of principles	4. Answer test questions that evoke higher-level use of these concepts.
Analysis of reasoning exercises	5. Analyze thought processes that lead to accurate interpretation and appropriate use of principles for the questions designed.
Diagnostic feedback	6. Self-diagnose learning difficulties and reasoning errors (see Fig. 4-2, diagnostic grid).
Correction	7. Perform cognitive exercises to self-correct erroneous patterns of learning.

FIGURE 6-1. A MODEL FOR LEARNING.

Reasoning exercises in the form of test questions are provided to give you practice on mastering these concepts and applying the nursing process. If you have trouble or difficulty understanding the content in the chapters, you may need to consult a textbook to strengthen your knowledge base in these areas.

Be sensitive and alert to your strengths and weaknesses as you review. Analyze your performance by using the diagnostic grid to detect patterns.

A systematic and logical approach to this learning challenge will gradually bring you to mastery. It has worked for hundreds of graduates. It *will* work for *you!*

OXYGENATION

MARYTHERESE BALSKUS

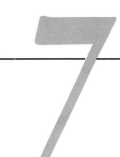

7

PRINCIPLE

TO MAINTAIN OXYGENATION, THE BODY REQUIRES A CONSTANT SUPPLY OF O_2 AND CO_2

Illustration of Principle

In order for the body to function, it is necessary that atmospheric oxygen (O_2) be inhaled and absorbed through the respiratory system. To understand this process, the nurse needs to be familiar with the structures involved in the respiratory system (see Fig. 7-1, The Respiratory System).

The nose is the respiratory system's air filter and humidifier. Atmospheric oxygen (O_2) enters the respiratory system and passes through the larynx. The larynx is at the top of the trachea and includes the vocal chords. When breathing occurs, the vocal chords open, allowing the free passage of O_2 through the larynx into the trachea. The trachea branches into two mainstem bronchi that direct O_2 into several bronchioles, which then branch off into millions of sac-like alveoli. It is at this point, where alveoli meet blood capillaries, that gas exchange occurs. Oxygen is transported from the respiratory system to the circulatory system by this process for use by the body's cells. By a reversal of this process, carbon dioxide (CO_2) moves out of the cells into the respiratory system, and excess CO_2 is exhaled.

Respiration is the process that enables the exchange of O_2 and CO_2. During inspiration, contraction of the diaphragm and intercostal muscles occur. The rib cage expands, creating a partial vacuum in the lungs. Because the pressure outside the body becomes greater than the pressure inside, air is drawn into the lungs.

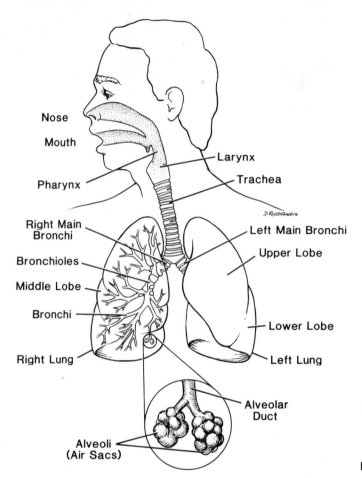

Nose

Mouth

Pharynx

Larynx

Trachea

D. ROSENZWEIG

Right Main Bronchi

Left Main Bronchi

Bronchioles

Upper Lobe

Middle Lobe

Bronchi

Lower Lobe

Right Lung

Left Lung

Alveolar Duct

Alveoli (Air Sacs)

FIGURE 7-1. THE RESPIRATORY SYSTEM.

When the body is in a state of equilibrium and is disease-free, the amount of O_2 in the cells is balanced by the amount of O_2 transported by the blood to the tissues. The CO_2 transported out of the lungs matches the volume produced by the tissues. This exchange of gases is necessary to maintain optimal body functioning and oxygenation.

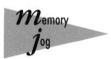

Memory Jog

In the healthy patient, adequate O_2 is inhaled, and excess CO_2 is exhaled.

This gas exchange can be measured by a blood–gas sample that will indicate the patient's blood pO_2, pCO_2, and pH. Both acid-base abnormalities and respiratory abnormalities can be demonstrated by blood–gas values, which are covered in detail in Chapter 10.

Principle

Illustration of Principle

Airway obstruction can pose a threat to a patient's oxygenation. Airway obstruction is characterized by an increased resistance to flow in the airways of the lungs. This can result in variable degrees of dyspnea (difficulty breathing), easy fatigability, wheezing, and often a cough productive of sputum. A disruption of oxygenation can occur upon acute airway obstruction (*e.g.,* asthma) or chronic airway obstruction (chronic bronchitis or emphysema). Nurses must always be aware of the patient's oxygenation and how it is affected by airway obstruction.

> Airway obstruction can be fully reversible in acute asthmatic attacks but may not be reversible in chronic bronchitis or emphysema.

Bronchial asthma is characterized by intermittent airway obstruction and narrowing. This obstruction involves constriction of bronchial smooth muscle and mucosal edema that results in bronchospasm. When this occurs, oxygenation can become impaired.

Asthma can be either intrinsic or extrinsic. Intrinsic asthma is generally considered to be the result of the autonomic nervous system's response to an inhaled irritant, weather changes, infection, emotion, or exercise. Intrinsic asthma is thought to result from an imbalance in the actions of the sympathetic and parasympathetic nervous systems. Sympathetic stimulation relaxes bronchial smooth muscle; parasympathetic stimulation constricts bronchial smooth muscle. Increased parasympathetic stimulation results in hypersensitivity of the airways, which can trigger an asthma attack.

> **Intrinsic asthma**
>
> Parasympathetic stimulation causes airway sensitivity and can trigger an asthma attack.

Extrinsic asthma can be caused by external factors such as allergens. Pollen, dust, and feathers can often precipitate an asthma attack. In many asthmatic patients, the attack begins with a nonproductive cough, wheezing, chest tightness, and shortness of breath. Wheezing may be prolonged during expiration, as a result of airway obstruction. In severe attacks, wheezing may decrease as dyspnea increases. This is a dangerous signal that complete airway obstruction may occur. The nurse must be constantly aware of the physical signs of hypoxia, which can include the use of accessory respiratory muscles, such as the sternocleidomastoid in the neck and the intercostal muscles between the ribs. Because O_2 to the brain may be diminished, symptoms of acute restlessness, anxiety, and confusion may occur. A sedative should never be given to an asthmatic patient to alleviate anxiety. The administration of a sedative could lead to further depression of the patient's respiratory status.

No sedatives in asthmatic patients!

Nonpharmaceutical measures should be taken by the nurse to reassure the patient. Asthmatic patients often become afraid that they will stop breathing and "need a tube to help me breathe." This is a genuine fear because many asthmatic patients can require intubation and may have been intubated previously for severe asthmatic attacks.

Nursing care of the asthmatic patient will often involve the administration of aminophylline, a bronchodilator. Aminophylline relaxes smooth muscle and dilates the bronchial tubes. This allows the patient to breathe easier, and oxygenation is improved. Aminophylline also stimulates the cardiac muscle and the central nervous system and can irritate the gastric mucosa. Palpitations, anxiety, restlessness, nausea, and vomiting are side-effects of aminophylline and may indicate a higher than therapeutic level.

Aminophylline dilates the bronchioles and improves oxygenation.

The nurse must be continually aware of the patient's oxygenation status. An ongoing assessment of the patient's respiratory function should occur. The nursing assessment should include the degree of shortness of breath, the duration and severity of the attack, and the duration, severity, and frequency of past attacks. The general appearance of the patient must be assessed to determine the presence or absence of respiratory distress, inspiratory or expiratory wheezing, and accessory muscle use. Auscultation of the lungs should reveal the severity of the attack. In severe attacks, many patients may be moving so little air through their lungs that they have barely audible breath sounds and may be unable to speak in complete sentences. Another clinical sign that can be easily identified by the nurse is pulsus paradoxus. A pulsus paradoxus of greater than 10 millimeters (mm) of mercury (Hg) indicates a severe attack. It is present when the systolic blood pressure during inspiration is more than 10 mm Hg above that of expiration.

SEVERE ATTACK

▷ Use of accessory muscles

▷ Barely audible breath sounds

▷ Pulsus paradoxus of >10 mm Hg

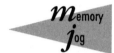

All patients with asthma must be carefully observed by the nurse to detect any decrease in oxygenation and worsening of hypoxemic signs and symptoms. The nurse's ongoing assessment can be invaluable in recognizing and preventing the progression of asthma attacks.

PRINCIPLE

OXYGENATION MAY BECOME IMPAIRED WHEN THE RESPIRATORY SYSTEM IS AFFECTED BY DISEASE, RESULTING IN DAMAGE TO LUNG FUNCTION

Application of Principle

In order for the cells and the tissues they comprise to function effectively, they must have adequate O_2. The adequacy of oxygenation, or the process by which O_2 is delivered to the cells and tissues, depends on three interrelated factors: O_2, hemoglobin, and cardiac output. The presence of O_2 requires sufficient cardiac output to deliver oxygenated blood and an adequate amount of functional hemoglobin.

NEEDS

Adequate oxygenation depends on:

Cardiac output

Hemoglobin

O_2

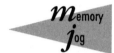

In chronic respiratory disease, a permanent alteration in O_2 delivery occurs. Chronic diseases of the respiratory system generally limit the O_2 supply to the tissues, creating a state of chronic hypoxia. Chronic hypoxia occurs slowly and continues over a long period of time. The body is able to adjust to this limited O_2 supply—to a point. In most cases, there are no obvious symptoms of chronic hypoxia. When acute exacerbations of chronic respiratory disease occur, however, signs and symptoms result. There may be fatigue, shortness of breath on exertion, and a general feeling of being less able to carry out the activities of daily living.

Chronic obstructive pulmonary disease (COPD) is the most common chronic respiratory condition in which chronic hypoxia occurs. COPD refers to a group of diseases (chronic bronchial asthma, chronic bronchitis, and emphysema) that are characterized by increased airway resistance. These result in varying degrees of dyspnea, easy fatigability, wheezing, and a productive cough. These symptoms may be the same as in acute obstruction but are much more ominous in chronic disease. The nurse must be alert for underlying chronic illness when confronted with acute symptoms.

Memory Jog

> **COPD is characterized by:**
>
> Increased airway resistance
>
> Dyspnea
>
> Fatigability
>
> Wheezing
>
> Productive cough

Chronic bronchitis is a continual inflammation of the lining of the respiratory bronchioles. Normally, the bronchioles are open and elastic. They allow and aid O_2 to move in and out of the lungs, ensuring proper oxygenation.

In chronic bronchitis, diseased bronchioles are narrowed by chronic inflammation. As a result of the inflammation, airway obstruction and excessive mucous production develop. Mucus replaces surfactant, a substance manufactured by respiratory cells, that is necessary to decrease the surface tension of the airways. Without surfactant, these airway passages lose their stability and tend to collapse easily. One of the first symptoms of chronic bronchitis is a recurrent productive cough. Shortness of breath on exertion progresses over years. Chronic airway narrowing and obstruction are the end results (see Fig. 7-2).

Emphysema is another chronic lung disease in which patients experience chronic hypoxia. Emphysema is defined in anatomic terms. It is present when there is a permanent abnormal enlargement of any part or all of the alveoli. Their many thin elastic walls are destroyed, leaving much larger air sacs and less surface area through which to exchange gases. (see Fig. 7-2). The result is that the lungs cannot deflate and expand as they should normally, and air trap-

Normal Breathing Tubes   **Bronchitis Diseased Tubes**

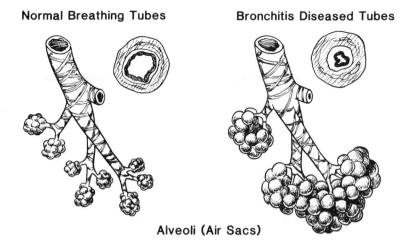

Alveoli (Air Sacs)

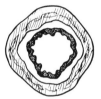

Air Passage Open   **Air Passage Closed**

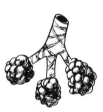
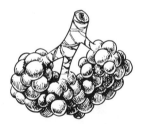

FIGURE 7-2. THE BRONCHI (BREATHING TUBES).

Normal Alveoli   **Emphysematous Alveoli**
(Air Sacs)   **(Air Sacs – Diseased)**

ping occurs. Patients are forced to breathe through pursed lips to try to eliminate the excess air. It becomes more difficult to blow air out than to breathe it in. Constant shortness of breath is the end clinical result.

Cigarette smoking is felt to be a major contributor to the development of chronic bronchitis and emphysema. Tobacco irritates airways and produces excess mucus and airway obstruction. Air pollution and occupational exposure may also be contributing factors.

While caring for the patient with chronic respiratory disease, nurses can take several therapeutic roles. First, they can encourage patients to stop smoking. Second, since nicotine in cigarettes is addictive, nurses must be aware of the signs and symptoms of a withdrawal: headache, nausea, anxiety, and restlessness. These symptoms can parallel symptoms of hypoxia; therefore, a good history and evaluation of the patient's respiratory status must be obtained. Third, they must understand and teach that smoking itself is an addiction for which the patient should not be blamed, but instead which he or she, with the help of health professionals and loved ones, can fight against and win.

Nursing management must include an assessment of the patient's ability to remove secretions. Adequate hydration and mobilization of secretions, by suctioning, by chest physical therapy, or by encouraging the patient to cough are all essential. Continual evaluation of the patient's vital signs and identification of the signs and symptoms of pulmonary infection are necessary for the patient with COPD. Frequent assessment of the rate of respirations, their pattern and depth should be noted. Any changes in breathing must be continually assessed.

PRINCIPLE

OXYGEN THERAPY IS NECESSARY TO RESTORE OXYGENATION WHEN OXYGENATION IS IMPAIRED

Illustration of Principle

Oxygen is essential for life. All cells require adequate oxygenation to remain viable. The purpose of O_2 therapy is to increase the percentage of O_2 gas in the alveoli and pulmonary capillaries. Goals of O_2 delivery should be to prevent or reverse cellular hypoxia, to decrease the work of breathing, and to decrease the myocardial workload. Oxygen is a drug that MUST be administered carefully, properly, and safely. Too much O_2 can cause damage to the body. In patients with COPD, too much O_2 can eliminate the patient's drive to breathe (*hypoxic drive*) and allow CO_2 retention and respiratory depression.

Memory Jog

Too much O_2 = decreased hypoxic drive

Nurses must have an adequate understanding of frequently used O_2 terms and modes of O_2 therapy.

Fraction of inspired O_2 (FiO_2) equals the percent of O_2 delivered to the lungs. Room air is a constant 21% O_2; therefore, room air is an FiO_2 of 21%. When patients require additional O_2, they can receive an FiO_2 from 24% to 100%. A blood–gas should always be obtained prior to O_2 administration unless it is a life-threatening situation.

High-flow O_2 is a system of O_2 delivery in which the total gas flow delivered to the patient is the only gas the patient is breathing. The advantage of high-flow O_2 systems is that they are reliable in delivering a precise amount of O_2. These systems cannot be influenced by the patient's breathing pattern.

Low-flow O_2 is a system that can deliver any O_2 concentration from 21% to 100%. These systems lack the accuracy and dependability of a high-flow O_2 system.

Nasal cannula is a low-flow O_2 system. Nasal prongs are placed in the nares of the patient. One to six liters of O_2 may be delivered to the patient. Oxygen delivery by nasal cannula should never exceed 6 liters because of nasal mucosal drying. The nurse must remember that because the patient also inhales room air, the precise fraction of inhaled O_2 is unknown. Therefore, the exact FiO_2 delivery cannot be determined when O_2 is given through a nasal cannula.

Simple O_2 mask is a low-flow system. A simple mask is placed over the patient's nose and mouth to deliver an FiO_2 at a range of 24% to 60%. This is the most common low-flow O_2 system.

Venturi mask is a high-flow system, a mask that fits over the patient's nose and mouth. It mixes O_2 and room air prior to delivery to the patient. It is the only mask available in which the exact amount of FiO_2 can be determined. This mask is indicated for the COPD patient.

Oxygen mask with a reservior bag is a high-flow system. This mask can deliver 70% to 90% O_2 for the patient with severe hypoxia that is not corrected by other O_2 systems. This system is used most commonly in patients who have smoke inhalation and CO_2 poisoning.

Endotracheal tube is a high-flow system. This requires that a tube be inserted into the trachea to the lungs to deliver as high as 100% O_2. Any concentration of O_2 can be delivered to the patient. In addition, intubation is the most effective method of O_2 administration for the severely hypoxic patient. Benefits of intubation include the prevention of aspiration and a direct route to suction patients.

Nurses must administer O_2 carefully because its effects can be damaging. It is critical that the nurse be knowledgeable as to the amount of O_2 that is appropriate for a given patient depending on the clinical situation. Accurate O_2 delivery can correct hypoxia and assist patient's recovery.

Reasoning Exercises: Oxygenation

Mr. John Jacobs is a 65-year-old retired factory worker who comes to the emergency room with complaints of progressive shortness of breath, dyspnea, fever, and productive cough.

1. The nurse caring for Mr. Jacobs should implement which of the following actions first?

    A. Assess vital signs

    B. Administer medication as ordered

    C. Apply O_2 as ordered

    D. Start an IV of normal saline and regulate to a keep open rate

The intended response is **A,** since airway, breathing, and circulation are essential in the determination of the respiratory status and the degree of observed respiratory distress. The vital signs are valuable measures of function and will assist in the determination of what therapy to implement first.

2. The physician orders Mr. Jacobs to receive 1 liter of O_2 per nasal cannula. The nurse should explain to the patient that the O_2 will

    A. Increase the work of breathing

    B. Treat the low levels of O_2 in his blood

    C. Reduce his blood pressure

    D. Increase his pulse rate

The intended response is **B.** Oxygen will help relieve the symptoms of hypoxemia and will decrease the work of breathing. By augmentation of his blood levels of O_2, the patient's vital organs will receive an increased O_2 supply.

3. After 30 minutes of treatment, Mr. Jacobs suffers sudden difficulty breathing. The nurse on duty observes that the rate of O_2 delivery is 6 liters per minute. The nurse knows that the increased O_2 intake can lead to a respiratory arrest by

    A. Increasing the respiratory rate

    B. Irritating the nasal mucosa

    C. Decreasing the total lung volume

    D. Eliminating the hypoxic drive

The intended response is **D.** Too much O_2 may overwhelm the patient's underlying cerebral mechanism for respiration, thereby eliminating hypoxic drive and causing respiratory arrest.

4. Mr. Jacobs required intubation because he stopped breathing. The nurse should explain to the patient that the endotracheal tube will

    A. Increase his oxygenation and allow suctioning of secretions

    B. Promote his fear and anxiety

    C. Improve the cardiac output

    D. Not allow hyperoxygenation

The intended response is **A.** Intubation allows the direct administration of medications, including O_2, into the respiratory and circulatory systems. Suctioning to clear the patient's secretions can be easily performed through the plastic tube. Intubation will improve the patient's ventilatory status.

5. Mr. Jacobs' family arrives and is surprised to find him on a respirator. They have brought his Living Will, which reads, "Do not intubate me under any circumstances." The nurse should

   A. Ignore the family and the Living Will

   B. Call the hospital ethics consultant

   C. Examine the document, noting the date, witnesses, and state of issue

   D. Explain to the family the therapies utilized in treating the patient's respiratory failure and notify the emergency room physician

The intended response is **D.** An adequate explanation to the family of the patient's emergency department course is necessary to allay their own fear and anxiety. It is not up to the nurse to check the validity of the document, and although an ethics consultant may be useful if problems arise, clear attempts at communication of the diagnosis, prognosis, and therapies are necessary before they are called in.

References

Cahill S, Balskus M. Intervention in Emergency Nursing: The First 60 minutes. Rockville, MD, Aspen Systems Corp, 1986

Snyder JV, Pinsky MR. Oxygen Transport in the Critically Ill. Chicago, Year Book Medical Publishers, 1987

CIRCULATION

NANCY B. CAILLES

8

PRINCIPLE

ALL HUMAN CELLS REQUIRE O_2 FOR LIFE

Illustration of Principle

A basic essential for cellular viability and function is O_2. Regardless of type, structure, or role of the cell, O_2 is *critical* to life. When cells are deprived of a ready and adequate supply of O_2, even for a brief period of time, cellular integrity and viability are compromised.

> Just as an automobile engine, even if in prime condition, cannot function without adequate input of gasoline as fuel, the human cell cannot function without adequate input of O_2.

*m*emory *j*og

Thus, nurses must always be concerned with the adequacy of the patient's oxygenation and be constantly aware of any factors that could interrupt O_2 transport by the extensive circulatory system. Such factors can range from prolonged placement of a forearm tourniquet during IV insertion to the more complex congestive heart failure with secondary circulatory collapse.

> Interruption of O_2 supply to body tissues will result in cellular damage or death.

*m*emory *j*og

87

The principle that all human cells require O_2 for life can be applied in a virtually limitless number of clinical situations. For example, the patient on complete bedrest, who cannot turn and reposition himself, will develop circulation-related complications, perhaps most obviously in the skin layers. Prolonged pressure on the patient's sacral or gluteal areas will result in an impairment of oxygen-rich blood flow. As the tissues of the skin layers are deprived of adequate O_2, degenerative changes and cellular damage occur, progressing through *ischemia* (temporary anemia) to eventual *necrosis* (tissue death). The formation of *decubitus ulcers,* then, is evidence of circulatory impairment.

*M*emory *J*og

> Decubitus ulcers are caused by prolonged pressure to an area of the body, which impairs circulation of O_2.

The same tissue death that occurs in decubitus ulcers occurs in *myocardial infarction.* The human heart uses O_2 at a greater amount and rate than any other organ in the human body. Any factor that interrupts oxygen-rich blood flow through the coronary arteries, then, will result in damage or even death to cells of the cardiac muscle. Similarly, brain cells deprived of essential O_2 as a result of thrombosis or rupture of a cerebral vessel will infarct, as in cerebrovascular accident. Thus, even though most signs and effects of cerebrovascular accident are *neurologic,* the process itself is very much *circulatory.*

A final illustration of this principle is the dependence of a developing fetus on adequate circulation of oxygen and nutrients by way of the maternal placental system. Should umbilical cord compression occur during labor, O_2 delivery by the placenta will be impaired, with resultant changes in fetal heart tones, indicating fetal distress or hypoxia. Prolonged decrease in fetal–maternal circulation can result in fetal cell damage, such as in the various syndromes of cerebral palsy. Awareness of this principle guides the nurse to closely monitor both progress of the female through her labor and response of the fetus to uterine contractions that might cause a decrease in fetal circulation or oxygenation.

*M*emory *J*og

> Impairment of the circulation of O_2 results in tissue damage.
>
> Skin: Decubitus ulcer
>
> Heart: Myocardial infarction
>
> Brain: Cerebrovascular accident
>
> Placenta: Fetal cell damage

PRINCIPLE

THE HUMAN HEART IS A TWO-SIDED OR "DOUBLE" PUMP GENERATED BY ELECTRICITY

Illustration of Principle

The heart serves as the mechanical pump for blood flow in the human body. Activation of the pumping of fluid by way of ventricular contraction occurs in response to electrical stimulation of the muscle fibers of the ventricles by the *sinoatrial (S/A) node* (pacemaker of the heart). The two sides of the heart, each composed of an atrial chamber and a ventricular chamber, allow blood flow from the body to progress through the oxygenation process in the lungs and then to be redistributed to the cells through simultaneous but separate phases of filling (*diastole*) and contraction/ejection (*systole*). The right heart receives blood from the body by way of the venous system, then sending blood to the lungs for oxygenation. At the same time, the left heart receives blood from the lungs by the pulmonary vein then sending oxygen-rich blood back to the body through the aorta. The heart, then, is a "double" pump, allowing for two separate but simultaneous pumping actions to occur.

The atria of the heart essentially serves as "waiting areas" for incoming blood, analogous to a waiting room in a busy physician's office. As more and more patients enter the waiting room with fewer chairs available, congestion occurs. This congestion is much like the pressure that increases in the atria as blood fills these chambers. When the waiting room becomes too crowded, patients are allowed through a door connecting the waiting room to the treatment areas, where the actual work with the patient will be done. Similarly, when the atria fills and pressure rises, a door between the atria and ventricles opens to allow blood to leave one chamber and enter the other. These "doors" are termed *valves*, which open and close to facilitate passage of blood in a continuous direction through the cardiac cycle. In our analogy, the treatment areas of the office where the work is carried out are like the ventricles, which receive the blood and, after attaining adequate filling, do the "work" of systole (contraction) causing blood to move either to the lung or to the aorta.

For the average adult patient with a heart rate of 70 beats/min, the above cardiac events occur in less than *1 sec.* It is very apparent, then, that each structure within the heart must function correctly in both its action and timing in order for the patient to maintain adequate cardiac output. *Cardiac output,* the volume of oxygenated blood ejected from the left ventricle every minute, is normally between 5 to 6 liters/min. Disease conditions or degenerative changes that interrupt the series of events occurring with each cardiac cycle will result in a compromised cardiac output, with subsequent loss of circulation of O_2 to the cells of the body.

For example, if the S/A node malfunctions or fails, regulation of the mechanical or pumping action of the heart is affected. Since the S/A node generates the electrical impulse that ultimately stimulates the muscles of the ventricles to contract, a deficit of S/A node function will result in decreased excitation of the cardiac muscle with a subsequent decrease in cardiac output.

Likewise, valves within the heart that are *stenosed* (narrowed and inflexible) or *insufficient* (unable to fully open and close) will impair the full filling and emptying of the chambers of the heart, influencing cardiac output. Narrowing or stenosing of the mitral valve, for example, will result in a decrease in the volume of blood leaving the left atrium with subsequent reduced filling of the left ventricle. With less blood filling, the left ventricle will contract, but less blood will be ejected, resulting in a decrease in cardiac output.

Finally, myocardial infarction provides another excellent example of how disease-related changes can negatively influence the critical activities of the heart. Myocardial infarction muscle damage occurring secondary to impaired oxygenation reduces the ability of the muscle to contract forcefully enough to eject blood effectively. The infarcted muscle is weakened and loses strength of contraction, resulting in a decreased stroke volume, or volume of blood ejected from the left ventricle with each heartbeat (or stroke). The reduced stroke volume results in a decreased cardiac output.

Since the heart pumps oxygenated blood to all tissues of the body, a decrease in cardiac output results in a decrease O_2 supply to the body's tissues. Since all human cells require O_2 for life, the effects of cardiac impairment can be noted in virtually every system of the body. For example, the kidneys are dependent upon an adequate perfusion of blood in order to sustain their activities of filtering, cleansing, and eliminating. When cardiac output is significantly decreased, so blood flow to the kidneys is decreased, with subsequent loss of kidney function that ultimately may result in renal failure. Likewise, a decrease in cardiac output of oxygen-rich arterial blood will result in inadequate oxygenation of brain cells. The patient will evidence this impairment with changes in mental status, becoming more disoriented, combative, and restless. As O_2 deficit continues, the patient will slip into unconsciousness and may suffer irreversible brain damage secondary to cardiac insufficiency.

$$\uparrow CO_2 \rightarrow \downarrow O_2 \rightarrow \text{function of organs}$$

It is obvious from this discussion that cardiac impairment can cause many undesirable and potentially life-threatening effects in the body. The nurse must always be conscious of the patient's status of circulation and oxygenation and should use ongoing assessment strategies to ensure adequate circulatory function. (See Assessment Guidelines in this chapter.)

PRINCIPLE

VEINS AND ARTERIES ARE THE PASSAGEWAYS FOR CIRCULATION OF O_2 TO THE CELLS OF THE BODY

Illustration of Principle

Adequacy of O_2 transport through the body's circulatory system is dependent upon the integrity of the veins and arteries—structures that serve as the passageways for blood flow. Thus, even though cardiac function may be adequate and cardiac output within normal parameters, circulation of O_2 may *still* be inadequate if these structures of blood flow are not functioning properly. The nurse, then, must be aware of any impairment of blood flow in veins or arteries, because these structures must function *with* the heart to ensure adequate circulation of O_2.

> Arteries carry oxygenated blood *away* from the heart to the body's cells. Veins carry deoxygenated blood back from the body *to* the heart and lungs.

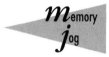

Memory Jog

Veins are thin-walled structures that carry blood toward the heart under low pressure. Each vein has a series of valves, which serve to prevent back-flow or pooling of blood in the structure as the blood courses through the body. Failure of these valves to function correctly will result in a pooling of blood in the vein, increasing pressure within the structure and resulting in the eventual development of *varicosities*—swollen, bulging, engorged veins with weakened walls. Such veins cannot support adequate circulation, resulting in notable signs of peripheral edema, extremity coolness, and aching or tenderness of the extremity. Blood that pools in the structures may form clots, or *thrombi*, which will further decrease blood flow within the structure and to the tissues the vein supplies. Thrombus formation within the venous passageway then presents an impairment of circulation even though cardiac function may be entirely adequate.

Changes within the structure of the arteries can likewise compromise oxygenation. Deposits of *plaque* (accumulated fats, cholesterols, and other elements) will cause an impairment of arterial blood flow to the cells of the body. Plaque deposits cause a narrowing of the arterial lumen, with subsequent decrease in blood flow and increase in pressure within the artery. The plaque formation in *atherosclerosis* may lead to hypertensive disease and impairment of oxygen transport to body tissues supplied by the arterial structure. Since all cells require oxygen for life, the effect of this disease becomes obvious. Atherosclerotic changes in the arteries that supply brain cells, for example, will cause decreased oxygenation of those cells, resulting in impaired mental alacrity and ability—as in Organic Brain Syndrome. Thus, the degeneration of mental processes noted in some elderly patients once attributed to old age and termed "senility" is more accurately attributed to impairment of cerebral blood flow and decrease in cerebral oxygenation secondary to changes within arterial structures.

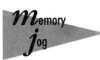

> Deposits of plaque (atherosclerosis) narrow arterial lumen. Rigidity of arterial walls (arteriosclerosis) increases arterial pressure. Both degenerative changes reduce arterial blood flow.

Similarly, *arteriosclerotic* changes in the arteries will result in an impairment of circulation or of oxygenation. In arteriosclerosis, the arterial wall loses its flexibility, becoming less and less able to expand and contract with corresponding changes in pressure from blood flow. As the artery becomes increasing rigid, pressure within the structure rises, resulting in hypertension and decreased arterial perfusion. Because the heart consumes O_2 at a very high rate, circulatory impairment from athero- and arterosclerotic changes within the arteries becomes the number one cause of *myocardial infarction,* necrosis or death of myocardial tissue secondary to cessation of arterial oxygen supply to the heart. Alteration in arterial blood flow, then, presents a hazardous, potentially life-threatening condition for the patient and must be considered by the nurse as important a concern as alteration in cardiac output.

PRINCIPLE

DELIVERY OF O_2 TO THE CELLS IS DEPENDENT UPON MICROSCOPIC BLOOD CELLS, WHICH "CARRY" O_2 GAS

Illustration of Principle

Essential to the delivery of O_2 *to* the cells and removal of CO_2 *from* the cells are adequate number and function of certain microscopic blood cells, principally erythrocytes or red blood cells (RBCs) and hemoglobin (Hgb), which serve to "carry" these gases in the blood stream. Reduction in the numbers of these circulating blood cells or defects in the structures of the cells may result in decrease in oxygenation of the cells of the body. Thus, even though cardiac output of oxygen-rich blood may be adequate, and arterial perfusion may be unrestricted, oxygenation can *still* be compromised by altered blood cell function.

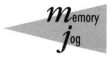

> Microscopic blood cells, such as RBCs and Hgb, carry O_2 to the cells and remove CO_2 from the cells. The heart pumps the blood, the veins and arteries are the passageways for blood, and the blood cells "carry" these gases through the passageways.

Patients with decreased *numbers* of these blood cells, such as those experiencing significant blood loss, will evidence signs of impaired oxygenation: pallor, dyspnea, shortness of breath, and fatigue. Other patients at risk for decreased numbers of RBCs and Hgb include those with poor dietary intake of iron, hematopoietic diseases, such as polycythemia vera and leukemia, or bone marrow depression secondary to cancer chemotherapy and radiation therapy.

Nursing Management

For this reason, numbers of these blood cells are routinely assessed to ensure adequate transport of O_2. The nurse should note depression of RBC and Hgb blood values that might suggest an impairment of O_2 transport. Patients experiencing surgical intervention, traumatic injury with blood loss, or labor and childbirth should be considered at risk for impaired oxygenation secondary to decreased numbers of these essential O_2 carriers.

> Any disease condition or clinical situation that involves loss of blood will likewise cause a loss of RBCs and Hgb, essential oxygen carriers in the blood. The nurse should monitor such patients for evidence of hypoexmia.

Patients with decreased RBCs and Hgb values may require nursing intervention in order for adequate oxygenation to be maintained. Such supportive measures include:

▷ Work in conjunction with medical intervention to arrest source of blood loss

▷ Administer transfusions of blood or blood products to increase number of circulating RBCs and Hgb

▷ Maintain the patient on bedrest to reduce O_2 need

▷ Administer O_2 therapy to increase cellular oxygenation (See oxygenation, Chapter 7, for discussion of oxygen therapy.)

▷ Continue to monitor blood values of RBCs and Hgb, oxygenation status, mental status and orientation

Defects in the *structure* of oxygen-carrying blood cells will also influence cellular oxygenation. In sickle cell anemia, for example, the shape of the red blood cell changes from its usual round shape to that of a sickle, with an elongated, hooked shape. Such misshaped cells cannot traverse easily through the circulatory passageways, resulting in impaired O_2 transport. Thus, symptoms of sickle cell anemia are very much like symptoms displayed by patients with decreased number of oxygen-carrying blood cells, including fatigue, shortness of breath, and so forth. It is apparent that both number and structure of oxygen-carrying blood cells significantly influence cellular oxygenation.

In the past few principles, then, we have reviewed the many structures of the circulatory system and their interrelated roles in the process of cellular oxygenation. In order for oxygenation to be adequate, the human body must have proper cardiac function and output, adequate and unrestricted venous and arterial blood flow, and sufficient number and function of oxygen-carrying cells in the blood.

PRINCIPLE

BECAUSE THE CIRCULATORY SYSTEM PROVIDES ESSENTIAL O_2 TO ALL CELLS OF THE HUMAN BODY, ALTERATIONS IN CARDIOVASCULAR FUNCTION ARE EVIDENCED BY MANY SYSTEMS

Illustration of Principle

It is apparent that the cardiovascular system supplies O_2 and nutrients to all cells of the human body in order to maintain their viability and function. Thus, impairments of circulation may be evidenced in a variety of ways in a variety of systems, depending upon the source and nature of the circulatory impairment. For example, chest pain would certainly be a typical cardiovascular symptom, indicating a circulatory impairment. But likewise, pain in the lower extremities associated with intermittent claudication would *too* indicate cardiovascular impairment, with both chest pain and extremity pain suggesting decreased oxygenation of that particular area of the body. Therefore, the nurse must observe carefully for symptoms suggesting cardiovascular impairment that would result in decreased circulation.

The nurse may find it easier to conduct assessments of cardiovascular function by examining for signs and symptoms of alterations *vis-a-vis* the following specific cardiovascular functions:

CARDIOVASCULAR FUNCTION	ASSOCIATED SIGNS AND SYMPTOMS
Oxygenation	Pain (such as chest pain, extremity pain) Loss of function of body part or parts (*i.e.,* hemiplegia following CVA) Rate, depth, and ease of respirations Color, warmth, and moisture of skin Abnormalities in arterial blood–gas values Abnormalities in arterial blood values Presence of abnormal findings, such as pallor, mottling, cyanosis, shortness of breath (SOB), dyspnea, syncope
Fluid circulation	Alterations in blood pressure Alterations in urine output Alterations in central venous pressure Rate and adequacy of apical and peripheral pulses Presence of abnormal findings, such as edema, distended jugular veins, lung congestion, decreased urinary output
Cellular nutrition	Presence and distribution of body hair Integrity of skin layers General physical vitality, energy, strength Presence of abnormal findings, such as body alopecia, decubitus ulcers, persistent fatigue, fatigue upon exertion

Reasoning Exercises: Circulation

Mr. Robert Bacchus is a 63-year-old retired business executive who comes to the emergency room with complaints of dyspnea, shortness of breath, and chest pain radiating to the left arm.

1. The nurse caring for Mr. Bacchus should implement which of the following actions FIRST?
   A. Administer prescribed pain medication
   B. Apply oxygen per nasal cannula as ordered
   C. Assess vital signs
   D. Apply electrocardiogram electrodes to the patient's chest

The intended response is **C**, since vital sign assessment will provide baseline data of vital cardiac and respiratory function, which will then serve as a guideline for diagnosis and therapy measures.

2. The physician orders Mr. Bacchus to receive 1 tablet of nitroglycerin sublingually every 3 min for chest pain. The nurse should explain to the patient that this medication will

   A. Reduce his blood pressure
   B. Increase the pulse rate
   C. Increase the oxygenation of the cardiac muscle
   D. Decrease the output of blood from the heart

The intended response is C. Nitroglycerin is a vasodilator, which will increase the flow of oxygen to the cardiac muscle by increasing the arterial blood flow through the heart's circulatory system. Since the cardiac muscle receives increased oxygen supply, pain associated with decreased oxygenation should decrease.

3. Following two doses of nitroglycerin, Mr. Bacchus reports that the chest pain has subsided. A diagnosis of angina pectoris is reached, and a coronary angiogram is scheduled for the following day. Mrs. Bacchus asks, "Has my husband had a heart attack?" The nurse should respond:

   A. "It is not possible to know that until the angiogram test has been performed."
   B. "Since the pain was relieved by the nitroglycerin, it's very likely that he *has* had a heart attack."
   C. "We will have to watch him closely for further symptoms before we know for sure."
   D. "Although it appears that he hasn't had a heart attack, the test is needed to help explain why he was experiencing the chest pain."

The intended response is D, since relief of pain with nitroglycerin and the subsequent diagnosis of angina pectoris effectively rules out the probability of myocardial infarction (heart attack). This response best allays the spouse's anxiety about her husband's condition but likewise stresses the importance of the ordered angiogram test.

4. The angiogram is performed, revealing extensive coronary artery occlusive disease secondary to arterial plaque formation. The nurse understands that this condition leads to anginal pain by

   A. Causing coronary arteries to be inflexible to arterial pressure changes
   B. Reducing the contractility of the cardiac muscle fibers
   C. Decreasing the diameter of the lumen of the coronary arteries
   D. Increasing the stroke volume of the heart

The intended response is **C.** The condition described in the item stem is atherosclerosis, characterized by a buildup of plaque deposits in the arterial network of the heart. Atherosclerotic deposits reduce the size of the arterial lumen, making a narrower pathway for the flow of oxygen-rich arterial blood. Decrease in O_2 supply to the cardiac muscle will result in the development of chest pain, or angina pectoris. Response **A** describes the effect of *arteriosclerotic* heart disease.

5. Care of Mr. Bacchus immediately following the coronary angiogram with femoral artery catheter insertion site would include all of the following actions *EXCEPT:*

    A. Maintain the patient on bedrest

    B. Frequently check pressure dressing to femoral artery for bleeding

    C. Assess vital signs every 4 hr

    D. Medicate patient discomfort with mild analgesics as needed

The intended response is **C.** Following a diagnostic procedure such as an angiogram the nurse should be alert for evidence of bleeding from the catheter insertion site, because blood loss will impair cellular oxygenation. The patient should be maintained on bedrest, since movement may encourage bleeding. The artery dressing should be assessed frequently so that any blood loss from the catheter insertion site can be identified. The patient may be medicated for pain after the procedure as needed. Vital signs must be assessed much more frequently than every 4 hr postprocedure, since changes in vitals may indicate bleeding. Rather, the nurse should assess vitals every 15 min during the first hr, every 30 min during the second hr, and every hr for the remaining 2 hr postprocedure.

FLUIDS AND ELECTROLYTES

Nancy B. Cailles

Diane M. Black

9

PRINCIPLE

WHERE SODIUM (Na^+) GOES, WATER (H_2O) GOES

Illustration of Principle

Sodium is an electrically charged ion (electrolyte), which has an intimate relationship with water or fluid in the human body. This basic principle is critical to one's understanding of fluid and electrolyte balance, since it helps to explain the processes and results of Na^+ excesses and losses that may result from inadequate Na^+ intake or Na^+ loss. Therefore, when planning care for the client with an Na^+ imbalance, it is likewise necessary to review the client's *fluid* status as well, since presentation of the Na^+ imbalance will be evidenced likewise in changes in the client's *fluid* balance.

> Although Na^+ as an electrolyte influences central nervous system (CNS) function, its primary action is on fluid balance in the body. Thus, when the patient experiences a Na^+ imbalance, the nurse must also anticipate an alteration in fluid balance.

*m*emory *j*og

PRINCIPLE

Na^+ IS WELL STORED IN THE HUMAN BODY

Illustration of Principle

Since a large percentage of the body is composed of fluid, and Na^+ and fluid are interrelated, there is usually ample storage of Na^+ in the human body. Additionally, the hormone aldosterone plays a role in Na^+ retention and excretion by its action on the kidneys.

The human body requires approximately 4 g of Na^+ per day, supplied principally by dietary intake. However, since the body stores Na^+ so well, a decrease in dietary intake of Na^+ will not immediately result in a Na^+ imbalance, since reserve stores of Na^+ are available.

Food sources rich in Na^+ are commonly addressed on the NCLEX licensure examination and can be easily remembered by the use of this simple acronym:

Prevent **M**ore **S**odium

The *P* in *Prevent* stands for *processed* foods, since Na^+ is often used as a preservative for such foods. Examples of processed foods include

▷ Frozen foods (*e.g.,* vegetables, dinners)

▷ Canned foods (*e.g.,* soups, gravies, fruits)

▷ Boxed pastry mixes (*e.g.,* cakes, breads)

▷ Prepared cereals and breads

▷ Processed meats (*e.g.,* bologna, sausage, corned beef, franks)

The *M* in *More* stands for *Moo* food, that is, dairy products. This group includes

▷ Milk and cream

▷ Cheese

▷ Butter

▷ Ice cream

Finally, the *S* in *Sodium* stands for *salty* foods, that is, foods with an obvious salty taste. These foods are rich in Na^+, because salt is used in the manufacture of the products. This group includes

▷ Potato chips and pretzels

▷ Pickles and olives

▷ Nuts

▷ Bacon

▷ Ham

The nurse should be aware that restrictions of these food groups will depend on the type of sodium-restricted diet ordered for the patient. Whereas some Na^+ restrictions only call for the avoidance of table salt, others will restrict salt in cooking and foods in these groups. Regardless of the type of restriction, the most common indication for Na^+ restriction is *fluid* imbalance. Patients placed on Na^+ restrictions are most often those suffering from conditions that involve fluid problems, such as congestive heart failure or renal disease. Once again, the intimate relationship between Na^+ and fluids in the body is underlined.

> Sodium-rich foods can best be categorized into three groups: processed foods, dairy products, and salty foods.

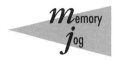

*M*emory *J*og

PRINCIPLE

HYPERNATREMIA   *(Hyper, "too much" or "excess")*
  (Na, symbol for sodium)
  (Emia, "serum," or "blood")

IS AN EXCESS OF Na$^+$ CONCENTRATION IN THE BLOOD, CHARACTERIZED BY A SHIFT OF FLUID FROM THE CELLS INTO EXTRACELLULAR FLUID, CAUSING SHRINKING OF THE CELLS

Illustration of Principle

Although hypernatremia can be caused by either an increased concentration of serum Na$^+$ or an excess loss of body fluid, the symptoms of this imbalance are the same. The hallmark feature of hypernatremia is *dehydration,* since the high concentration of serum Na$^+$ "pulls" fluid from the cells, resulting in cell shrinkage. The classic symptoms of dehydration, and thus, of hypernatremia, include the following:

▷ Hot, dry, flushed skin with poor turgor

▷ Thirst

▷ Dry mucous membranes

▷ Absence of tears (particularly in children)

▷ Soft, sunken eyeballs

▷ "Doughy" abdomen

▷ Increased body temperature

The vascular effects of hypernatremia cause fluids to shift from intracellular to extracellular, thereby initially raising pressure in the arteries (increased BP) and causing tachycardia and increased urinary output. The body then compensates from fluid shift and loss to oliguria and decreased BP in an effort to retain needed fluid. Since Na$^+$ as an electrolyte influences the transmission of nerve impulses, CNS symptoms may also appear, including irritability, excitability, restlessness, and convulsions.

Laboratory data will evidence hypernatremia with an elevated serum Na$^+$ value, greater than normal range of 132 to 142 mEq/L.

Patients at risk for hypernatremia are principally those experiencing a decreased intake or excess loss of fluid. For example, in the disease diabetes insipidus, excessive loss of fluids in urination may result in a hypernatremic state. Likewise, patients experiencing severe diarrhea have excessive loss of fluids, which may result in hypernatremia. Patients experiencing kidney failure, congestive heart failure, or shock can experience hypernatremia owing to reduced glomerular filtration.

The primary goal of treatment for a patient with hypernatremia is the administration of fluid replacement therapy and continuation of fluid maintenance therapy. Supportive measures are needed with continued close assessment of the patient's condition in terms of fluid balance.

PRINCIPLE

HYPONATREMIA   *(Hypo, "too little" or "decreased")*
                (Na, symbol for sodium)
                (Emia, "serum," or "blood")
IS A LESS THAN NORMAL CONCENTRATION OF SODIUM IN THE BLOOD

Illustration of Principle

Hyponatremia may result from two causes: excess loss of Na^+ from body serum or excess retention of body fluids.

In hyponatremia, there is a low serum level of Na^+—132 mEq/L or lower. Since Na^+ is an electrolyte that influences the transmission of nerve impulses, decreased serum Na^+ will demonstrate symptoms of headaches, abdominal cramps, and muscular weakness. Due to excess fluid accumulation, nausea and vomiting are common symptoms.

Clients at risk include those who experience loss of Na^+ through the skin: excessive sweating as a result of increased environmental temperature, fever, or muscular exercise. Great quantities of Na^+ are also lost through burn wounds, postoperative wound drainage, bleeding, a combination of low-Na^+ diet and potent diuretics, excessive plain H_2O intake. With adrenal cortex dysfunction, hyponatremia can present itself as Addison's disease with loss of Na^+ across renal tubules, caused by decreased mineralocorticoid production. Hyponatremia can result from SIADH (syndrome of inappropriate antidiuretic hormone), which causes more H_2O to be absorbed and extracellular fluid to become diluted.

The goal of therapy with hyponatremia is to restore sodium levels. If there is an excess of fluid with decrease of Na^+ levels, therapy is aimed at restricting fluids. If fluid balance is normal with decreased Na^+ levels, an isotonic saline solution is given.

PRINCIPLE

OVERHYDRATION IS AN EXCESS OF H_2O IN THE EXTRACELLULAR COMPARTMENT WITH A NORMAL AMOUNT OF SOLUTE
OR DEFICIENT AMOUNT OF SOLUTE

Illustration of Principle

Water is the primary body fluid. It serves many functions from the transport of nutrients and temperature regulation to the removal of waste products.

The adult human body is approximately 55% to 70% fluid, while the infant is 70% to 80% fluid composition. Therefore, the infant and young child are at risk for fluid imbalance problems as a result of the large percentage of body weight that is H_2O. Likewise, the elderly are also at risk, because they have less fluid reserve as their body H_2O content averages 45% to 50%.

When discussing hydration, our assessment of clients pertains to extracellular fluid composition, which consists of interstitial (fluid between cells or in tissues) and intravascular (plasma).

Many terms have been identified for excess extracellular fluid volume, such as overhydration, H_2O excess, and hypervolemia. In essence, there is an excess of fluid volume, which causes the following symptoms:

▷ Weight gain and edema

▷ Dyspnea ⎤

▷ Cough ⎬————— Fluid congestion in lungs

▷ Moist rales ⎦

▷ Puffy eyelids

▷ Increased central venous pressure ⎤

▷ Bounding pulse ⎬——— Fluid excess in vascular system

▷ Neck vein engorgement ⎦

▷ Bulging fontanelles

▷ Decreased hemoglobin and decreased hematocrit (hemodilution)

▷ Nausea, vomiting

Many types of clients are at risk for development of overhydration, particularly kidney failure caused by retention of Na^+ and H_2O and congestive heart failure (clients have backflow of fluids as a result of a weakened pump). Cushing's syndrome can create fluid overload because of increased production of adrenal corticoid hormones.

Massive generalized edema may also be called anasarca, which is fluid retention for an extended period of time, usually of cardiac or renal origin.

The primary goal of treatment is to restrict fluids to lower fluid volume. Diuretics or hypertonic saline may be used. The nurse is cautioned to make continuous skin assessments to prevent skin breakdown and daily weights to assess progress of treatment.

PRINCIPLE

DEHYDRATION IS A LOSS OF BODY FLUIDS, PARTICULARLY FROM THE EXTRACELLULAR FLUID COMPARTMENT

Illustration of Principle

Water moves from an area of lesser concentration to an area of greater solute concentration until both are equal. With dehydration, the excess loss of body fluids occurs in the extracellular compartment, thereby creating a hyperosmolar dehydration. The signs and symptoms of dehydration are then closely related to those of hypernatremia.

Included in signs and symptoms are:

▷ Thirst

▷ Dry mucous membranes

▷ Sunken eyeballs

▷ "Doughy" abdomen

▷ Dry skin with poor turgor

▷ Elevated temperature

▷ Body weight loss

As dehydration progresses, vascular effects become noticeable. The hyperosmolar dehydration causes a state of hypovolemia leading to tachycardia and increased respiratory rate and decreased blood pressure. Behavioral changes lead to

▷ Restlessness, irritability

▷ Disorientation and delirium

▷ Convulsions

▷ Coma evolves with fatal dehydration of 22% to 30% loss of body H_2O

Loss of body fluids can occur from fever or insufficient water intake as in clients that are NPO or comatose. Dehydration can also occur from losing body fluids from the gastrointestinal system (diarrhea, vomiting), renal system (excess urine output from diabetes insipidus or diuretics), integumentary system (excessive perspiration, burns). Clients in hypovolemic states may have great loss of body fluids from hemorrhage, shock, or metabolic acidosis.

The treatment for dehydration is primarily to administer fluid replacement therapy and continue with fluid maintenance therapy. This fluid replacement is especially crucial in children because their body is approximately 70% to 80% body H_2O. The formula to guide by in infants is 100 cc/kg of body weight per 24 hr.

PRINCIPLE

POTASSIUM (K^+) IS AN ESSENTIAL ELECTROLYTE IN BODY FLUIDS WHOSE PRIMARY FUNCTION IS TO *IRRITATE*.

POTASSIUM SERVES TO IRRITATE NERVE CELLS, WHICH ULTIMATELY INFLUENCES MUSCULAR FUNCTION

Illustration of Principle

As an electrically charged ion, K^+ plays a critical role in neuromuscular function through the excitation, or *irritation,* of nerve cells, resulting in muscular contraction. Both smooth and skeletal muscle and especially the human heart are dependent upon K^+ for proper and regulated contraction and function.

Unlike sodium, K^+ is poorly stored in the human body with approximately 90% being excreted in urine. Therefore, imbalances of K^+ can occur rather quickly, when an insufficient supply of K^+ is ingested or an excessive loss occurs, such as in potassium-wasting diuretic therapy.

Since K^+ is poorly stored, the human body requires a daily intake of potassium-rich food sources in order to maintain adequate K^+ levels and thus maintain proper neuromuscular function. Food sources rich in K^+ are perhaps most easily remembered by the word *fruit,* since many fresh fruits are potassium-rich.

Fruits rich in K^+ include:

Peaches

Figs

Bananas

Oranges/orange juice

Strawberries

Pears

Prunes

Raisins

Watermelon

Dates

Cantaloupe

Apricots

Although many may mistakenly believe tomatoes to be vegetables, they are, in fact, fruits, and tomato juice is likewise potassium-rich. Finally, instant coffee and many salt substitutes currently on the market are relatively high in K^+. The human body requires approximately 40 mEq of K^+ per day, but this need is usually met with dietary intake alone.

PRINCIPLE

WHERE Na^+ GOES, K^+ DOESN'T

Illustration of Principle

Sodium and K^+ have an inverse relationship in the human body. Thus, when an imbalance of Na^+ occurs in the serum, the opposite imbalance of K^+ frequently occurs. For example, if excess Na^+ is retained as in *hyper*natremia, a corresponding excess of K^+ will be excreted, resulting in *hypo*kalemia. This principle illustrates the fact that electrolyte imbalances will infrequently occur in isolation, and therefore the nurse should monitor *all* electrolyte values of a client experiencing a singular electrolyte imbalance.

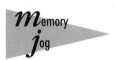

> Potassium (K^+) is an electrolyte whose primary action in the body is excitation of nerves which influences muscular function. Potassium is poorly stored in the body, and dietary intake of potassium-rich foods such as fruits must meet the need for 40 mEq of K^+ per day.

PRINCIPLE

HYPERKALEMIA IS AN INCREASE IN SERUM K^+ LEVELS CHARACTERIZED BY MUSCULAR IRRITABILITY AND TENSION

Illustration of Principle

In hyperkalemic states, increased levels of serum K^+ circulate to body cells, resulting in an increased irritability of nerves and muscles. The symptoms of hyperkalemia, then, are those of *hyperexcitability* of the target body system. For example, when the gastrointestinal tract is overstimulated by excess K^+, symptoms of gastrointestinal hyperexcitability, including nausea, colic, and diarrhea, result. Muscular cramping, pain, and weakness are evidence of overstimulation of muscle cells by excess K^+. As with hypokalemic states, the impact of K^+ imbalance on the function of the human heart is *most* critical and thus the priority concern for the nurse. Since hyperkalemic states lead to increased irritation of the cardiac muscle, tachycardia and potentially life-threatening dysrhythmias, which may ultimately lead to cardiac arrest, can result.

Treatment of hyperkalemic states must be prompt in order to forestall alterations in cardiac function and possible cardiac failure. If the patient evidences a serum K^+ in excess of normal parameters (3.5 to 5 mEq/L), the nurse in conjunction with the physician must take aggressive steps to achieve the goal of reducing serum K^+ levels. These steps include:

▷ Withdrawal of all potassium-rich foods, supplements or IV additives

▷ Administration of IV fluids and Lasix diuretic therapy to "flush out" excess K^+ through urine (only *if* the hyperkalemic patient has adequate renal function)

▷ Administration of Kayexalate solution (most often via rectal instillation) to hasten removal of excess K^+

The nurse should carefully monitor serum K^+ values for evidence of efficacy of treatment measures as well as assessing cardiac function by electrocardiograph tracings. Safety measures, such as placing the side rails in upright position and having someone in attendance with the hyperkalemic patients, should be employed to reduce the risk of injury to the patient in his hyperexcited state.

> *Hyper*kalemia results in *hyper*excitability of nerves and muscles. The nurse should place greatest priority on cardiac function, since the heart is overstimulated and may evidence life-threatening changes in rate and rhythm.

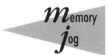

PRINCIPLE

HYPOKALEMIA IS A DECREASE IN SERUM K$^+$ LEVELS CHARACTERIZED BY MUSCULAR WEAKNESS AND FATIGUE

Illustration of Principle

In hypokalemic states, there is an insufficient supply of K$^+$ to body cells, causing insufficient stimulation or irritation to nerves and muscles. Therefore, muscular weakness is a cardinal feature of this electrolyte imbalance.

Since K$^+$ is poorly stored in the human body, reserves of K$^+$ are limited. Patients who are unable to take in adequate amounts of K$^+$ (40 mEq/day) by mouth are at risk for hypokalemia. Additionally, patients who are experiencing K$^+$ loss, secondary to taking oral diuretics or severe diarrhea, may also risk this imbalance.

> Patients need daily intake of K$^+$. Those with limited or restricted oral intake of foods and fluids should be monitored for hypokalemia. These would include:
>
> ▷ Surgical patients with NPO status
>
> ▷ Patients with pronounced anorexia (cancer chemotherapy)
>
> ▷ Patients with impaired chewing or swallowing (post-CVA)
>
> ▷ Patients undergoing gastric suction or surgery

Because hypokalemia results in decreased irritation to nerves and muscles, symptoms of this imbalance are related to neuromuscular function. Symptoms would include

▷ Muscular weakness

▷ Fatigue

▷ Decreased muscle tone

▷ Decreased cardiac rate

▷ Dysrhythmia

It is important to note that the end product to either K^+ deficit or excess is cardiac arrest, or asystole, in response to changes in stimulation to the cardiac muscle. Thus, the effects of either potassium imbalance on the human heart can best be summarized as "K^+ kills," underlining the critical effects of K^+ imbalance.

Serum K^+ levels below the normal range of 3.5 to 5 mEq/L indicates hypokalemia. Since hypokalemia may be related to either an insufficient intake or an excess loss of K^+, K^+ *replacement* is the key to management of this imbalance. Potassium may be administered orally via potassium-rich foods or K^+ supplements, such as K-Lyte or K-Lor. If K^+ is to be added via an intravenous route, it *must* be added to an IV drip, and never by direct IV route, since this route will cause rapid irritation of cardiac muscle with potential dysrhythmia and asystole. Supportive nursing measures include careful monitoring of the IV insertion site, if IV drip route is being utilized, since K^+ infusions may cause venous irritation and subsequent extravasation. The nurse should closely monitor the client's cardiac function, best observed via a continuous ECG monitor. Since the client's muscles are weak and fatigued, the nurse should monitor client safety and prevent accidental falls by keeping the bed rails up and the call light within easy reach of the client. Finally, the nurse must carefully monitor the client's urinary output, since K^+ supplements are being administered and must be able to be excreted to avoid a potential K^+ excess from therapy.

Reasoning Exercises

1. Baby Jones, 6 weeks old, is admitted with a diagnosis of hypertonic dehydration after 24 hr of vomiting and diarrhea. Clinical manifestations would include all of the following, except

   A. Rough, dry tongue

   B. Doughy abdomen

   C. Elevated temperature

   D. Bulging fontanelles.

The intended response is **D**, since dehydration causes loss of body fluids, therefore leading to depressed fontanelles. Bulging fontanelles are indicative of overdehydration. **A, B,** and **C** are clinical manifestations of loss of body fluids.

2. Nursing assessment of Baby Jones' dehydration status would indicate particular attention to baby's

   A. Height

   B. Weight

C. Pulse

D. Respirations

The intended response is **B,** since dehydration refers to loss of body fluids. Weight is the best indicator of the amount lost. **C** and **D** are important assessments to make since dehydration will alter these values, but they are not indicators of the amount of the loss of body fluids. Very often height is used with weight with infants, but it has no value to assess loss of body fluids.

3. Nursing care of Baby Jones would place immediate priority on
    A. Replacing fluids
    B. Growth and development needs
    C. Maintaining vitals within normal range
    D. Maintaining patent airway

The intended response is **A,** since dehydration is loss of body fluids and this loss of body fluids has created the clinical manifestations, priority is placed on replacement therapy. **B** is a general need of all children, but does not become a priority of sick children. **C** is incorrect because vitals will return to normal range when fluid replacement has occurred. **D** is incorrect since the priority is fluid replacement without a problem with airway obstruction.

4. Fluid replacement therapy has been given, and maintenance therapy of fluids has continued over 24 hr. Baby Jones becomes listless, cyanotic, with good skin turgor and bulging fontanelles. Respirations are 68 and pulse rate is 180. The nurse assesses the infant and analyzes the situation and immediately should
    A. Start O_2
    B. Decrease intravenous drop rate
    C. Assess vital signs in 15 min to observe for further change
    D. Stimulate the infant

The intended response is **B.** The infant has now developed bulging fontanelles, a clear indicator of fluid overload or overhydration. Immediate priority would be to decrease fluids. **A** is incorrect as a priority, but would be included in the care of the cyanosis. The cyanotic condition is caused by the overhydration condition. **C** is incorrect as a priority but would be an intervention to be done after the IV rate is decreased. **D** is incorrect as stimulus would have no effect on hydration status.

Reasoning Exercises: Fluids

Mr. Smith is a 44-year-old iron worker, who is admitted through the emergency room with a flushed face, irritability, and the following vital signs:

Temp . . . . 99.1 °C

Resp 20

Pulse 108

BP 280/114

A diagnosis of hypertensive crisis is made.

1. Signs and symptoms of hypernatremia would include all of the following, except
    A. Restlessness
    B. Muscular weakness
    C. Tachycardia
    D. Thirst

The intended response is **B,** since high Na^+ levels cause excitability of nerve transmission, creating restlessness and tachycardia. Thirst is included as high salt levels create a need for fluids. **C** or muscular weakness is evident in hyponatremia because of low levels of Na^+ in the blood causing decreased nerve transmission.

2. Mr. Smith is placed on a sodium nitroprusside and chlorothiazide. The purpose of chlorothiazide with this client is to
    A. Promote excretion of H_2O, Na^+ and chloride in the body
    B. Reduce the pulse rate
    C. Relax the client
    D. Lower the blood pressure through vasodilation of arteries

The intended response is **A** as chlorothiazide is a diuretic that can help lower BP by reducing body fluid and sodium chloride levels. **D** is incorrect as it has no primary effect on arteries. **C** and **B** are erroneous as these are not purposes of this drug.

3. Nursing intervention of this client would place great importance on maintaining the client
    A. Near a busy nursing station under close observation
    B. Ambulating to the bathroom frequently
    C. In a quiet nonstimulated environment
    D. In education sessions on hypertension immediately on admitting him

The intended response is **C**, since this client has a dangerously high BP with high Na^+ levels. The client needs to be in a nonstimulated environment to decrease already dangerously high CNS transmission and reduce BP through reduction of stress and stimulus. **A, B,** and **D** suggest activities that increase nerve impulses and added stress to the body, which would further elevate a blood pressure.

4. Mr. Smith is placed on a low-sodium diet. Which of the following diets would be appropriate?
   A. Tuna fish sandwich, potato chips and dip, lettuce salad, glass of ice tea
   B. Veal parmesan, broccoli, baked potato, milkshake
   C. Breast of chicken, peas, lettuce salad, 1 slice of bread, glass of 2% milk
   D. T-bone steak, cauliflower with cheese sauce, green beans, instant chocolate pudding, cup of hot tea

The intended response is **C** as there are no processed foods or salty foods. **A** contains salty food, such as potato chips and processed foods such as tuna fish. **B** contains dairy food, such as cheese and tomato sauce on the veal parmesan and dairy food, such as the milkshake. **D** contains high Na^+ concentration in the cheese sauce and the instant chocolate pudding.

Reasoning Exercises: Fluids & Electrolytes: Potassium

Molly Flannery is a 67-year-old female with chronic congestive heart failure and hypertension. She is being evaluated for complaints of muscular weakness and general fatigue.

1. Molly's serum electrolyte studies reveal a K^+ level of 2.9. Which of the following medications taken by the patient at home contributed *most* to her hypokalemic state?
   A. Digoxin, .125 mg, PO, daily
   B. Lasix, 80 mg, PO, daily
   C. Aldomet, 250 mg, PO, tid
   D. Aspirin, 10 grains, bid

The intended response is **B**, since Lasix, in addition to its diuretic action, also wastes K^+ by increasing urinary excretion. Digoxin, response **A**, contributes to K^+ loss by enhancing urinary output, but Lasix is much more directly related to the development of hypokalemia. Response **C** is an anti-hypertensive that is not related to K^+ loss. Response **D**, aspirin, may have been prescribed as myocardial infarction prophylaxis, and is not related to K^+ loss.

2. In addition to receiving IV fluids with K^+ additive, Molly is to increase her intake of potassium-rich foods. Which of the following menu selections indicates that Molly has a knowledge of potassium-rich food sources?

   A. Scrambled eggs, bacon, toast, apple juice
   B. Chicken noodle soup, saltines, fresh lettuce salad, milk
   C. Fresh melon salad, hamburger steak, strawberry shortcake, instant Decaf coffee
   D. American cheese sandwich, green beans, baked potato, tea

The intended response is **C,** since both melon, such as canteloupe, and strawberries are potassium-rich as well as the instant decaffeinated coffee selected by the patient. Responses **A, B,** and **D** are not potassium-rich and are additionally relatively high in Na^+, which would likely be contraindicated for this patient because of her impaired cardiac status.

3. The nurse caring for Molly should place special emphasis on the assessment of which of the following vital signs?

   A. Temperature
   B. Pulse
   C. Respirations
   D. Blood pressure

The intended response is **B,** since hypokalemia may cause the patient to experience bradycardia and arrhythmia.

ACIDS AND BASES 10

NANCY B. CAILLES

ARTERIAL BLOOD pH IS THE MEASURE OF ACID-BASE BALANCE IN THE HUMAN BODY

Illustration of Principle

The human body has an incredible ability to maintain itself in equilibrium, or balance, in order to maintain optimal functioning.

It is able to utilize its own resources, its own compensatory mechanisms, in order to keep its systems operating at optimal levels of efficiency. Perhaps in no other area of bodily function is this maintenance of balance more evident than in the balance of acids and bases.

Normally, acid ions and base ions are retained and excreted by the body in such a way as to preserve a delicate balance between the two. This balance is indicated by an arterial blood pH value, which is normally between the extremes of 7.35 and 7.45. When an excess or deficit of chemicals and gases occurs in the body, the balance between acids and bases is disrupted, resulting in a change in the pH of arterial blood. For example, if an individual is unable to expire adequate amounts of CO_2, an excess accumulation of this gas occurs in arterial blood. Since carbonic acid is formed when CO_2 is combined with water, the acid nature of the blood increases. Correspondingly, the arterial blood pH value drops, eventually falling below the low normal value of 7.35. This lowered blood pH, then, is an index of an acid-base imbalance. The body's compensatory mechanisms attempt to reestablish balance by altering retention or excretion of acids and bases as an automatic response to an alteration in blood pH. Compensatory mechanisms are limited, however, and thus a change

113

in the arterial blood pH from normal range presents an immediate concern for the nurse, since maintenance of pH within the narrow range of 7.35 to 7.45 is essential for life.

*M*emory
*j*og

> Normal arterial blood pH range is 7.35 to 7.45. A pH value below 7.35 indicates acidosis or accumulation of acids in the bloodstream. A pH value above 7.45 indicates alkalosis, an excess of base. Compensatory mechanisms are available in the body to help maintain balance between acids and bases.

PRINCIPLE

CONDITIONS THAT INVOLVE HYPOVENTILATION LEAD TO RETENTION OF CO_2 AND POTENTIAL RESPIRATORY ACIDOSIS

Illustration of Principle

The key to understanding respiratory acidosis is to focus on its symptomatic cause—hypoventilation. Although respiratory acidosis is associated with a variety of diseases, the hallmark feature of these diseases is a depression of respirations with a decrease in O_2–CO_2 gas exchange. Since hypoventilating clients have decreased rate and depth of respirations, they are unable to release necessary amounts of CO_2 with expiration, thus increasing the CO_2 level of arterial blood. Carbonic *acid* forms when CO_2 mixes with water in serum, resulting in increased *acidity* of arterial blood. Increased acid levels, termed *acidosis,* cause a decrease in arterial blood pH. The evidence of respiratory acidosis, then, is a decrease of arterial blood pH below 7.35 with an accompanying increase in CO_2. The symptoms of respiratory acidosis are directly related to its cause, which is hypoventilation. These symptoms include

▷ Slow, shallow, weak respirations
▷ Declining levels of consciousness, stupor
▷ Mental lethargy, confusion, disorientation
▷ Associated signs of impaired oxygenation: *e.g.,* pallor, cyanosis

*M*emory
*j*og

> Accumulation of acids in the bloodstream is evidenced by a decrease in pH value. A lowered pH with an accompanying elevated CO_2 value suggests respiratory acidosis. Patients with conditions involving hypoventilation are prone to developing this condition.

Diseases or conditions associated with hypoventilation and acidotic states include

▷ Emphysema (retention of CO_2)

▷ Pneumonia (interference with alveolar gas exchange)

▷ Head trauma (damage to respiratory center of the brain)

▷ Overdose (depression of respiratory center)
  Barbiturate
  Narcotic
  Anesthetic

▷ Respiratory or cardiac arrest (loss of O_2, accumulation of CO_2)

Nursing Management

Nursing interventions for the patient with any acid-base imbalance should be focused on first addressing the underlying cause of the imbalance, and then secondly treating the related symptoms. In respiratory acidosis, the nurse needs to address first the underlying problem, hypoventilation and hypoxemia, by providing sources of O_2 (cannula, mask, endotracheal intubation, or mechanical ventilation). Second, the nurse may be ordered to administer sodium bicarbonate injection in an effort to increase the blood pH by increasing the bicarbonate ion (HCO_3) content of the blood. The nurse should monitor the patient's mental status and provide for safety needs as indicated. In order to ensure that these interventions are successful in reversing the acidotic condition, the nurse should consistently monitor serial arterial blood–gas readings to identify changes in pH and CO_2 values that would mark patient progress. An increase in blood pH and a decrease in CO_2 level would indicate reversal or correction of the acidotic condition.

> Since hypoventilation causes respiratory acidosis, the nurse should provide O_2 and support for ventilation, such as intubation, if needed. Sodium bicarb injection may be used to "buffer" the excess acid in the bloodstream.

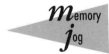

PRINCIPLE

CONDITIONS WHICH INVOLVE *HYPERVENTILATION* LEAD TO EXCESSIVE LOSS OF CO_2 AND RESPIRATORY ALKALOSIS

Illustration of Principle

The key to understanding respiratory alkalosis is to focus on its symptomatic cause—hyperventilation. Whereas respiratory acidosis is caused by *retention* of CO_2, respiratory alkalosis is caused by an excessive *loss* of CO_2 as a result of *hyperventilation*. Since a hyperventilating patient has increased rate and depth of respirations, he begins to lose CO_2 by "blowing it off" with expiration. The excessive loss of CO_2 then causes a decrease in acid, disrupting the balance between acids and bases. This results in an increased arterial blood pH, indicating an alkalotic condition.

The evidence of respiratory alkalosis, then, is an increase in arterial blood pH above 7.45 with an accompanying decrease in CO_2. The symptoms of respiratory alkalosis are directly related to its cause—hyperventilation—and are very similar to a common *cause* of hyperventilation, acute anxiety.

▷ Rapid, deep, "blowing" respirations

▷ Acute excitation, trembling, nervousness

▷ Neuromuscular irritability

▷ Numbness and tingling of extremities

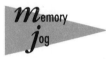

Excessive loss of acid with hyperventilation (loss of CO_2) may result in respiratory alkalosis. Anxiety often causes a patient to hyperventilate. Symptoms of acute anxiety are very like symptoms of alkalosis.

Diseases or conditions associated with hyperventilation and alkalotic states include

▷ Asthma (acute bronchial constriction)

▷ Brain injury (stimulation of respiratory center)

▷ Overdose
    Aspirin (attempt of body to eliminate ASA acids)
    Cocaine (stimulation of respiratory center)

▷ Acute anxiety ("fight or flight" response)

Additionally, women in active labor, who have been trained in Lamaze delivery techniques, but who are losing control over their breathing patterns with increased intensity of uterine contractions, may begin to hyperventilate, placing them at risk for the development of respiratory alkalosis as well.

Nursing Management

In order to correct the source of this imbalance, the nurse needs to take actions to increase the CO_2 level of the patient's arterial blood. This can readily be achieved by

▷ Coaching the patient's breathing pattern to slow, deep respirations (especially valuable in labor and delivery settings)

▷ Encouraging the patient to hold his breath for several seconds in between respirations

▷ Instructing the patient to breathe into a paper bag, allowing him to reinhale his own exhaled CO_2

Antianxiety or sedative medication may be administered both to calm the patient and to depress his rate and depth of respiration, thus increasing the retention of CO_2. Finally, the nurse should utilize reassurance and supportive skills in an effort to reduce the patient's anxiety and irritability, which will in turn regulate the rate and rhythm of his respirations. The nurse should attempt to identify any underlying issues or problems that may have precipitated the alkalotic episode, including fear, anxiety, or acute stress reaction with impaired coping. A decreasing pH with elevated CO_2 and return to normal respiratory rate and depth signal improvement in the alkalotic state.

PRINCIPLE

METABOLIC ACIDOSIS IS CHARACTERIZED BY AN *INCREASED LOSS* OF HCO_3 OR AN *INCREASED RETENTION* OF ACID IONS, RESULTING IN A *DECREASED* ARTERIAL BLOOD pH

Illustration of Principle

Metabolic acidosis is associated with a variety of disease conditions without a hallmark characteristic or feature. Each, however, involves an imbalance of metabolism of foods or fluids, making this acid-base imbalance easily discernible from *respiratory* acidosis. Clients with renal failure may develop this imbalance in response to the kidney's inability to excrete phosphate and sulfate acid ions. Thus, in renal failure, inability of the body to metabolize and excrete fluids also causes an inability to excrete acid, resulting in an increased acid concentration of arterial blood. The lungs may attempt to compensate for the increasing levels of acid by increasing rate and depth of respiration in order to "blow off" CO_2. This type of respiratory pattern is termed "Kussmaul breathing," and is often associated with diabetic ketoacidosis, another example of metabolic acidosis. (Discussed in detail in Chapter 14, Diabetes).

The evidence of metabolic acidosis is a decrease in arterial blood pH below 7.35 with an accompanying decrease in HCO_3. The symptoms of metabolic acidosis are related to the drop in arterial blood pH, and are typified by signs of central nervous system depression, including cardiac dysrhythmia, apathy and lethargy, disorientation, and eventually, coma. Other symptoms of the acidosis will be related to its underlying cause, such as acetone odor to the breath in diabetic ketoacidosis, or oliguria or anuria in the patient with renal failure.

> Decreasing arterial pH with decreased HCO_3 is indicative of metabolic acidosis. The respiratory system may try to compensate the imbalance by "blowing off" CO_2 by hyperventilation, reducing blood acidity.

Additional disease or conditions associated with metabolic acidosis include

▷ Severe or prolonged diarrhea (loss of bicarbonate ion in stool)

▷ Prolonged fasting (anorexia nervosa; anorexia associated with cancer chemotherapy)

▷ Diabetes mellitus (rapid metabolism of fats with accumulation of acid by-products in diabetic ketoacidosis [DKA])

Nursing Management

Since the causes of metabolic acidosis are so varied, the nurse must take steps to correct the underlying problem causing the acidosis *first,* and then provide for other supportive strategies to deal with the acidotic state. For example, the nurse caring for the client who is becoming acidotic as a result of prolonged diarrhea must *first* take measures to control the diarrhea, and *then* provide for reversal of the acidotic state by administration of sodium bicarbonate, if needed. The client in diabetic ketoacidosis must first receive an infusion of regular insulin to halt the rapid metabolism of fats, which produces ketone acid bodies. The nurse should also keep a close watch of client's vital signs and level of consciousness, since central nervous system depression is a feature of metabolic acidosis. Continuous cardiac monitoring is an essential intervention, since cardiac dysrhythmias are common in acidotic states.

The nurse can evaluate the patient's progress through the acidotic condition by monitoring serial arterial blood–gas values, noting an increase in pH and an increase in HCO_3 levels. The patient should show steady improvement in level of consciousness and alertness, but should still have safety precautions maintained during the recovery process.

PRINCIPLE

METABOLIC ALKALOSIS IS CHARACTERIZED BY A DECREASED LOSS OF HCO_3 OR A DECREASED RETENTION OF ACID RESULTING IN AN INCREASED ARTERIAL BLOOD pH

Illustration of Principle

Like metabolic acidosis, metabolic alkalosis is associated with a number of different disease conditions without a hallmark characteristic or feature. However, metabolic alkalotic conditions most commonly involve disorders of the gastrointestinal tract, making them easily discernible from respiratory alkalosis states. In metabolic alkalosis, there is an increase in the level of serum bicarbonate or a loss of acid resulting in decreased levels of serum acid. This causes an increase in arterial blood pH accompanied by an increased serum HCO_3 level. For example, if a client diagnosed with peptic ulcer overmedicates himself with antacid medications in a desperate effort to reduce abdominal discomfort, he may develop an increase in serum bicarbonate levels, since antacids are highly alkaline. Likewise, if a client suffers a loss of acids from the body, such as one would with prolonged vomiting or gastric suction, the acid levels of the serum will decrease from loss of hydrochloric acid (HCl) from the stomach, resulting in an alkalotic state.

> Metabolic alkalosis can be caused by excess HCO_3 or loss of acid ions, such as HCl from the stomach. This imbalance is most associated with disturbances of the gastrointestinal tract.

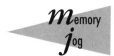

The evidence of metabolic alkalosis, then, is an increase of arterial blood pH above 7.45 with an accompanying increase in HCO_3.

The patient experiencing metabolic alkalosis will demonstrate symptoms of central nervous system *excitement,* the exact opposite of the patient with metabolic acidosis, who evidences signs of central symptoms of central nervous system *depression.* Symptoms include irritability, disorientation, muscular twitching, and seizures. The heart is likewise overstimulated, resulting in dysrhythmia.

Patients at risk for the development of metabolic alkalosis are those whose disease conditions or treatments involve the loss of acid ions or the increase of base ions. In addition to the patients identified above, patients who have acid loss secondary to the irrigation of a nasogastric tube with sterile water rather than the accepted sterile saline solution will undergo loss of acid with the loss of HCl from the stomach, resulting in metabolic alkalosis. For this reason, gastric irrigation must always be performed with an isotonic solution, such as 0.9 normal saline, to prevent loss of acid ions.

Nursing Management

First, the nurse should focus on correcting the underlying cause of the alkalotic condition so that acid-base balance may be restored. The nurse should be sure to monitor blood–gas values on patients with upper gastrointestinal disturbances, so that excess loss of acid ions would not go undetected, as it could in prolonged vomiting or improper gastric suction and irrigation. Likewise, the nurse should instruct patients with gastrointestinal problems, such as gastritis or peptic ulcer, to follow medication schedules carefully to prevent antacid overdose that could lead to alkalosis.

The nurse can evaluate for a reversal of the metabolic alkalosis by serial arterial blood–gas values that would indicate a decrease in pH and a decrease in HCO_3 values. A more detailed explanation of arterial blood–gas interpretation and its value and use in monitoring acid-base imbalances follows in this chapter.

PRINCIPLE

WHEN ATTEMPTING TO IDENTIFY AN ACID-BASE IMBALANCE, THE NURSE SHOULD FIRST CONSIDER THE *ARTERIAL BLOOD pH*

Illustration of Principle

The pH is the cardinal indicator of acid-base balance in the human body. A decrease in pH from normal range indicates an acidotic state. An increase in pH from normal range indicates an alkalotic state. A pH that falls within normal range of 7.35 to 7.45 indicates that the acids and bases of the body are in balance or that excesses or deficits of acids and bases in the body are being compensated.

> **Normal Values: Arterial Blood Gas**
> pH: 7.35–7.45
> CO_2: 35–45
> HCO_3: 25

Consider the example below:

A patient is admitted to the emergency room following a motor vehicle accident. She is visibly anxious, hyperventilating, and tremulous. Respiratory rate is 36. Arterial blood pH is 7.52.

In this example, the patient's symptoms would certainly suggest a respiratory alkalosis, but only through review of the arterial blood pH does the nurse know conclusively that the patient is alkalotic.

PRINCIPLE

THE SECOND STEP IN IDENTIFYING ACID-BASE IMBALANCES IS TO CONSIDER THE CO_2 LEVEL OF ARTERIAL BLOOD

Illustration of Principle

The arterial blood pH gives the nurse evidence that an acid base imbalance is occurring. The CO_2 level will give information about which system is *causing* the imbalance, either respiratory or metabolic. Consider these examples:

Example 1

pH: 7.30
CO_2: 50

In this example, the pH value indicates an acidotic state, since the value is below the normal range for arterial blood pH. The CO_2 level is elevated above the normal range of 35 to 45, indicating an increased amount of CO_2 and thus an increased amount of acid. The CO_2 value, being elevated, indicates that the patient is in *respiratory acidosis.* The respiratory system is causing the imbalance.

Example 2

pH: 7.31
CO_2: 32

In this second example, the pH is again decreased, indicating acidosis. But the CO_2 level is *decreased,* reducing the amount of acid in the blood. Thus, the decreased CO_2 is *compensating* for the decreased pH. This patient then is likely in *metabolic acidosis,* and is utilizing deep, rapid respirations (Kussmaul) to "blow off" CO_2 in the body's compensatory effort to decrease arterial blood acidity.

PRINCIPLE

THE FINAL STEP IN IDENTIFYING ACID-BASE IMBALANCES IS TO CONSIDER THE HCO_3 LEVEL OF ARTERIAL BLOOD

Illustration of Principle

Like the CO_2 value, the level of HCO_3 provides information about the cause of the acid-base imbalance. Likewise, its relationship to CO_2 levels will reflect the body's compensation for the imbalance. Consider the examples below:

Example 1

pH: 7.57
CO_2: 36
HCO_3: 29

In this example, the pH indicates an excess of base, an alkalotic state. The HCO_3 level is elevated, indicating an increase of HCO_3 in the serum, causing the alkalosis. The CO_2 level is within normal range, indicating that no compensation for this imbalance is occurring. If compensation were occurring, the CO_2 level would be increasing to raise the acid level of blood to "buffer" the elevated base level.

Example 2

pH: 7.29

CO_2: 54

HCO_3: 29

In this second example, the pH indicates an acidotic state. The CO_2 level is increased, indicating greater retention of CO_2 in the body with resultant respiratory acidosis. The HCO_3 level is likewise elevated above the normal value of 25, indicating that the kidneys are attempting to compensate the high acid levels in the body by releasing bicarbonate to "buffer" the acids and restore balance.

Reasoning Exercises: Acids and Bases

Jean Thomas is a 25-year-old secretary admitted to the emergency room with diaphoresis, hyperventilation, palpitations, and trembling. Jean tells the nurse that she has been "very upset and nervous" over a poor employment evaluation. A tentative diagnosis of acute anxiety episode is made.

1. Which of the following acid-base imbalances would likely occur as a result of Jean's hyperventilation?

   A. Respiratory acidosis

   B. Respiratory alkalosis

   C. Metabolic acidosis

   D. Metabolic alkalosis

The intended response is **B,** since hyperventilation will cause an increased loss of CO_2, leading to a decrease in acid in arterial blood, resulting in an alkalotic state.

2. Which of the following arterial blood–gas values would likely occur with continued hyperventilation?

   A. pH 7.30, CO_2 32

   B. pH 7.34, CO_3 46

   C. pH 7.48, CO_2 31

   D. pH 7.50, CO_2 48

The intended response is **C,** since these two values are associated with the CO_2 loss and subsequent increase in pH that result from hyperventilation. Responses **A** and **B** are incorrect, since the pH values indicate an acidotic state. Response **D** is incorrect, because the CO_2 level is higher than the normal range, which would not occur with a hyperventilating patient.

3. Which of the following nursing interventions should the nurse employ *first* with Jean?

    A. Administer oxygen per nasal cannula at 2 to 3 L/minute

    B. Administer sedative medication as ordered

    C. Instruct the client to breathe into a paper bag

    D. Place the client in a quiet, nonstimulating room

The intended response is **C,** since this intervention would be most valuable in increasing the CO_2 content of the patient's arterial blood, thus helping to reverse the alkalotic state. Response **A** is incorrect, since the patient needs CO_2. Responses **B** and **D** are also important interventions in respiratory alkalosis, but should be employed *subsequent* to the initial response of having the patient reinhale her exhaled CO_2 using the paper bag technique.

Leslie Burns is a 32-year-old known diabetic brought to the Urgent Care Clinic by her husband. Leslie is conscious, but lethargic, complaining of excessive thirst, hot and dry skin, and frequent urination. Immediate blood glucose, ketones, electrolytes, and blood gases are performed.

1. Which of the following laboratory data would indicate that Leslie is in a diabetic-related acid-base imbalance?

    A. Blood glucose 860

    B. Potassium 5.9

    C. Urine ketones large

    D. Arterial blood pH 7.29

The intended response is **D,** since pH is the cardinal indicator of acid-base balance in the human body. Although the remaining laboratory data are pertinent to the client's physical status, they are reflections of her diabetes and cannot provide conclusive information about her acid-base state.

2. The nurse notes that Leslie's pH value and HCO_3 values are both decreased. Leslie is in which of the following types of acid-base imbalance?

    A. Respiratory acidosis

    B. Respiratory alkalosis

    C. Metabolic acidosis

    D. Metabolic alkalosis

The intended response is **C,** since a decreased pH and HCO_3 indicate an acidotic state with a metabolic origin.

3. Which of the following CO_2 values would indicate that Leslie is Kussmaul breathing to compensate for her decreased bicarbonate value?

   A. 32
   B. 35
   C. 40
   D. 47

The intended response is **A**, since a decrease in CO_2 level of arterial blood from the normal range would indicate that the patient is "blowing off" CO_2 by Kussmaul breathing in an effort to compensate for the decreased serum bicarbonate levels.

ELIMINATION

WAYNE NAGEL

11

PRINCIPLE

ELIMINATION HAS DIRECT BEARING ON THE BODY'S ABILITY TO BALANCE FLUIDS AND ELECTROLYTES

Illustration of Principle

Elimination is the process by which waste products are removed from the body. The principle systems include the gastrointestinal system and the urinary system. Alterations in gastrointestinal elimination such as diarrhea or constipation affect the body's balance of electrolytes and fluids. For example, diarrhea manifests as frequency of defecation producing watery, loosely formed stools. During episodes of diarrhea the organs associated with absorption are in a hypermotile state. Ingested foods pass quickly through the system, thereby decreasing the amount of time for nutrients and electrolytes to be absorbed. Since fluids and electrolytes essential to metabolic balance are primarily obtained from the foods and fluids that we ingest, alterations occur.

Constipation, a condition characterized by hard, dry stools and irregularity, results from hypomobility. Passage of ingested fluids and foods is slowed. Increased absorption of the nutrients occurs. Constipation can be a very uncomfortable condition for the client. Client knowledge deficits related to low-fiber intake is a frequent nursing finding.

125

> The key to assessing client regularity is whether the client's bowel patterns have changed.

Regularity can be defined as one bowel movement per day at the same time. Not everyone is "regular."

The urinary system–renal system organs function directly on the composition and the volume of extracellular fluid. In addition to producing urine, these structures interact with the excretion and absorption of water and electrolytes. Renal insufficiency potentially can produce fluid volume excess. This volume excess is related to an excess of Na. Renal nephron damage produces an inability to filter Na and to excrete water. Water is held in the extracellular compartments because Na is so osmotically active. This Na excess produces an excess of water and is observable in such conditions as hypertension, volume overload, and pulmonary edema. Excess fluid volume also increases the work load of the heart.

Potassium is another key electrolyte related to alterations in elimination. Potassium excess is related to alterations in tubular secretory function. Rises in K related to altered excretion are responsible for a hyperkalemic state. Hyperkalemia can result from acute or chronic conditions affecting renal function or from traumatic tissue injuries such as burns.

Hypokalemic condition can occur secondary to alterations in elimination when a hyperexcretory state exists. Rapid movement of fluid through the system minimizes the time in which K can be absorbed. Diuretics increase the elimination of fluids from the body; subsequently, K is lost with the increased urinary elimination. Client teaching regarding kalemic balance including signs and symptoms and diets rich in K is a significant nursing intervention.

> Potassium has a very narrow normal range. Clients with conditions producing hypo- or hyperkalemic states should be monitored closely.

Alterations in renal tubular function affects Mg balance. Episodes of oliguria tend to increase Mg levels, and polyuric states that produce diuresis decrease Mg levels. The client who has been burned sustains Mg losses secondary to hypermobility of the gastrointestinal system.

Alterations in calcium–phosphate balance occurs when vitamin D is not activated. Calcium is absorbed from the intestines. The kidneys are responsible for activating exogenous vitamin D within the body. Renal disease decreases this response allowing Ca to be lost. Hypermobility in the gastrointestinal system permits Ca to be lost in feces. Renal dysfunction inhibits the excretion of phosphates, resulting in elevated phosphate levels. The calcium–phosphate interaction is essential in maintaining healthy bone tissue.

PRINCIPLE

THE RETENTION OF METABOLIC WASTES RELATED TO INADEQUATE ELIMINATION AFFECTS MULTIPLE BODY SYSTEMS

Illustration of Principle

The food and fluids that we ingest provide the body with the essentials to maintain structure, function, health, and balance. The body breaks down the ingested substance into substances that can be used. Substances that cannot be used are therefore eliminated. By-products of metabolism become the wastes that are eliminated. Conditions producing alterations in elimination, for example, inadequate elimination, result in retention of these waste products. Renal and gastrointestinal dysfunctions result in the inadequate elimination of electrolytes and metabolic waste products. As the disease processes become increasingly more severe, balance is more affected, and the consequences to the body are more profound. The buildup of nitrogenous waste products, electrolytes, and other substances produces a toxic condition in the body.

Inadequate nutrition is frequently seen in clients experiencing retention of waste products. The by-products of ingested foods and fluids, as stated earlier become these toxic substances when their ammonium exceeds what is required for balance. In a uremic toxic state, as the blood urea nitrogen level (BUN) elevates, a metabolic acidosis occurs. This condition occurs because the metabolic processes of the body are unable to produce buffers in sufficient quantity to keep up with the rising acidic state of the body. As the metabolic acidosis worsens, the client becomes increasingly more anorexic. Protein substances seem to not taste good to the client with an elevated BUN. Foods high in K are to be watched carefully because of the narrow range of normal limits of this electrolyte. Conditions such as renal failure may call for fluid restrictions; subsequently the client may feel very thirsty. Other associated conditions such as pain, elevated temperature, or immobility may decrease the client's desire for food.

Protein limitations or deficiencies can lead to muscle wasting. Small, frequent feedings are indicated in conditions where intake intolerance is the identified problem.

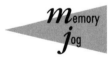

Memory jog

Inadequate wound healing is frequently seen in clients experiencing retention of metabolic wastes. The buildup of intracellular waste products secondary to inadequate elimination of these substances results in the cells' inability to synthesize, differentiate, and multiply. Meticulous skin and wound care is essential to prevent complications. Buildup of metabolic wastes such as uric acid crystals on the skin are irritating and can produce integument breakdown. The client should be assessed frequently of signs and symptoms of skin breakdown. Clients who are bed bound or experiencing alterations in mobility are especially susceptible to skin breakdown.

Septicemia is a common complication in clients experiencing retained metabolic wastes. The toxic substance overwhelms the body. Because normal metabolism promotes the function of all body systems, alterations related to retained waste products place the client in a state of imbalance. The immune system suffers, in that it is unable to keep up with the increasing demands to protect the body from the aggressor pathogens. Pathogens then spill into circulating volume and are transported throughout the body. Multiple system injury can ensue.

Memory jog

Meticulous care of invasive devices, intravenous lines, and catheters is important. These are direct portals of pathogenic entry into the body.

A buildup of metabolic waste products in the body can produce alterations in mental neurologic status. Waste products and their by-products can cross the blood brain barriers. As this phenomenon occurs the central nervous system is affected. Substances like ureas are osmotically active substances that attract abnormal amounts of body water into the central nervous system. The buildup of water produces swelling, which produces neuronal displacement or compression, which can produce disorientation, confusion, and seizures.

Activity intolerance is frequently seen as conditions become more chronic. The buildup of waste products, altered nutritional status, lack of energy requirements and calories can and do impede a client's ability to participate in activities of daily living. Pain associated with the underlying pathological condition may produce malaise and even fear of increasing discomfort. Anemias can occur producing weakness and fatigue.

Sexual dysfunctions occur secondary to alterations in libido, potency, ovulation, and menstruation. These conditions result from the toxic effects of the circulating high levels of metabolic wastes that directly and indirectly interact negatively with the system associated with sexual function.

Memory jog

Clients and families should be encouraged to discuss conditions affecting their sex lives and to seek counseling. Clients often feel that their sexual dysfunction is unique to them alone.

Chronic conditions producing alterations in one's ability to eliminate body wastes may be responsible for ineffective coping. A condition, for example, requiring ongoing dialysis certainly calls for significant life-style changes. These changes can produce feelings of powerlessness, require financial adjustments that can be burdensome, and limit one's physical stamina, thereby making life's dealings difficult to handle. Support groups, community resources, individual counseling, and therapy are just some of the interventions available to promote effective coping. The buildup of metabolic wastes over a period of time can alter the client's ability to reason. This condition may require alternative long-term client placement.

PRINCIPLE

PATTERNS OF ELIMINATION ARE AFFECTED BY PSYCHOSOCIAL AND PHYSIOLOGICAL FACTORS

Illustration of Principle

Alterations in pattern of elimination can be affected by functional disorders. Disorders such as tumors requiring bowel resection that result in a colostomy may produce needs for dietary changes. The client who has to undergo hemodialysis secondary to kidney failure will be required to adhere to a dialysis regimen. These functional disorders may be temporary or permanent but will require client compliance in order to maintain balance.

Clients may develop feelings of emotional stress, secondary to feeling different. This stress may decrease the client's ability to reintegrate into society, family, or profession. Stress interrelates to overall balance, because it increases the demands on the multiple systems to function in an optimal fashion. Hypermetabolic states can occur. These states increase the production of wastes, which increases the need for optimal elimination.

A client experiencing stress in continence, for example, may be fearful of going shopping or out to dinner because she may become embarrassed. Alterations in body image often times produce a feeling of being "different." That sense of being out of the ordinary may produce withdrawal from social behaviors.

Discussing the client's feelings with the client may relieve some client discomfort. The goal is to promote client emotional comfort.

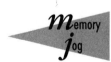

Reasoning Exercises: Elimination

Assessment/Analysis

Stephanie Leeder is a 46-year-old diabetic diagnosed with nephrosclerotic kidney disease and renal failure. She is to begin continuous ambulatory peritoneal dialysis (CAPD).

1. Which of the following statements by Stephanie in her admission history most strongly supports the diagnosis of renal failure?

   A. "I just got to feeling tired all the time, could hardly do anything around the house."

   B. "I was keeping watch over what I ate, but my sugar was always high when I checked on it."

   C. "I started noticing that I was gaining weight and my clothes were getting tight around the middle."

   D. "I knew I should be passing urine, but I couldn't. Nothing would come out, you know?"

** The intended response is **D.** Although fatigue, weight gain, and fluctuations of serum glucose are associated with renal failure, the symptom that *most* strongly supports a diagnosis of renal failure is the absence of urine production or excretion, indicating a failure of the kidneys to maintain fluid balance within the elimination system.

2. Which of Stephanie's lab values should the nurse assess as most significant to the diagnosis of renal failure?

   A. BUN 53

   B. K^+ 6.2

   C. Uric acid 8.0

   D. Creatinine 9.0

** The intended response is again **D.** Although elevation of BUN is suggestive of renal disease, this laboratory value may also increase in dehydrative states. The elevation of creatinine is specific to renal disease and failure, and the value listed is substantially elevated over the norm, indicating decreased renal function.

Planning

3. The nurse preparing Stephanie's plan of care should identify which of these nursing diagnoses as the highest priority?

   A. Activity intolerance as a result of anemia and impaired renal function

   B. Alteration in nutrition: less than body requirements owing to impaired renal function

   C. Alteration in fluid volume: excess or deficit owing to impaired renal function

   D. Alteration in glucose metabolism: hyperglycemia caused by impaired renal function.

** The intended response is **C.** Since the kidneys function in fluid balance by excretion and reabsorption functions, failure of the kidneys causes an imbalance in fluid balance, predisposing the patient to serious fluid overload or deficit, depending upon the actual phase of renal failure. The remaining responses are associated with renal failure but are of less priority than response **C.**

Implementation (update)

Surgical insertion of a Tenckhoff catheter is performed and Stephanie is now receiving CAPD treatment.

4. When performing an outflow dialysate solution bag change for Stephanie, the nurse should consider which of these as the most important nursing action?

   A. Measurement of total return volume of dialysate

   B. Assessment of postdialysis weight and vital signs

   C. Use of astute aseptic technique when handling catheter and dressing

   D. Measurement of postdialysis blood glucose by use of a glucometer.

** The intended response is **C.** Maintenance of aseptic technique is critical in the handling of dialysis treatments (whether peritoneal or hemodialysis) because these treatments involve the entry into a *sterile* body area, in this case, the peritoneum. The nurse must utilize sterile technique in order to prevent the complication of infection for the patient receiving dialysis treatment.

Evaluation

5. Which of the following findings would indicate to the nurse that CAPD has been effective for Stephanie?

   A. Sodium decreasing, creatinine increasing

   B. BUN increasing, blood glucose increasing

   C. Blood glucose decreasing, K increasing

   D. BUN decreasing, creatinine decreasing

** The intended response is **D.** The primary purpose of CAPD treatment is to stimulate kidney functions of fluid balance and waste removal and excretion. The decreases in BUN and creatinine levels evidence that these functions are being achieved by the CAPD treatments.

INFECTION AND INFLAMMATION

WAYNE NAGEL

PRINCIPLE

THE IMMUNE SYSTEM DIFFERENTIATES BETWEEN SELF AND NONSELF

Illustration of the Principle

This system protects the body against pathogenic organisms and other foreign bodies through a series of complex biochemical interactions. Humoral immune response produces antibodies to react with specific antigens that fight viral and bacterial infections. Through complex biochemical activity, this component of the immune system stimulates B cells to produce invader-specific antibodies. Humoral response may vary from immediate reaction to the invading organism or virus to 48 hours. Cellular immunity, also known as the cell-mediated response, produces T-lymphocytes that mobilize tissue macrophages. These macrophages then attack invading foreign bodies. The cellular immune system directly attacks the invading organism by producing appropriate numbers of white blood cells to identify, engulf, and destroy the invader. This system is also involved in what we commonly refer to as "resistance" to infection. Together, humoral and cellular immunity work as self in order to protect the body from the nonself pathogenic organisms and cancers.

Memory **J**og

> *Antibodies* are immunoglobins essential to the immune system. They are produced by lymphoid tissue in response to bacteria, viruses, or other antigenic substances. An antibody is specific to an antigen. *Antigens* are proteins that cause the formation of antibodies. Antigens react specifically with an antibody. The *antibody–antigen* reaction is the process by which specific B-cells recognize the invader or antigen, stimulating antibody production, thereby protecting the body from infection.

The immune response, therefore, becomes a defense function of the body that produces antibodies to destroy invading bacteria, viruses, and malignancies. The physiologic weapons of self, therefore, become the antibody–antigen reaction. Immunity can be created by immunizing a client through vaccinations, for example, polio, tetanus, rubella. Natural immunity, on the other hand, is a genetically inherited resistance to specific infectious organisms. Natural immunity can and is affected by components of health such as mental health metabolism, diet, environment, and the strength of the invading organism. Balance is maintained when the self is able to effectively check the nonself.

Memory **J**og

> *Vaccines* are produced from attenuated or killed microorganisms and inoculated into clients to stimulate the immune system to induce active immunity. *Antibiotics, bacterials,* and *fungals* are synthesized chemically or produced from specific organisms. This group is effective in interfering with the production of the cell wall, interfering with protein synthesis, nucleic acid synthesis, or membrane synthesis. They also can and do inhibit critical biosynthetic pathways in the invading organism.

It is important, therefore, to summarize the physiology associated with the immune system. Relating back to our principle, *the immune system differentiates between self and nonself,* it is essential to understand that all components of the immune system work together. Through complex biochemical and physiological interactions, the immune system serves as the body's main defense against infections and cancers. As we later discuss inflammation, you will see the interplay in this system.

White blood cells (WBCs) are the main defense of the immune system working to destroy invading organisms or cancer cells. Lymphocytes are a specific type of white blood cell considered the intelligence of the immune system. Lymphocytes possess the ability to recognize infectious agents and cancer cells. These lymphocytes direct the other white blood cells to destroy those agents. Humoral and cellular immunity work together to first produce antibodies and secondly to produce T-lymphocytes in order to combat infections and cancer cells through direct cellular contact. The T-lymphocytes consist of two

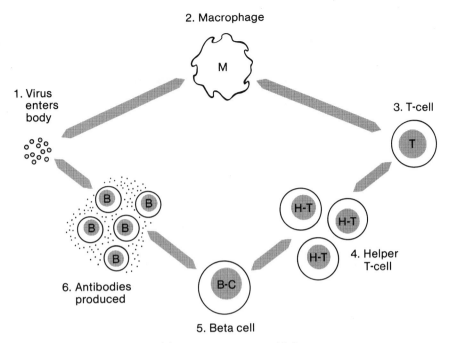

FIGURE 12-1. THE NORMAL IMMUNE SYSTEM. (*1*) INVADING *VIRUS* ENTERS THE BODY. (*2*) *MACROPHAGES* ACT AS THE ALARM SYSTEM. THEY IDENTIFY THE INVADING VIRUS AND BIOCHEMICALLY NOTIFY THE T-CELLS. (*3*) AFTER BEING NOTIFIED OF THE INVADER, THE *T-CELL* ACTIVATES THE IMMUNE SYSTEM AND BEGINS PRODUCING HELPER T-CELLS. (*4*) *HELPER T-CELLS* ACTIVATE BETA CELLS (B-CELLS). THE B-CELLS BEGIN PRODUCING ANTIBODIES. (*5*) IN RESPONSE TO THIS DIRECTION, THE *BETA CELLS* INCREASE IN NUMBER, MULTIPLYING TO MEET THE NEED FOR ANTIBODY PRODUCTION AND FIGHT THE ATTACKING VIRUS. (*6*) THE *ANTIBODIES,* WARRIORS OF THE IMMUNE SYSTEM, SEEK OUT AND ATTACK THE INVADING VIRUS. ONCE IT IS DETERMINED THAT THE VIRUS HAS BEEN CHECKED, *T-8 (SUPPRESSOR CELLS),* ARE PRODUCED. THESE CELLS CALL OFF THE ATTACK, ALLOWING THE IMMUNE SYSTEM TO BECOME BALANCED ONCE AGAIN.

subsets: T-4 helper cells and T-8 suppressor cells. For optimal balance of the function of the immune system, T-4 helper cells and T-8 suppressor cells must be present in sufficient quantities.

Consider three terms relating to the immune system:

Immunomodulators: These substances act to alter the immune response. They are naturally present in the body or are pharmacologically reproduced.

Immunosuppression: This represents a significant interference with the ability of the immune system to respond to antigenic stimulation.

Immunoglobins: These are antigenically distinct antibodies that are present in the serum and external secretions of the body.

*m*emory *j*og

Clients experiencing immunologic deficits will exhibit signs and symptoms related to the etiology of the deficit. These etiologically specific deficits manifest in many different ways depending upon which component of the immune system is being affected or inactivated. Pathogenic organisms, the non-self, produce unique and varied effects to which the immune system, the self, must respond. Because the immune system is made up of many components, diseases will require more activity from one component as opposed to another. Balance of this system requires that all components are able to function fully and optimally.

Consider the affect on the immune system when attacked by the AIDS virus.

*M*emory *J*og

> AIDS is a condition reflective of immunologic deficits. This condition is caused by the *human immunodeficiency virus* (*HIV*), which alters the balance between T-4 helper cells and T-8 suppressor cells. Skewing is in favor of the T-8 suppressor cells. This causes immune system suppression and increased susceptibility to infection.

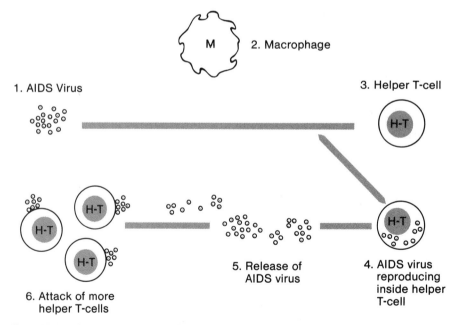

FIGURE 12-2. AIDS AND THE IMMUNE SYSTEM. (*1*) WHEN THE AIDS VIRUS ENTERS THE BODY, THE MACROPHAGE IS BYPASSED, AND HELPER T-CELLS ARE ATTACKED. THE MACROPHAGE IS INEFFECTIVE AS AN ALARM SYSTEM, RESULTING IN ALTERED IMMUNOLOGIC RESPONSE. (*2*) THE HELPER T-CELL IS INVADED BY THE AIDS VIRUS. THE AIDS VIRUS REMAINS IN THE HELPER T-CELL BUT IS INACTIVE FOR A PERIOD OF TIME. WHEN THE HELPER T-CELL IS ATTACKED BY ANOTHER VIRUS OR BACTERIA, THIS STIMULATES THE AIDS VIRUS TO BEGIN REPRODUCING ITSELF. (*3*) THE AIDS VIRUS REPRODUCES ITSELF WITHIN THE HELPER T-CELL. THE INFECTED HELPER T-CELL DIES AND THE AIDS VIRUS IS RELEASED TO INFECT OTHER HELPER T-CELLS. (*4*) NEWLY RELEASED AIDS VIRUS. (*5 & 6*) AIDS VIRUS ATTACKS OTHER HELPER T-CELLS.

PRINCIPLE

THE FIRST BARRIER TO INFECTION IS THE EPITHELIAL LAYER COVERING THE BODY KNOWN AS SKIN

Illustration of the Principle

Not only the skin but also hair, mucous membranes, and secretions provide barriers to infection. The external and internal environments of man are teaming with microorganisms. Internally microorganisms are controlled by overall good health of man and a functional immune system. Exposure to microorganisms in the external environment is dependent upon several factors.

A break in the integrity of the skin or epithelial covering of the body is a major source of exposure to environmental microorganism. Subsequent to this interruption, infections can and do develop. Such interruptions can occur in the urinary tract, gastrointestinal tract, and respiratory tract. Once a disruption occurs, microorganisms thriving in the external environment can enter the body. Microorganisms, bacteria, and viruses have the ability in some cases to escape the natural defenses of the host. Because of this lack of detection the invading organisms are able to generate infection and/or inflammatory responses.

Mechanisms of defense related to the integument differ from site to site. Characteristics reflective of this phenomenon relate to the specialized functions of surface cells: macrophages and cilia; flora that normally is present at the site and is able to inhibit pathogens to colonize; the skin and mucous membranes that act as a physical barrier to invading microorganisms; and secretions such as gastric acid, mucus, and saliva.

In general, the skin does not provide an optimal environment for microbial development. Epithelial cells are tightly compacted, thus providing a dense mechanical barrier. This barrier exists because of the multilayered structure that is created by the densely packed epithelial cells. The horny outer layer of the skin is being shed and replaced constantly. This phenomenon helps in the elimination of externally attacking pathogens. Moist areas of the body promote the growth of microorganisms. Most microorganisms require a nonacidic environment to promote their growth. The acidic pH of the skin repels this growth.

The skin consists of two layers: the outer (epidermis) and the deeper (dermis).

The epidermis (outer layer) functions as a barrier to protect inner tissues from injury, chemicals, organisms; as a receptor for a range of sensations (touch, pain, heat, cold); as a regulator of body temperature through radiation, conduction, and convection.

Carpenito, p 424.

Impairment of skin integrity, either actual or potential, places the client at risk. Many factors can contribute to this state. It is important to consider that pathogenic organisms may contact the body in various ways, and the disease does not always result. Contributing factors related to the disruption of skin integrity can be due to inadequate personal hygiene, which permits a medium for pathogens to grow and promotes excoriation of the skin. Inadequate nutrition does not permit optimal cellular growth and differentiation of this protective barrier. Other pathological conditions such as impaired oxygen transport related to such conditions as anemia or cardiovascular disorders, metabolic conditions such as diabetes mellitus and cancer, and medications such as steroids can and do contribute to skin disruption.

Obvious other conditions such as penetrating traumatic injuries, burns, and surgical incisions open the way for organisms to enter the internal environment of man. Coupled with other compromising conditions such as shock, malnutrition, or previously existing pathology, the microorganisms can go on to reproduce and compromise man's balance.

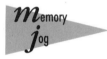

Dressings are mechanical barriers of the skin. Dressings absorb drainage, protect wounds from injury, control bleeding, apply medication, and keep the wound clean. Types of dressings include pressure dressings, occlusive dressings, absorbent dressings, wet dressings, and antiseptic dressings.

PRINCIPLE

THE INTERACTIONS AMONG HOST DEFENSE MECHANISMS, MICROBIAL VIRULENCE, AND ENVIRONMENTAL CONDITIONS ARE THE DETERMINANTS FOR DEVELOPING INFECTIONS

Illustration of the Principle

Microorganisms find their way into the body in many ways. They can be ingested, as in the case of salmonella, inhaled, as in the case of mycobacterium tuberculosis, or from other modes not known such as cytomegalovirus. Natural resistance to infection relates to the overall health of the body in producing secretory or circulating immune globulins. Therefore, in addition to the physical barriers consisting of skin and mucous membranes, there exists a series of chemical barriers.

Chemical barriers include all of the secretions or excretions of the stomach in the form of hydrochloric acid, digestive enzymes, bacteriostatic agents present in the plasma, products released or activated by antigen–antibody reaction, and waxes and other fatty acids with bacteriostatic properties such as cerumen.

Front line phagocyctic cells, which are part of the reticuloendothelial system, are continuously filtering the circulating blood. These cells are able to clear entering particles of bacteria from the bloodstream.

To keep in mind an understanding of this principle, the nurse must be aware that a series of events is necessary for an infection to occur. Required are a disease-producing agent, a reservoir, a mode of transmission, a portal of entry, and a susceptible host. Susceptibility is not well understood, but relationships exist between the virulence and number of organisms attacking the host, the immune system's ability to destroy invading organisms, and the overall health and nutritional status of the host. Susceptibility to disease is known to be influenced by factors such as psychosocial and life-style practices, the general environment that the host is exposed to, finances, recreation patterns, and stress.

Nursing application in the form of promoting prevention through community education plays a major role in keeping infections in check. Nurses should assess clients' attitudes regarding infectious diseases, promote adequate personal and environmental hygiene practices, instruct clients regarding adequate nutrition and food handling, storage, and preparation practices, and assist clients in maintaining balance with regard to psychosocial and stress relationships.

Isolation: These practices are employed to prevent cross-contamination. Contamination can occur from an infected client to care providers or from care providers to the compromised client. The form of isolation employed should be specific to the needs of the client.

Important to keep in mind is that the isolation of clients places physical barriers between the client and the rest of the world. Barriers in the form of restricted access to the client's room and the use of gowns, gloves, and masks may lead to behaviors associated with withdrawal and sensory deprivation.

Hand washing: This practice continues to be one of the most effective mechanisms in the prevention of transmission of microorganisms. Inattention to this very important detail is unsafe nursing practice.

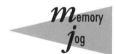

PRINCIPLE

INFLAMMATION WORKS TO LIMIT THE TISSUE DAMAGE, REMOVE THE INJURED CELLS, AND REPAIR THE TRAUMATIZED TISSUE

Illustration of the Principle

Inflammation is a defensive response against cellular injury wherein the body attempts to restrict the injurious agent, neutralize the agent, and repair tissue that has been damaged by the harmful agent. Cellular damage can result from various causes. Without regard to the causative agent, the dynamics of the inflammatory response remains constant and is essential.

Damage that occurs in the body is of course dependent upon the invader and the condition of localized immune response. If the local reaction to the invader is weak or absent, the invading organism can enter the bloodstream and the lymphatic system. When the organism enters the systems, heat and pain are produced as signs of inflammation. Tissue damage occurs.

If the host has been exposed previously to the invading organism, antibodies may have been formed. This prior exposure provokes the immune system

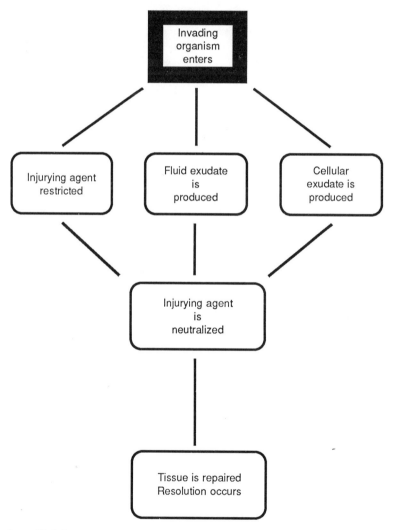

FIGURE 12-3. THE INFLAMMATORY RESPONSE.

to respond more efficiently to rid the body of the invading organism. Immune system memory cells are responsible for this phenomenon. When the invading organism is new to the body, the inflammatory response is less efficient.

Inflammation is characterized by three phases: the vascular stage, the exudative phase, and the reparative stage. Look closely at the schematic of the inflammatory response (Fig. 12-3), and you will see these phases. The end result of this response is to promote tissue healing and regeneration.

A healthy body has the ability and capacity to protect and restore itself. In order to handle tissue trauma, the body is influenced by the extent of the damage and the individual's overall state of health. The body responds systematically to trauma in any of its parts and transports beneficial substances to the site of injury and harmful substances away. Circulating blood is the means of transport. Both open and closed wounds of soft tissue or bone can be invaded by pathogens resulting in an inflammatory response. Normal healing is promoted when the wound is free of foreign substances such as bacteria. Wound healing occurs by first and second intention. Maladaptive responses to the invading organism include the symptoms associated with systemic inflammation, such as fever, chills, myalgias.

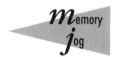

Reasoning Exercises: Infection and Inflammation

Jerry is a 32-year-old white male. He has been married for 10 months, and he and his wife, Sue, are expecting their first child in 6 months. Prior to marrying Sue, Jerry was sexually active and nonmonogamous. He has been sexually active since the age of 18. Recently Jerry has complained of persistent dry cough, night sweats, and a temperature over 100°F. Although Jerry is concerned about his weight and watches his diet, he has lost 15 pounds without even trying. Upon assessing Jerry, he admits to having had sexual intercourse with prostitutes, both male and female, during the last 10 years.

1. Jerry's symptoms of elevated temperature, chills, and dry cough are probably related to which undiagnosed condition?

   A. Alteration in tissue perfusion

   B. An infection, etiology unknown

   C. Indigestion from too frequent traveling

   D. Lack of knowledge related to frequent travel

The intended response is **B.** Classic signs and symptoms of infection are fever, chills, loss of appetite, generalized myalgias, or localized pain and discomfort. The dry cough that Jerry experiences can be associated with the system of involvement. Pulmonary etiology should be assessed and evaluated.

1. Jerry is admitted to your unit. His admitting diagnosis is fever of unknown origin. He is required to be placed in strict isolation. As the nurse caring for Jerry you would explain this intervention best by

   A. Telling Jerry that he is so sick that other patients would be at risk if he were not in isolation.

   B. Reading Jerry the hospital policy regarding isolation and explain how he is affected

   C. Recognizing that isolation is a mechanical barrier separating Jerry from the rest of the world and spending as much time as possible with him

   D. Explaining to Jerry that isolation is only temporary and that he can always reach help by pushing the call light.

The intended response is **C.** Isolation has a dual purpose. First isolation is used to protect the client from contamination from the external environment. Such contaminants can be introduced through contact with care-givers, family, and friends. Secondly, isolation is used to protect the external environment, and those persons in it, from a particular type of infection that the client may have. Isolation is not a punitive measure, it is therapeutic. By recognizing that Jerry's freedom to interact with the external environment is mechanically limited, the nurse should view herself as the bridge to this gap. Spending as much time as possible with Jerry supports his interaction with the external environment.

1. Jerry undergoes a number of diagnostic tests. His testing reveals that he is HIV positive. This lab result indicates

   A. Jerry's immune system is showing signs of immunodeficiency.

   B. He has a definitive diagnosis of AIDS.

   C. Jerry is experiencing an inflammatory response that can be erradicated with antibiotics.

   D. This result is normal and requires no cause for concern.

The intended response is **A.** AIDS is a condition that reflects immunodeficiency. A positive HIV indicates the client has been exposed to the virus known to cause AIDS and has produced antibodies. In addition, the immune system indicates a skewing in favor of the suppressor cells. This skewing indicates an underlying immunodeficiency.

1. In planning nursing care for Jerry, one must keep in mind the holistic needs that Jerry has. An appropriate expected outcome for Jerry would be

   A. Client will learn to deal with an acceptable discomfort level.

   B. Client will verbalize commitment to sexual abstinence.

    C. Client will maintain self-care ability according to physical psychological condition.

    D. Client will accept the loss of security and social acceptance.

The intended response is **C.** Consider the client's needs for independence and sense of control. Powerlessness can seriously limit one's ability to participate in one's own care. This feeling can be demoralizing and self-limiting. By considering the client as an individual in regard to his physiological and psychological condition, encouraging appropriate self-care will promote independence and control.

1. On the third day of Jerry's hospitalization, he develops the following symptoms: temperature 101.2°F, pulse 110, chills, and white blood cell count of 14,000. These symptoms are reflective of

    A. Hyperbola immuno sensitivity

    B. Skewing of T-8 suppressor cells in favor of T-4 cells

    C. Untoward reaction to antibiotic therapy

    D. An underlying infection

The intended response is **D.** An elevated temperature is reflective of the body's response to some infection. Many organisms cannot survive in temperatures above normal body temperature. Temperature elevations assist the fighting off of invading organisms by speeding up cellular and biochemical responses. The cellular component of the immune system responds to infection and inflammation by producing more white blood cells. These cells are then available to combat invading microorganisms. The pulse rises to improve circulation of blood and all of its cellular components, carrying oxygen and nutrients throughout the body. Because infections and inflammations produce body stress, metabolic needs are higher. Waste materials and by-products associated with the invading organisms are carried away in the circulating blood.

1. Jerry is finally diagnosed as having AIDS. He and his wife, Sue, are very concerned for their unborn child. Jerry asks what the risks are to Sue and the developing child. What would your best response be?

    A. Viruses rarely cross placental barriers.

    B. It would be wise for your wife to be tested for exposure to the virus.

    C. You should have thought about your life-style before you put innocent people at risk.

    D. You should indicate that there is no reason to worry until Sue develops signs or symptoms of inflammation.

The intended response is **B.** Baseline information in the form of HIV testing could indicate exposure to the virus known to cause AIDS. Once that information is obtained, additional counseling regarding Sue's pregnancy could be discussed. Since HIV testing reveals that the client has been exposed to the virus and that the immune system has produced antibodies, it is valuable in considering transmission to the developing fetus. This virus has demonstrated that ability to cross the placental barrier and infect developing infants *in utero*. In the event that Sue tests negative, she would be followed closely by her obstetrician. A positive HIV test does not mean that the client will definitely go on to become symptomatic for AIDS. However, Sue is at risk because of the sexual history that her husband Jerry relates. It would be valuable to elicit a sexual history from Sue also, in order to determine any additional risk factors.

Reference

Carpenito L: Nursing Diagnosis: Application to Clinical Practice, 2nd ed. Philadelphia, JB Lippincott, 1987

Doenges M, Moorhouse M: Nurse's Pocket Guide: Nursing Diagnoses with Interventions. Philadelphia, F A Davis, 1985

Elhart D et al: Scientific Principles in Nursing. St. Louis, CV Mosby, 1978

Harvey A et al: Principles and Practice of Medicine. New York, Appleton-Century-Crofts

Kneisel C, Ames S: Adult Health Nursing: A Biopsychosocial Approach. Massachusetts, Addison-Wesley Publishing, 1986

Mosby's Medical and Nursing Dictionary. St. Louis, CV Mosby, 1986

Patrick M et al: Medical Surgical Nursing: Pathophysiological Concepts. Philadelphia, JB Lippincott, 1986

MOVEMENT, SENSATION, AND COGNITION

13

MARIAN B. SIDES

PRINCIPLE

THE NERVOUS SYSTEM IS A COMMUNICATION NETWORK THAT CONTROLS AND COORDINATES ACTIVITIES THROUGHOUT THE BODY

Illustration of Principle

The nervous system plays a key role in man's ability to interact meaningfully with his environment. Movement, sensation, and cognition are normal bodily processes that result from effective communication between the nervous system and the various parts of the body that it serves.

A key function of this system is to receive information from the environment, interpret it, and transmit electrical impulses to precise locations of the body for action. Thus, it controls and coordinates man's interactions and behaviors and is largely responsible for his adjustments in life.

PRINCIPLE

THE FLOW OF COMMUNICATION TO VARIOUS BODY PARTS DEPENDS UPON THE STRUCTURAL AND FUNCTIONAL INTEGRITY
OF THE NERVOUS SYSTEM

Illustration of Principle

The nervous system conforms closely to the bony structure of the body. The skull and vertebral column contain the brain and the spinal cord and is known

145

as the central nervous system. The cerebrospinal and autonomic nerves are located outside the bony structure and together form the peripheral nervous system.

Functionally, the nervous system is divided into the voluntary and the involuntary systems.

Voluntary Function

Both the central nervous system and the peripheral nervous system have voluntary functions. The central nervous system is responsible for conscious behavior and includes all processes activated by the individual. The cerebrum is the largest part of the voluntary system.

The peripheral nervous system conducts and controls movement and sensation. The perception of muscle contraction, for example, or pain and temperature is transmitted by fibers along the pathway to its destination.

Memory Jog

STRUCTURAL INTEGRITY

a. Central nervous system
   1. Brain and spinal cord
   2. Inside bony structure
b. Peripheral nervous system
   1. Cerebrospinal and autonomic nervous system
   2. Outside bony structure

FUNCTIONAL INTEGRITY

a. Voluntary
   1. Brain and spinal cord, cerebral nerves, spinal nerves
   2. Control of cognition, movement, and sensation
b. Involuntary
   1. Autonomic nerves/sympathetic and parasympathetic nerves
   2. Control of visceral function

Involuntary Function

The involuntary autonomic nervous system consists of a series of nerve fibers and ganglia that extend from each side of the vertebral column. They form the sympathetic and parasympathetic divisions that act in an apparently opposite but cooperative manner on the organs of the body. In concert, they either accelerate, dilate, or stimulate bodily functions or contract, relax, or retard bodily functions.

These systems form a communication network and provide a mechanism for the transmission of impulses and stimuli to appropriate body parts. Internal balance and homeostasis depend upon the precision, synchronization, and patency of these systems.

PRINCIPLE

Illustration of Principle

The neuron is the most fundamental unit of the nervous system. It consists of a nerve cell that transmits impulses and stimuli to all parts of the body. Each cell has an energy-producing nucleus, a process called a dendrite that brings impulses to the cell, and an axom that sends impulses away from the cell.

The major systems of the brain and spinal cord that contain these cells are interconnected by a complex network of sensory and motor tracts that provide pathways for the relay of nerve impulses to designated body parts.

A disturbance in the integrity of these structures or an interruption in the flow of nerve impulses will result in a loss of sensation, cognition, or muscular activity.

This brief description of the nervous system conveys its basic principles of operation in a simple and easy to understand manner. The concepts provide an adequate foundation for understanding the impact of structural and functional breakdown on human functioning as well as implications for nursing care.

Several common neurological disorders can further demonstrate the phenomena related to the neurophysiology of the system and how they affect the performances of people.

Edema, or inflammation of peripheral or cranial nerves, with degeneration of the axons and myelin as seen in Guillain-Barré syndrome results in paralysis of affected body parts. Thus, movement and sensations are affected; cognition is not.

Amyotrophic lateral sclerosis (ALS) produces degeneration of the cell bodies of the lower motor neurons of the spinal cord and cranial nerves and results in muscle atrophy. Movement is affected, but cognition and sensation are not.

Spinal cord injury resulting from trauma can cause compression or severance of the spinal cord cells. Loss of function and sensation results.

Multiple sclerosis is a degenerative disease of the central nervous system that causes a breakdown of the myelin sheath in scattered areas of the brain and spinal cord. It causes interference in motor, sensory, and cognitive abilities, much like a lamp that has a frayed cord, causing a short or interruption in the connection between the source of electrical impulse and the light bulb itself.

These and other neurological disorders show common disturbances to movement, sensation, and cognition resulting from structural or functional breakdown in the nervous system.

The nurse's role in managing the patient-care problems resulting from these neurophysiological deficits starts with recognizing clinical patterns as a basis for nursing care.

PRINCIPLE

A COMMON ILLNESS PATTERN CHARACTERIZES MOST NEUROLOGICAL PROBLEMS AND ESTABLISHES THE FRAMEWORK FOR MANAGEMENT OF CARE

Illustration of Principle

The exact etiology of many neurological problems is unknown. It varies, however, from developmental, degenerative, traumatic, infectious, neoplastic, and vascular. Regardless of cause, most neurological problems present a clinical portrait or common illness pattern. These manifestations along with specific individualized behavior establish the framework for the management of care.

In preparing for state boards you should try to grasp the common, fundamental behavior patterns and the nursing care measures that are truly important in correcting these patterns. Don't memorize a lot of meaningless details.

Some of the common neurological problems and their conceptual origins are shown below.

Common Neurological Problems	Conceptual Origin
Spina bifida	Developmental
Multiple sclerosis	Degenerative
Spinal cord injury	Traumatic
Guillain-Barré syndrome	Infectious/degenerative
Brain tumor	Neoplastic
Aneurysm	Cerebrovascular
Meningitis	Infectious

Nursing management begins with a neurological assessment. The approach to data collection is guided by the location of the neurological lesion, if known, and the illness portrayal of the patient. For example, the patient with Guillain-Barré syndrome may have cranial nerve involvement that can pose a threat to respiratory status. Because many disorders involve the central nervous system, efforts will be directed at protecting the airway, breathing, and circulation.

> 90' Neurological assessment
> General observations
> Airway · breathing · pulse
> Cognitive functions
> Motor function
> Sensory function
> Pupillary response

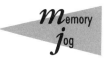

Analysis of data includes establishment of problem definitions or nursing diagnoses. Goals of care are directed at reducing life threats, maintaining body functions, preventing hazards of immobility, detecting changes in status, facilitating communication, providing emotional support, and promoting rehabilitation.

Nursing intervention in pursuit of these goals can be guided by the acronym SUPPORT:

S pecialize

U nderstand

P rotect

P revent

O bserve

R ehabilitate

T each

Specialize

Because neurological involvement can affect many bodily functions, general nursing measures must be maintained. In addition, these patients require specialized procedures and care measures determined by their individual needs. Be prepared to respond to unique, special, or additional needs presented in certain neurological problems.

Understand

These patients often face a serious threat to their self-esteem, autonomy, and independence. They often reflect on their youth and more healthy years (see Fig. 13-1). Show acceptance and understanding of their limitations. Provide emotional support, be a good listener, and show respect.

Prevent

Patients with neurological disorders are at great risk for hazards of immobility. Meticulous nursing care is the most effective preventive measure.

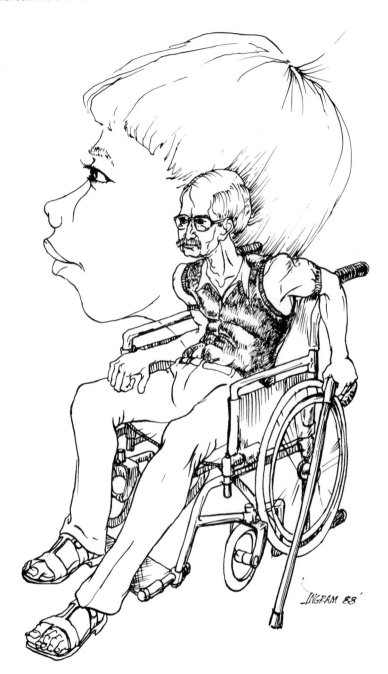

FIGURE 13-1.

Protect

Safety is a fundamental goal of patient care. Safety measures span a broad range of activities and include giving good skin care and proper positioning to prevent skin breakdown; providing assistance in ambulation to prevent falls from unsteady gait; protecting the pathway of an airway to prevent respiratory failure; protecting the personal integrity of a patient who has suffered a loss of self-worth.

Observe

Appropriate monitoring and observation are essential to detect changes in patient status. Certain conditions, for example, patients with epidural hematoma, can change rapidly, requiring immediate intervention. Changes in level of consciousness may be subtle but critical evidence of life threats.

Rehabilitation

Bringing a patient back to health can be a timely and arduous task. In certain degenerative problems, as in ALS, rehabilitation is limited and highly supportive. Conditions such as CVA and Guillain-Barré can have a good prognosis given extensive rehabilitative measures. An important objective is to promote self-care and independence and assist the patient only in those activities he is unable to perform.

Teach

Patient and family education are important for effective and optimal rehabilitation. Critical teaching areas include

1. Understanding of the illness
2. Diet and nutrition
3. Drugs, expected actions, and side-effects
4. Rest and exercise

Each aspect of care should be evaluated on an ongoing basis to determine effectiveness in meeting patient-care goals. The ultimate goal is to assist the patient in returning to the highest level of wellness possible, within the limitations of the illness and the patient's own abilities.

Reasoning Exercises: Movement, Sensation, and Cognition

Avery Stone is a 47-year-old corporate lawyer admitted for diagnostic evaluation of progressive lower extremity weakness and loss of mobility. Guillain-Barré syndrome is the suspected diagnosis.

1. Which of the following comments by Avery should the nurse consider most closely associated with a diagnosis of Guillain-Barré Syndrome?

   A. "I've had bad hay fever and allergies since I was a child."
   B. "I've been taking high blood pressure pills for the last 2 years or so."
   C. "I was off from work for 3 days with a cold about a week ago."
   D. "My father died of a stroke when he was 52 years old."

** The intended response is **C.** Although the actual cause of Guillain-Barré syndrome is unknown, it *is* known to be often preceded by a viral infection. The other three responses are unrelated to this diagnosis. In answering this question, the reader might focus on an *acute* onset neurologic problem.

2. The nurse assessing Avery would expect to find which of the following signs and symptoms related to Guillain-Barré?

   A. Nuchal rigidity, fever, hyperreflexia.
   B. Resting tremors, masklike facial expression, emotional liability
   C. Muscle weakness, incoordination, and pulmonary congestion
   D. Tetany, tachycardia, and diplopia

** The intended response is again **C.** Since Guillain-Barré syndrome involves an inflammatory degeneration of the myelin sheath, loss of muscle strength and control is a hallmark feature. Pulmonary congestion develops as a result of weakness of the respiratory musculature resulting in impaired breathing patterns.

3. A diagnosis of Guillain-Barré syndrome is confirmed, and Mr. Stone's neurologic status deteriorates rapidly, evidenced by advancing paralysis and increased respiratory difficulty. The nurse planning care for Mr. Stone should identify which of the following goals as the *highest* priority?

   A. Prevention of further paralysis by use of bedside P.T. and muscle-strengthening exercise
   B. Prevention of joint contracture by range of motion exercises
   C. Maintenance of adequate oxygenation by O_2 therapy and ventilation if needed
   D. Maintenance of adequate urinary output by fluid therapy

** The intended response is **C.** Since progressive muscular weakness can lead to respiratory depression and failure, the priority of care is maintenance of adequate oxygenation. Response **A** is incorrect, since paralysis results from the syndrome pathophysiology and is thus unpreventable. Responses **B** and **D** may be appropriate but are not the priority.

4. Mr. Stone demonstrates difficulty in swallowing and nearly continually drools saliva. In order to ensure adequate nutritional intake, the nurse might implement all of the following nursing actions EXCEPT

   A. Position Mr. Stone supine for oral feedings

   B. Insert a nasogastric feeding tube for formula feedings

   C. Offer small bites of soft foods and allow extra time for chewing

   D. Consider the possibility of hyperalimentation therapy as indicated

** The intended response is **A.** Because of his generalized weakness and difficulty swallowing, the nurse should position Mr. Stone in Fowler's position for feedings in order to decrease the risk of aspiration. All other responses in this except question would be appropriate.

HORMONES

NANCY B. CAILLES

14

PRINCIPLE

THE PRIMARY ROLE OF THE ENDOCRINE SYSTEM IS TO MAINTAIN BALANCE OF VARIOUS PROCESSES OCCURRING IN THE HUMAN BODY

Illustration of Principle

The various glands that make up the endocrine system perform different and diverse tasks that influence a number of processes in the human body. The thyroid gland, for example, releases hormones that directly affect metabolic processes in the body; the pituitary gland releases gonadotropin-stimulating hormones that influence reproductive cycles in the body. Even though the actions of the glands and the hormones produced in each gland differ, the primary role of each gland of the endocrine system is to maintain *balance* within the body. This balance, or homeostasis, is accomplished in the endocrine system essentially via the *feedback mechanism,* a communication network that signals glands to either release or inhibit hormone secretion. Through this feedback mechanism, the hormonal balance of the body can be ensured.

The following is a brief review of how the feedback mechanism works.

The *hypothalamus,* located in the brain, receives messages from the body's central nervous system, and it subsequently sends a message to the appropriate gland for either hormone release or inhibition. When hormone release has had its effect on the body's processes, feedback is sent to the gland and hypothalamus, so that balance may be maintained.

For Example

An individual who is exercising metabolizes carbohydrate more rapidly, and thus develops hypoglycemia.

155

↓

The central nervous system sends a message to the hypothalamus that the individual is hypoglycemic.

↓

The hypothalamus sends a message about the hypoglycemia to the pituitary gland, stimulating the pituitary to release growth hormone. The release of growth hormone increases the glucose level of the blood.

↓

Once the glucose level begin to rise because of the release of growth hormone, a feedback message is sent to the pituitary and hypothalamus to inhibit further release of growth hormone. Thus, a balance of glucose metabolism is maintained via the function of the feedback mechanism of the endocrine system.

In this example, the reader can see how the communication of bodily messages via the feedback mechanism of the endocrine system serves to maintain balance or homeostasis of bodily processes. An excellent illustration of this communication network and the results of failure in the communication network is provided in the following discussion of the endocrine disease, diabetes mellitus.

PRINCIPLE

INSULIN IS REQUIRED BY THE BODY FOR THE METABOLISM OF CARBOHYDRATE, FAT, AND PROTEIN

Illustration of Principle

Although we tend to think of diabetes mellitus just as a disease characterized by an incomplete metabolism of carbohydrates, it actually involves the metabolism of fats and proteins as well. In the nondiabetic, insulin serves in nutrient metabolism in a number of ways, including assisting glucose to enter fat and muscle cells to be used as energy, stimulating the production of fat cells, inhibiting the release of stored fat cells into the bloodstream, and stimulating the liver to make and store unused simple carbohydrates in the form of glycogen, a complex carbohydrate.

Therefore, in the absence of insulin, normal metabolic processes cannot be maintained. Since the diabetic patient's pancreas does not manufacture and release insulin, energy needs of the body cells cannot be met by carbohydrate metabolism. Because insulin is not available to control the rate of fat metabolism, the diabetic patient is prone to rapid destruction of fat cells in order to provide for cellular energy needs. This rapid metabolism causes the release of free acid bodies (ketones) into the serum, precipitating an acidotic state in the body called *diabetic ketoacidosis,* (an acidosis caused by accumulation of ketone acid bodies in the serum), a serious complication of *hyperglycemia* and lack of insulin.

It is evident, then, that a principle management of the insulin-dependent, or Type I, diabetic patient is the administration of insulin. Because insulin is primarily a protein, it would be metabolized too quickly by salivary enzymes of the mouth, and thus must be administered by injection, typically into subcutaneous (fatty) tissues of the body. The goal of insulin administration is to provide this essential hormone in order to balance glucose levels in serum, promote glucose metabolism for cellular energy, and encourage glucose storage in the forms of glycogen and fat for future energy needs.

> In the absence of insulin, the diabetic patient metabolizes body fat rapidly for energy. This releases acidic by-products that accumulate in the serum, causing *acidosis.*

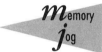

PRINCIPLE

GLUCAGON IS A HORMONE OF THE PANCREAS THAT SERVES TO INCREASE SERUM-GLUCOSE LEVELS

Illustration of Principle

In the nondiabetic, the alpha cells of the islets of Langerhans of the pancreas manufacture the hormone *glucagon,* whose primary action is to *increase* blood-glucose levels, when those levels drop below generally accepted normal parameters (60 to 100 mg/100 ml). Thus, insulin and glucagon work "hand-in-hand" to maintain *balance* of serum glucose, which then supports metabolism energy requirements of the cells. In the diabetic patient, however, the pancreas does not manufacture insulin, creating a disturbance in the "hand-in-hand" balance between insulin and glucagon.

Thus, as the diabetic patient will require injection of insulin to lower blood-glucose level, he may also require intermittent injection of glucagon to counteract abnormally low blood-glucose levels that have brought about symptoms of *hypoglycemia.*

> The pancreas manufactures two hormones that affect glucose serum levels. Insulin lowers blood glucose; glucagon raises blood glucose. Balance between insulin and glucose is essential.

Principle

Insulin, in the nondiabetic individual, is released on a p.r.n. basis

Illustration of Principle

This basic principle highlights a major difference between the nondiabetic individual and his diabetic counterpart. Normally, insulin is released from the beta cells of the islets of Langerhans of the pancreas on an as-needed or prn basis as foodstuffs are ingested or as glucose levels of serum rise. The process of timely insulin release is controlled by the feedback mechanism of the endocrine system with its secretory and inhibitory properties. Because the insulin-dependent diabetic's pancreas is *not* functioning properly, the feedback mechanism of the endocrine system that guides insulin secretion and inhibition, likewise, is nonfunctional, resulting in a lack of control over glucose levels and metabolism.

Since the insulin-dependent diabetic does not manufacture insulin in his own pancreas, he must receive his needed insulin by injection. Insulin injections, whether administered subcutaneously or for more rapid absorption by IV route, cannot simulate the prn release of insulin of the nondiabetic pancreas. Rather, the peaks and diminuations of insulin levels in the diabetic are dependent upon the *type* of insulin administered, with regular or crystalline insulin having a much more rapid peak than NPH insulin, for example.

> Each type of insulin the diabetic uses in the management of his disease has a different "peak" action. Whereas regular insulin acts on blood glucose levels and peaks rapidly, the longer-acting NPH insulin peaks at a much later time after injection. Thus, glucose levels of a diabetic patient may vary throughout the course of a day, depending upon the type of insulin being administered.

Nursing Management

Because of this fact, patients receiving insulin injections must be consistently monitored to ensure adequate and appropriate "coverage" by the administered insulin for the body's metabolic needs. As metabolic needs of the body change, such as with exercise or fever, insulin requirements of the body likewise change, calling for adjustment of insulin type and dose. It is impossible, then, for the diabetic patient to achieve a preset insulin requirement and maintain that same coverage level all throughout life. An important nursing intervention with the diabetic patient, then, is to provide teaching about what processes may alter metabolic needs and thus insulin coverage requirements, so that the diabetic patient learns to be flexible and sensible about providing insulin injections in relation to body need.

A time-honored method of helping the diabetic patient to recognize changes in his insulin coverage requirements is through routine testing of urine samples for the presence of glucose and acetone bodies. If the patient is "spilling" glucose or acetone into his urine, it is recognized that blood levels of glucose or acetone are elevated, and additional insulin coverage is needed.

Ever-advancing technology has allowed nurses and diabetics alike to utilize much more accurate methods of evaluating glucose levels and insulin needs by blood-glucose chemstrips and blood glucometers, and thus urine testing is progressively used less and less often. Regardless of the method used, the nurse should be aware that ongoing evaluation of blood-glucose and acetone levels is essential to the management of the diabetic patient.

> It is essential that the diabetic patient monitor his blood-glucose values in conjunction with insulin therapy. Since injected insulin cannot enter into the bloodstream on an "as needed or prn basis, the patient and nurse should anticipate fluctuations in glucose levels and corresponding insulin requirements.

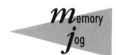

PRINCIPLE

THE GOAL OF MANAGEMENT OF THE INSULIN-DEPENDENT (TYPE I) DIABETIC IS TO ACHIEVE BALANCE AMONG THREE CRITICAL FACTORS: INSULIN, DIET, AND ACTIVITY OR REST

Illustration of Principle

Once the suspected diabetic patient has been differentially diagnosed by means of classic signs and symptoms of hyperglycemia (polyphagia, polydipsia, and polyuria) coupled with diagnostic results of a glucose tolerance test, the goal of management is to achieve balance among three critical factors: insulin, diet, and activity or rest.

The glucose tolerance test involves the administration of a set concentration of glucose with sequential blood-glucose value analysis. If the patient is a Type I diabetic, glucose levels of the blood will not decrease with sequential blood samples, indicating a lack of insulin production. With this information in mind, nurse and physicians must work together to find the correct plan of management of the patient, focusing on the following points:

▷ Type, amount, and frequency of insulin administration
▷ Dietary requirements for calories, carbohydrates, proteins, and fats

▷ Metabolic needs of the body and changes occurring with altered patterns of rest and activity

Insulin

Each type of insulin has a different effect on blood glucose because of varying peak action. Patients are often maintained on an intermediate-acting insulin (such as NPH) or a long-acting insulin (such as ultralente) in order to get adequate around-the-clock coverage of serum-glucose values. Regular insulin, with its rapid, peak action, would be indicated for an acutely elevated blood-glucose value and should not be used in routine diabetic management.

Unit amounts of insulin are gauged on serum-glucose values as well, until ideal dosage is identified for the individual patient. Dosage and frequency of insulin injections, then, may vary quite a bit from day to day until the patient's insulin needs are ascertained. If, for example, a morning injection of NPH humulin insulin, 40 units, causes the patient to experience hypoglycemic reactions, the dosage may be lowered, or the injections may be altered in frequency.

*M*emory *J*og

> Insulin needs of each diabetic patient are highly individualized. Type of insulin and the frequency of administration will depend on a number of factors, including age, metabolic rate, caloric intake, and activity level. Periodic adjustment of insulin coverage should be expected.

Diet

Although the diabetic patient has difficulty with carbohydrate metabolism, carbohydrates are essential for energy production, and thus are included in the diabetic diet. In fact, the American Diabetic Association (ADA) diet is composed of food exchange selections to match the prescribed caloric intake that represent approximately 60% carbohydrates. The nurse should explain to the diabetic patient that, although carbohydrates make up over half of the total caloric allotment, they must be *complex* forms of carbohydrate, such as breads and fruits. The diabetic patient must avoid simple forms of sugar, such as candies or sweetened carbonated beverages, because simple sugars cause rather rapid and unpredictable elevations of blood glucose. The diabetic patient can readily maintain optimal nutrition as well as diabetic management by adhering to the prescribed food exchanges per category of nutrient (carbohydrates, fats, and proteins). Only when the diabetic patient is experiencing acute hypoglycemia should simple forms of sugar (*e.g.,* table sugar, candies) be taken in small amounts. The patient should be advised of the importance of eating regularly scheduled meals to maintain optimal balance of glucose/insulin levels, and should be cautioned to avoid skipping meals or overeating at one meal, making caloric and nutrient distribution unequal for the day.

> The diabetic patient is allowed a substantial amount of carbohydrates in his diet. He should avoid simple carbohydrates, such as candies or carbonated beverages, though, since these will cause rapid fluctuations in blood glucose.

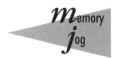

Activity and Rest

Activity levels will affect diabetic management and required insulin administration, because activity requires energy, acquired through glucose metabolism by the cells. Regular activity or exercise plans are desirable for the diabetic patient, since these will increase circulation and may even reduce requirements for insulin. Since the diabetic patient is prone to the development of atherosclerotic deposits in his arteries as a result of deposits of unmetabolized glucose and other solids, exercise is indicated and should be encouraged to stimulate improved circulation. However, the diabetic should plan exercise and activity under the guidance of a physician, since increased activity levels may bring about a hypoglycemic episode, if proper insulin and diet management have not been enacted prior to the exercise. The nurse should instruct the patient to follow the physician's prescription for activity and rest closely and to report any unusual signs or symptoms during or following activity and exercise that might indicate a precipitous change in blood-glucose values.

PRINCIPLE

AN IMBALANCE OF GLUCOSE ABOVE OR BELOW NORMAL SERUM-GLUCOSE PARAMETERS RESULTS IN THE DEVELOPMENT OF HYPERGLYCEMIC OR HYPOGLYCEMIC STATES WITH ASSOCIATING SYMPTOMS AND SIGNS

Illustration of Principle

Since the Type I diabetic patient does not manufacture insulin, balance of serum-glucose levels is often difficult to maintain. When a diabetic patient receives too much insulin per injections, or when he takes his usual dosage of insulin but does not take in adequate food supply, serum-glucose levels will fall, because pancreatic control of insulin production and release is not functional. Similarly, if the diabetic patient takes his usual dosage of insulin but experiences changes in body metabolism as would occur after vigorous exercise, carbohydrates will be too rapidly metabolized, and blood glucose decreases. As serum-glucose levels fall below the normal or accepted parameters of 60 to 100 mg/100 ml, the patient shows evidence of a *hypoglycemic* (hypo—little, glycemic—serum glucose) state, manifested by characteristic symptoms, including:

▷ Headache

▷ Slurred speech

▷ Disorientation

▷ Nervousness

▷ Tremor

▷ Convulsion

▷ Loss of consciousness

The hypoglycemic state should be treated as an emergency, with prompt and expedient action. It is critical that the nurse readily identify symptoms of hypoglycemia and respond in conjunction with the physician with appropriate administration of some form of rapidly metabolized glucose, per IV administration of glucose solution, if the patient is unresponsive or by oral administration of simple sugars, such as in orange juice, candy, or table sugar, if the patient is able to swallow without difficulty.

Memory jog

> The symptoms of hypoglycemia are primarily those of CNS changes. Hypoglycemia can rapidly result in loss of consciousness and must be treated as a medical emergency. If unsure of the diabetic patient's status, it is wisest to treat the condition as hypoglycemia until diagnostic values can confirm hypoglycemia *versus* hyperglycemia.

Following the administration of some form of glucose, the patient should show rapid improvement in CNS functioning, and blood-glucose values should begin to elevate toward normal parameters. When the opposite phenomenon occurs, and the diabetic patient receives too little insulin per injection, or when metabolic needs of the body are changed causing an increased *need* for insulin, serum-glucose levels will rise, resulting in a *hyperglycemic* state. Since circulating insulin levels are not adequate enough to allow glucose to enter into body cells to be metabolized and used as an energy source, the glucose remains in the serum, causing blood-glucose levels to rise and leading to characteristic symptoms. The nurse should assess the patient for indications of hyperglycemia, including elevated blood glucose, polyuria, polydipsia (excessive thirst), and polyphagia. The nurse may note a "spilling" of glucose into the patient's urine per urine-glucose testing. If the hyperglycemia goes unchecked, the patient may begin to evidence signs of ketoacidosis, an acid-base imbalance that occurs when glucose cannot be metabolized for energy by the cells, and fats are metabolized at a rapid and uncontrolled rate, releasing fatty acids into the bloodstream. Symptoms of diabetic ketoacidosis (DKA) are those of a metabolic acidosis and are accompanied by signs of acute dehydration: warm, dry, flushed skin; soft, sunken eyeballs; poor skin turgor; increased body temperature, pulse, and respirations; decreasing blood pressure. In response to the compensatory efforts of the body, the nurse will note an acetone odor to the patient's breath, sometimes described as fruity or sweet.

Arterial blood gases will reveal a decrease in pH, because of the accumulation of fatty acids in serum, with an accompanying drop in HCO_3 values, signifying a metabolic acidosis. The CO_2 may be decreased in a compensatory effort as the ketoacidotic patient begins to breathe rapidly and deeply in an effort to "blow off" CO_2 to reduce acidic content to arterial blood. Thus, the presence of Kussmaul respirations described above indicate the body's drive towards compensation.

The hyperglycemic or ketoacidotic patient requires immediate administration of a rapid-acting form of insulin in order to correct the elevated blood-glucose value and halt the subsequent rapid metabolism of fats that leads to ketoacidosis. The nurse should plan for administration of regular (crystalline) insulin to the patient. Arterial blood gases should be assessed for evidence of metabolic acidosis. Administration of sodium bicarbonate may be necessary to reverse or "buffer" the excess acid bodies in the serum. Vital signs and urine output should be measured so that a fluid and electrolyte imbalance secondary to polyuria does not progress unchecked. Since insulin is required to allow K into cells, hyperglycemic states may result in hyperkalemia with associated increase in cardiac irritability. Thus, the patient's apical pulse and cardiac rhythm should be monitored for evidence of tachycardia and dysrhythmia.

The nurse will evaluate progress of the patient through the hyperglycemic episode as serum-glucose levels begin to diminish back to normal or to more acceptable levels. The patient will become more responsive and mentally alert and will no longer evidence excessive thirst or polyuria. If the patient's hyperglycemic state advanced into ketoacidosis, the nurse should note both a decrease in glucose and ketone levels following administration of insulin. Arterial blood gases would evidence an increasing blood pH and a corresponding increase in HCO_3, demonstrating reversal of the metabolic acidosis. The patient's respiratory pattern should return to normal with cessation of Kussmaul respirations. Vital signs should return to normal ranges, and evidence of dehydration should begin to reverse. The nurse should continue to monitor the patient's cardiac function carefully, since the administration of insulin will force serum K into the cells, with resultant drop in serum levels precipitating hypokalemia. Serum-glucose levels should be continuously monitored after the hyperglycemic or ketoacidotic episode to ensure that insulin treatment has not caused a precipitous *fall* in blood glucose that could result in a hypoglycemic reaction. For this reason, patients recovering from hyperglycemic reactions may be given intermittent orange juice to ensure adequate glucose values following insulin therapy.

Reasoning Exercises: Hormones, Diabetes Mellitus

Loberta Jackson, a 21-year-old college student, is admitted to a medical unit with diagnosis of uncontrolled diabetes, acute hypoglycemic reaction.

1. Loberta explains to the admitting nurse that she had been feeling "sick to my stomach, like I was coming down with the flu" for the past 48 hours. She has continued to take her usual daily dosage of insulin. Noting that Loberta has been admitted with a blood-glucose value of 46, which of the following assessment questions would provide the most valuable information about Loberta's status?

   A. "Have you been under a great deal of stress lately, Loberta?"

   B. "Were you having difficulty sleeping after this illness started?"

   C. "Have you eaten anything in the past 48 hours?"

   D. "Did you take any medications for this illness other than your insulin?"

The intended response is **C,** because it is highly probable that Loberta, feeling "sick to her stomach," has not taken in adequate foods and fluids, and coupled with taking her usual dosage of daily insulin, has brought about an acute hypoglycemic reaction. (Higher than normal circulating levels of insulin with insufficient food intake of essential nutrients will result in acute decreased blood-glucose levels). Response **A,** focusing on increased stress, would more than likely stimulate a hyperglycemic reaction, since stress causes elevations of blood glucose. Response **D,** focusing on other medications the patient has taken, would probably not trigger a hypoglycemic reaction. Response **B** is unrelated to her present status.

2. Which series of symptoms would Loberta most likely display, because of her hypoglycemic state?

   A. Hot, dry skin; thirst

   B. Polyuria; poor skin turgor

   C. Fruity odor to breath; tachycardia

   D. Faintness; headache

The intended response is **D,** since faintness and headache are classic signs of acute hypoglycemia related to the central nervous system. Responses **A, B,** and **C** are all incorrect, because these responses strongly suggest the opposite serum-glucose imbalance, *hyper*glycemia.

3. Which of the following nursing actions would be most appropriate in managing Loberta's blood-glucose value of 46?

   A. Encourage Loberta to take frequent sips of water.

B. Instruct Loberta to eat a few saltine crackers and drink additional water.

C. Offer Loberta orange juice or sugar water.

D. Offer Loberta her choice of several sugar-free snacks.

The intended response is **C**, because orange juice or sugar water will provide the hypoglycemic patient with rapid-acting simple sugars, which will then quickly elevate her low blood-glucose levels. Responses **A** and **D** will not provide any needed sugar source. Response **B** is incorrect, because saltine crackers and water, though possibly desirable for the nauseated patient, do not provide a simple form of sugar needed to raise the decreased blood-glucose value.

Margaret O'Hara, a 30-year-old known diabetic, is brought to the emergency department by ambulance. The paramedic team reports symptoms of apparent hyperglycemia. Stat blood glucose is 640.

1. The nurse is aware that excess serum glucose acts to draw fluids osmotically with resultant polyuria. In addition to increased urinary output, the nurse should expect to observe which of the following sets of symptoms in Margaret?

   A. Polydipsia, diaphoresis, bradycardia

   B. Thirst, dry mucous membranes, hot dry skin

   C. Hypotension, bounding pulse, headache

   D. Nervousness, rapid respirations, diarrhea

The intended response is **B**, because these are all symptoms associated with the dehydration that occurs in hyperglycemia. Although polydypsia is expected (response **A**), diaphoresis does not occur in the body's effort to compensate by holding back fluid. The patient would experience tachycardia as a cardiac compensatory mechanism, causing a rapid, thready pulse. Headache and nervousness (responses **C** and **D**) are symptoms associated with *hypoglycemia.*

2. Arterial blood-gases indicate that Margaret is experiencing acidosis secondary to her hyperglycemic state. Which of the following blood-gases would indicate an *improvement* in her acidotic condition?

   A. pH 7.23

   B. HCO_3 18

   C. pH 7.39

   D. HCO_3 20

The intended response is **C**, since a pH of 7.39 is within normal parameters and is not indicative of an acidotic condition. The remaining blood gases all indicate a continuing state of acidosis for the patient.

CELL DIVISION

BARBARA ETLING MURPHY

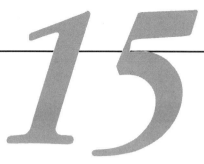

15

PRINCIPLE

THE CELL IS THE BASIC STRUCTURAL AND FUNCTIONAL UNIT OF THE HUMAN BODY

Illustration of the Principle

A cell is the smallest, intact component of a living organism. It is life in its simplest form, a nucleus floating in cytoplasm, encased in a membrane. Yet the cell is not a simple structure. Each individual cell in a living organism is a complex unit of information, activity, and function.

The nucleus of the cell acts as its control center. It is the "brains" of the operation, directing all the cell's activities. The nucleus also contains the cell's genetic information. Chromatin material, made up of deoxyribonucleic acid (DNA) and protein, develops into threadlike structures known as chromosomes. Segments of the DNA strands, the genes, contain coded information that ultimately determines the individual characteristics of the organism (*e.g.,* eye color, hair texture). In humans, all this information is organized into 23 pairs of chromosomes. Each individual cell nucleus is actually a blueprint of the entire organism.

> The nucleus is the cell's control center.
>
> It directs and coordinates all intracellular activities.
>
> It influences how the cell interacts with the extracellular environment.
>
> It contains the cell's genetic information.

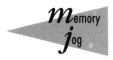

*M*emory *J*og

In order to survive and function, the cell must have some means to meet its own metabolic needs. It must be able to nourish itself. It must be able to synthesize the materials it needs to perform its various functions. It must have some means of transporting these materials throughout the cell. Finally, it must have access to a power source capable of keeping all these mechanisms running. These activities occur in the cytoplasm of the cell. The cytoplasm lies between the nucleus and the cell membrane. It houses a number of different structures, known as organelles, that perform the actual work of the cell. Organelles are distinct, self-contained systems, working together to maintain balance within the cell.

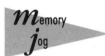

Under the direction of the nucleus, the organelles in the cytoplasm perform the actual "work" of the cell.

The nucleus and the cytoplasm of the cell are held together by the cell membrane, which serves to protect the cell from the outside environment. The membrane itself is composed primarily of lipid and protein and contains openings or "pores" that allow the internal mechanisms of the cell to communicate with the outside environment. However, the cell membrane does much more than just separate the cell from the outside world. Under the direction of the nucleus, it performs a number of critical functions that are essential to the survival and proper functioning of the cell.

The cell membrane participates in certain chemical reactions occurring within the cell. Digestive enzymes, located in the membrane, initiate the processes by which necessary nutrients are made available for use by the cell. The cell membrane also acts as a site for the activation of adenosine triphosphate (ATP), the cell's fuel, into a form of energy the cell can utilize to carry out its various chemical reactions. However, one of the cell's most significant functions involves its control over the passage of materials into and out of the cell. This mechanism is essential for maintaining balance within the cell. The ease with which this is accomplished depends on how permeable the cell membrane is. Most cell membranes are considered semipermeable, which means that certain substances, like water, can pass freely into and out of the cell, whereas other substances cannot. Some of the factors that influence membrane permeability include the following:

The molecular size of the substance attempting to enter the cell, in relation to the size of the pores in the membrane.

The composition of the substance attempting to enter the cell. The cell membrane has a high lipid content, so lipid-soluble substances have an easier time passing through the membrane than nonlipid soluble substances.

The electrical charge carried by the substance attempting to enter the cell, as compared with that carried by the cell membrane. Two like charges repel each other and make passage through the membrane difficult.

The presence of active transport mechanisms within the cell membrane. Using energy, these "carriers" transport substances into the cell that might otherwise not be able to enter.

If this system were perfect, the cell membrane would be permeable to the substances that the cell needs for growth and reproduction and impermeable to the substances that could harm it. Unfortunately, the system is not that specific. Because of these properties of cell membrane permeability, appropriately prescribed medication is able to reach its target tissues and perform its functions appropriately. However, if this situation is occurring in a pregnant female, these are also the properties that are allowing the drugs to cross the placental membranes and potentially result in damage to the developing fetus.

> The cell membrane separates the intracellular environment from the extracellular environment and controls the passage of substances into and out of the cell.

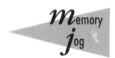

The cells of living organisms all go through similar processes in performing their individual functions. They take in and process nutrients, they eliminate wastes, and most of them reproduce. A single-cell organism, like the protozoa, is just that—a single cell. This one cell must independently perform all of the activities necessary to ensure its survival. It is by necessity a relatively simple organism. As the number of cells in an organism increases, they become less able to perform all functions independently. Therefore, the various cells tend to specialize in whatever function they are best suited for, counting on their fellow cells to fill in the gaps. For example, nerve cells are capable of absorbing nutrients but are primarily involved in transmitting impulses back and forth between the brain and other parts of the body. These cells depend on the cells in the intestinal mucosa to process nutrients for use by the entire body. The end result is an effective division of labor. Groups of specialized cells function interdependently to meet the needs of the organism as a whole.

> Multicellular organisms, like human beings, are made up of groups of specialized cells, functioning interdependently to meet the needs of the organism as a whole.

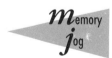

Human cells come in a variety of shapes and sizes, depending upon the kind of work they do. Muscle cells are long, so that they can shorten and create a force when they contract. Red blood cells are round and flat to provide an increased surface area over which O_2 and CO_2 can cross. Nerve cells are long and spiderlike because they cover extensive ground connecting all the body's tissues with the brain and spinal cord. In health, the functions of these and all the other cells in the human body are coordinated so that balance is maintained within the organism. However, if part of this system fails, the balance is disrupted. The impact that this has on the individual human being depends on what cells are involved and to what extent.

PRINCIPLE

IN ORDER TO FUNCTION APPROPRIATELY, CELLS MUST GROW AND DIVIDE IN AN ORDERLY, SYSTEMATIC MANNER

Illustration of the Principle

Human life begins as a single cell, the product of the union between a female egg and a male sperm. Each of these parent cells offer their offspring 23 chromosomes, one-half the full human complement of 46. The mechanism by which this occurs is known as meiosis. The human sex cells, the ova and the spermatozoa, are the only cells in the human body capable of this type of cell division. The result of their union is a new life, a single cell with a full complement of 46 chromosomes in a unique combination of the best and the worst characteristics each individual parent cell has to offer.

> Meiosis is a form of cell division in which the full human complement of 46 chromosomes is halved. The ova and the spermatozoa are the only human cells capable of this type of cell division.

This single cell, the zygote, spends its first few days of life dividing and increasing in number. It accomplishes this through a mechanism known as mitosis. This process allows the cell to make exact, genetic duplicates of itself. It is a continuous process that involves dissolution of the nuclear membrane and division of the 46 chromosomes into two identical sets, which migrate to opposite ends of the cell. The cell membrane constricts, dividing the cytoplasm in half. Finally, the nuclei reorganize around their respective chromosomes, and the division is complete.

> Mitosis is a mechanism of cell division whereby the cells of living organisms are able to make exact, genetic duplicates of themselves.

Once the zygote reaches the uterus, it has developed into a mass composed of several hundred cells. It then begins a process of differentiation. The physical properties and functions of the cells change as they begin to develop into the different structures in the body. Initially, this process involves a separation between the developing embryo and the placenta. Eventually, the cells will differentiate into the germ cell layers from which all body tissues and structures develop. If all goes well, that one single cell will develop into a complex system of specialized tissues and organs, the human body.

When problems occur at this point in development, they usually arise from one of two possible origins, either a genetic defect in the zygote or a failure of the zygote to differentiate appropriately.

When a zygote inherits a defect from either or both parent cells, the eventual outcome and the impact it has on the developing offspring depend on the nature of the defect. For example, cystic fibrosis is a chronic metabolic disease that results in defective exocrine gland function. Although its victims are usually of normal intelligence, they suffer from a variety of respiratory and digestive complications and frequently die in early adulthood. This disease can be traced to a single, defective gene, directly transmitted from parent to offspring. Down's syndrome, or trisomy 21, occurs when a zygote inherits an extra twenty-first chromosome from either of the parent cells. The syndrome includes a number of physical abnormalities, mental retardation, and occasionally heart and intestinal defects. However, with appropriate care, these individuals can live near-normal life spans. Not all genetic defects have as significant an impact on their victims as these two disorders have. However, it is important to understand that any genetic defect is an inherent part of the individual's entire cellular structure, and no technology currently available can correct these defects once they have occurred. Therefore, intervention is aimed at supporting the individual and his family and counseling them as to their chances of having more similarly affected offspring.

> Genetic defects originate somewhere in the female egg cell or in the male sperm cell or in both. The defect is inherent in the newly formed organism from the time it is a single-cell zygote.

Hydatidiform mole is an example of what occurs when a zygote fails to differentiate appropriately. Instead of developing into the specialized tissues and structures that become a fetus, trophoblastic cells proliferate wildly into a cluster of fluid-filled, grapelike structures. Although this mass is composed of gestational tissue, it will never develop into a human being. Treatment involves evacuation of the tissue and support of the family who has experienced the loss. Since hydatidiform mole has also been associated with subsequent malignancy, follow-up of these women is extremely important.

Most cells do not live forever, but their life spans vary. Certain blood cells may only live a few hours or days, whereas nerve cells may live as long as the human being does. In order for a living organism to survive, its cells must be able to grow and reproduce. This mechanism allows the body to replace dead cells with cells that are identical in structure and function, thereby preserving the integrity of the tissue and the balance within the entire organism. Cell reproduction also allows the body to grow and develop, as the infant grows to adulthood.

The rate of cell growth and reproduction varies among cell types and is genetically regulated. Skin and blood cells reproduce rapidly, because their average life span is short. If there happens to be a deficiency of these cells in the body, they will reproduce even more rapidly until an appropriate balance is regained. It is for this reason that a surgical wound heals in a relatively short period of time. Skin cells, damaged by the scalpel, are quickly replaced by newly generated tissue. Similarly, a healthy individual can tolerate donating a unit of blood without compromising his circulatory status, because replacement blood cells are rapidly produced by the bone marrow. Nerve cells, on the other hand, do not reproduce at all, which is why no amount of time or effort can fix a spinal cord once it has been transected.

Memory jog

> The rate of cell growth and reproduction is genetically regulated in the nucleus of the cell and varies among cell types.

With the exception of highly differentiated cells, like the nerve cells, a deficiency in the number of any kind of cell in the body triggers an increase in the rate of that particular cell's reproduction. The impact this has on the entire system depends on what cells are involved and how many. For example, if an individual cuts himself and loses 100 cc of blood, he has fewer red blood cells available to deliver O_2 to all the tissues in his body. However, since 100 cc is a relatively small percentage of his total blood volume, this blood loss should have little effect on his overall health. In an attempt to achieve a balance, his body will reproduce red blood cells until his normal red blood cell count is regained. However, if this individual happens to cut an artery and loses most of his total blood volume, the consequences are considerably more significant. If blood isn't circulating, O_2 is not being delivered to the tissues, which can lead to significant tissue damage and death. Since the body can't possibly reproduce enough red blood cells quickly enough to reverse the situation, this individual will need outside intervention in order to survive. The goal of treatment is to help him regain balance by augmenting his body's own efforts. This will involve controlling the bleeding, replacing the fluids, and providing supportive therapy.

Memory jog

> In an attempt to maintain balance within the organism, a deficiency in the number of almost any kind of cell in the human body will trigger an increase in the rate of that particular cell's reproduction.

PRINCIPLE

CELL GROWTH AND REPRODUCTION REQUIRE O_2 AND NUTRIENTS

Illustration of the Principle

It is an indisputable fact that human beings must eat and breathe in order to survive. Since the human body is actually a complex organization of specialized cells, it follows that each individual cell must also eat and breathe in order to survive. Nutrients are acquired through digestion of foodstuffs in the gut and transported to the various tissues by means of the circulatory system. Oxygen is acquired through respiratory activity in the lungs and is also transported to the various tissues by means of the circulatory system. Once these products are available at the cellular level, the cells assimilate them through either active or passive processes.

> Just as human beings must eat and breathe in order to survive and thrive, each individual cell in the human body must be able to acquire nutrients and O_2 to perform its specific function.

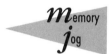

Passive processes occur as a result of concentration gradients and pressure differences. They are referred to as passive, because no energy is required for these processes to take place. The cell utilizes several passive mechanisms to acquire necessary nutrients.

Osmosis is the passage of water across a membrane, from an area of higher water concentration to one of lower water concentration. Water concentration is determined by how much material, or solute, is present on either side of the membrane. The greater the concentration of solute, the lower the concentration of water. In an attempt to establish a balance of water and solute on both sides of the membrane, water is drawn through the membrane to the side with the higher concentration of solute. If there is a greater concentration of solute inside the cell, water will enter, causing the cell to swell. If there is a greater concentration of solute outside the cell, water will leave, causing the cell to shrink. The ability of the human body to deal with either of these extremes depends on how many cells are affected, for how long, and to what extent. For example, many commercially prepared infant formulas come in a condensed form that requires dilution before they can be fed to an infant. An error in the appropriate dilution of this formula could result in a preparation that is either too concentrated or not concentrated enough. A single feeding of this preparation probably won't affect a healthy newborn significantly. However, if this error persists over a period of time, it may have very serious consequences. Highly concentrated formula in an infant's gut will draw water out of his bloodstream and tissues, resulting in diarrhea and dehydration. A formula that is too dilute will provide the infant with inadequate nutrients per volume of fluid, resulting in cellular malnutrition. If these conditions are not corrected, they may result in serious fluid and electrolyte imbalances and even death. The implications for nursing's role in parent education are obvious.

Diffusion refers to the mechanism by which substances move from an area of higher concentration to one of lower concentration in an attempt to distribute the substances evenly. A membrane is not required for this process to occur. For example, in the lungs, the air drawn into the alveoli during inspiration has a relatively high concentration of O_2. The blood vessels surrounding the alveoli have a low concentration of O_2. Therefore, O_2 will diffuse into the bloodstream from the alveoli and will be carried away for delivery to the various body tissues. Conversely, blood returning to the lungs from the rest of the body is loaded with CO_2, the waste product of respiration. Since the concentration of CO_2 is higher in the blood than it is in the alveoli, it will diffuse into the alveoli and be expelled through expiration.

Filtration occurs when substances are forced across a membrane because the pressure on one side of the membrane is higher than the pressure on the other side of the membrane. This process only works when the substance attempting to cross the membrane is small enough to pass through. The passage of waste products from the bloodstream into the kidneys, under the influence of the body's blood pressure, is an example of how this mechanism operates in the human body.

> The cell acquires some of the materials necessary for its survival through passive processes that depend on concentration and pressure gradients instead of energy. They include
>
> ▷ Osmosis
>
> ▷ Diffusion
>
> ▷ Filtration

When the materials necessary for the growth and reproduction of a cell are unable to enter passively, the cell facilitates their entry by utilizing active processes. They are referred to as active, because they require an energy expenditure on the part of the cell.

Active transport is the principle mechanism by which the cell acquires essential components, like amino acids, electrolytes, glucose, and vitamins. Because of their size, composition, and electrical charge, these substances would otherwise not be able to pass through the cell membrane. This process requires a coordinated effort by certain cellular components, including a carrier molecule, specific enzymes that assist the substance in attaching to and detaching from the carrier molecule, and an energy source. With this mechanism intact, substances entering the cell can overcome the passive barriers of both concentration and pressure gradients.

Pinocytosis is an active process by which the cell acquires very large molecular substances, like proteins. These large particles attach to indentations in the outer surface of the cell. The cell membrane folds around the molecule, allowing it to sink in toward the inner aspect of the cell. As the cell membrane closes around it, the particle finds itself floating in an intracellular compartment, and may then be dealt with by the appropriate structures within the cell.

The cell also uses an active mechanism to dispose of the waste products of cellular metabolism. This process is known as phagocytosis. Organelles, known as phagocytes, digest the cellular debris, which is then transported out of the cell by various active and passive mechanisms. Phagocytosis is also one of the mechanisms by which the cell attempts to rid itself of bacteria and other foreign substances.

Certain materials necessary for the cell's growth and development, which cannot enter the cell passively, are acquired through active processes that require an energy expenditure. These include

▷ Active transport

▷ Pinocytosis

▷ Phagocytosis

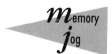

When an individual is healthy, his intracellular and extracellular environments are balanced. This means that sufficient amounts of O_2 and appropriate nutrients are available to the cell, and the cell is capable of utilizing them. When one or more components of this system fail, the balance is disrupted, which may result in cellular damage or death. As always, the impact that this has on the health of the individual depends on what cells are affected and to what extent.

In considering the concepts of cellular oxygenation and nutrition in humans, it is tempting to view them in black and white. If an individual is adequately nourished and oxygenated, he survives and thrives. If he is not, he dies. However, in reality, there is an enormous gray zone between these two extremes. Problems with cellular oxygenation and nutrition usually arise from one of the three following sources:

1. An inadequate supply of O_2 and nutrients available for use by the body

2. An ineffective mechanism for transporting O_2 and nutrients to the various tissues of the body

3. An inability of the individual cells to utilize O_2 and nutrients appropriately

If O_2 and nutrients are not available to a living organism, its cells cannot survive. For example, the individual who is in the process of drowning is anoxic. He has been cut off from his supply of O_2. His body will continue to function only as long as the O_2 remaining in his system lasts. Similarly, the individual who has no food to eat will eventually starve. Less dramatic examples include the individual with COPD, whose O_2 intake is limited by the condition of his lungs, and the infant with failure-to-thrive, whose nutritional intake is limited by various physiological and psychological factors. These individuals may have enough O_2 and nutrients to sustain vital functioning, but probably do not have enough of a reserve to maintain a normal activity level or to grow and develop. No matter what the cause, the goal of treatment is the same. Adequate oxygenation or nutrition must be restored, or when that is not possible, attempts must be made to help the individual make the best possible use of what he has.

The ineffective transport of O_2 and nutrients to the tissues of the body can also show as either an acute or a chronic condition. For example, the trauma victim who is hemorrhaging has a defect in his O_2 transport system. His lungs are capable of supplying adequate amounts of O_2, but he has no means of delivering it to the tissues. As the blood pours out of his body, it takes the O_2 with it. Similarly, the individual with a bowel obstruction may have access to an adequate supply of appropriate nutrients but is unable to deliver them to the intestines where they would ordinarily be processed for use by the body. Unless these conditions are remedied in a timely fashion, these individuals will die.

A child with cyanotic heart disease illustrates how a chronic deficiency in O_2 transport affects a living organism. Because of a defect in the circulatory system, the body is unable to deliver adequate O_2 to all its tissues. Subsequently, O_2 is shunted to the vital organs at the expense of the rest of the body. This results in a stunting of the child's physical and developmental growth.

Regardless of the cause, intervention is aimed at correcting the defect in O_2-nutrient transport, whether this involves suturing an arterial laceration or surgically correcting a congenital heart defect. When this is not possible, treatment focuses on supporting the individual and potentiating whatever function is intact.

Adequate cellular oxygenation and nutrition depends on three factors:

1. An adequate supply of O_2 and appropriate nutrients
2. An effective transport mechanism to deliver these materials to the bodily tissues
3. The ability of each individual cell to utilize these materials appropriately

Assuming that adequate amounts of O_2 and nutrients are available and that they've been appropriately transported to the various tissues in the body, cell growth and reproduction will continue only if the individual cells are capable of utilizing these materials appropriately. Consider the individual who has suffered tissue necrosis secondary to a temporarily inadequate blood supply, which has been corrected. In spite of the fact that adequate amounts of O_2 and nutrients are available and have been delivered directly to the tissues, the cells can't utilize them because they are already dead. Treatment is therefore aimed at removing the dead tissue and promoting the growth and development of surrounding tissue, with the hope that the healthy cells can make up for those cells that were destroyed. Although this mechanism works effectively for many tissues in the body, certain cells cannot be replaced once they are destroyed (*e.g.,* nerve cells). The impact this has on the individual will depend on what tissues are involved, over what period of time, and to what extent.

PRINCIPLE

WHEN CELLS GROW AND REPRODUCE TOO RAPIDLY, THEY ARE UNABLE TO PROVIDE FOR THEIR OWN NUTRITION

Illustration of the Principle

Cell growth and reproduction in the healthy human body are organized and controlled. Each individual cell, within the context of its own particular function, life span, and rate of reproduction, participates in the dynamic processes required to assure a balanced state of health. When cells grow and reproduce rapidly, they can't always nourish themselves adequately, because most of their energy and effort are involved in cell division. They must therefore rely on other cellular systems to provide this nourishment for them.

> When cells grow and reproduce rapidly, they are frequently unable to nourish themselves adequately and must rely on other cellular systems to provide this nourishment for them.

Memory Jog

Very rapid cell division in the human body can be of either a physiological or a pathophysiological origin. For example, the developing fetus is undergoing cell growth and reproduction at a rate that is unparalleled at any other point in human life. The fetus depends on the pregnant female to supply the O_2 and nutrients necessary to support this growth. This is accomplished by way of the placenta, which is the functional unit for cellular growth and metabolism in the developing fetus. Subsequently, all of the cellular systems in the pregnant female readjust to accommodate the growing fetus. However, when rapid cell division is the result of a pathologic condition, like cancer, adaptive mechanisms are not in place. Cancer is cell division out of control. These cells seize the available O_2 and nutrients at the expense of the body's healthy cells.

SUBPRINCIPLE

THE PLACENTA IS THE FUNCTIONAL UNIT FOR CELLULAR GROWTH AND METABOLISM IN THE DEVELOPING FETUS

Normal cell growth and reproduction in the developing fetus is explosive. In approximately 40 weeks, a single-cell organism evolves into a trillion-cell, highly differentiated, living, breathing human being. Adequate nutrition and oxygenation are of paramount importance if this phenomenon is to occur. However, these fetal cells are so busy growing into a baby that they don't have the time or the means to acquire these necessary materials independently. This is a job for the placenta.

Placental development begins in the third week of life, at the site of embryo implantation. It is divided into two parts, a maternal segment and a fetal segment. The maternal side of the placenta has a red, fleshy appearance. It is composed of a tissue layer known as the *decidua basalis* and its corresponding circulation. The fetal side of the placenta comprises a tissue layer known as the chorion and its corresponding circulation. An adherent, amniotic membrane covers the fetal side of the placenta giving it a shiny, gray appearance and making it easy to distinguish from the maternal side. Within the placenta, these two separate tissue layers interlock by means of a series of fetal chorionic villi that project into intervillous spaces formed by the maternal decidua, similar to the way the teeth of a zipper fit together. Fetal and maternal circulatory systems are separated by a chorionic membrane layer, which is only a few cells thick. Under normal situations, nutrients and gases can pass through this membrane without allowing the two separate blood supplies to mingle.

By the fourth week of life, the placenta has completely taken over the responsibility for metabolic exchange between the fetus and mother. The maternal circulatory system delivers O_2 and nutrients to the placenta by means of the spiral uterine arteries. This blood spurts into the intervillous spaces, under the influence of the maternal blood pressure. Through various active and passive mechanisms, O_2 and nutrients cross the chorionic membrane and enter the fetal circulation, where they are delivered to the fetus by means of a single umbilical vein. Carbon dioxide and other fetal waste products return to the placenta in reverse fashion by means of two umbilical arteries, where they are delivered to the maternal circulation for disposal.

*m*emory
*j*og

> The placenta is the functional unit for cellular growth and metabolism in the developing fetus.
>
> ▷ It supplies the fetus with O_2 and nutrients.
>
> ▷ It disposes of the waste products of cellular metabolism.
>
> ▷ It produces hormones essential to the continued growth and development of the fetus.

In addition to the mechanisms previously discussed, the placenta participates in a number of other metabolic activities, including endocrine and immunologic functions. The placenta produces hormones (*i.e.,* progesterone, estrogen, human chorionic gonadotropin [HCG], human placental lactogen [HPL]) that are essential for maintaining fetal well-being and promoting appropriate fetal growth and development. It is also thought that certain hormones produced in the placenta interfere with cellular immunity during pregnancy. This may be the reason why the maternal immune system does not seem to recognize the fetus as foreign and attempt to reject it.

When the maternal-placental-fetal unit is intact and functioning appropriately, it would seem reasonable to assume that the fetus has an excellent chance of growing and developing normally. Indeed, appropriate fetal growth and development is dependent on this maternal-fetal relationship. However, this fact alone can not guarantee a good fetal outcome. In fact, the very nature of this relationship may put the fetus at significant risk in situations where teratogenic substances are involved. The placenta's major function is to provide the fetus with O_2 and essential nutrients, but it is not particularly selective about what substances are allowed to pass to the fetus. Countless drugs, chemicals, viruses, and bacterias have been proven to cross the placental membranes to enter fetal circulation, often with tragic results. Prenatal counseling and appropriate education play a significant role in minimizing these hazards.

> Placental membranes are not particularly selective about the substances they allow to pass from the maternal circulation into the fetal circulation. Substances that do not adversely affect the mother may have teratogenic effects on the developing fetus.

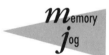

When the maternal-placental-fetal unit is not intact, both the developing fetus and his mother may be in jeopardy. The disrupting factors may be either acute or chronic. The effect it has on both mother and fetus depends on the extent of the problem, how long it persists, and at what point in fetal development it occurs. For example, placental abruption is the premature separation of the placenta from the uterine wall, which disrupts the supply of O_2 and nutrients to the fetus. If the separation is minimal, the rest of the placenta can usually accommodate fetal needs adequately. However, if the abruption involves the entire placenta, the mother hemorrhages into the uterus, and the fetus' lifeline is cut.

An example of a more chronic form of placental compromise is the uteroplacental insufficiency that frequently accompanies pregnancy-induced hypertension. In addition to the classic symptoms of hypertension, edema, and proteinuria, patients with pregnancy-induced hypertension experience generalized vasoconstriction and hypovolemia. This results in a decreased blood supply to the placenta, with a subsequent compromise in fetal oxygenation and nutrition. These infants are frequently growth retarded and may have a difficult time tolerating the stress of normal labor. Management of the patient with pregnancy-induced hypertension is aimed at improving uteroplacental blood flow by means of physical rest, stress reduction, and medication, while monitoring the condition and growth of the developing fetus. The final "cure" for pregnancy-induced hypertension is delivery of the infant. The route of delivery (*i.e.,* vaginal versus cesarean section) will depend on whether or not there is enough placental reserve to support the fetus adequately during the stress of labor.

Memory jog

> Disruption in the function of the placenta interferes with the delivery of O_2 and nutrients to the fetus. A deficiency in essential nutrients may result in intrauterine growth retardation.

SUBPRINCIPLE

CANCER IS CELL DIVISION OUT OF CONTROL

Cell division in the healthy human body is organized and controlled, so that the various cell types will grow and reproduce at an appropriate rate. Cancer is a disease that attacks the nucleus of the cell, causing genetic mutations that destroy these control mechanisms. The result is a rapid, uncontrolled reproduction of mutated cancer cells.

An occasional mutated cell is not unusual in an organism composed of trillions of cells. Under ordinary circumstances, it has no effect on the human body. The immune system views it as abnormal and eliminates it. How and why these isolated cells develop into cancer is not well understood. However, certain predisposing factors have been identified, including radiation exposure, chemical carcinogen exposure, chronic tissue inflammation, and various hereditary factors.

Once cancer cells have established a foothold in the human body, their nuclei are no longer able to control the growth process, and they reproduce rapidly and aggressively. They also tend to separate from each other and travel throughout the body by way of the circulatory and lymphatic systems. This tendency results in metastasis of the cancer to additional sites in the body.

Like any other cell in the human body, cancer cells require O_2 and nutrients to survive. They compete with the body's normal cells for these materials. Because their growth and reproduction are so rapid, they consume the available nutrients, at the expense of the rest of the body's tissues. Eventually, the body's healthy cells starve to death.

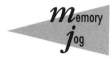

Malignant cells compete with healthy cells for available nutrients. Because malignant cells reproduce so rapidly, they consume these nutrients at the expense of the rest of the body's tissues.

The goal of treatment in cancer patients is to stop the growth and reproduction of these mutant cells and eliminate them from the body. Surgical excision, in combination with chemotherapy and radiation therapy, is commonly employed to achieve this goal. In general, chemotherapy and radiation therapy attempt to interfere with the metabolism and reproduction of the malignant cells. However, since these malignant cells mutated from healthy cells and are still quite similar in form and function, it is frequently impossible to kill the cancer cells without wiping out a significant number of healthy cells as well. Killing the patient in order to kill the cancer is not an acceptable treatment outcome. Subsequently, chemotherapy and radiation doses are tailored to kill as many cancer cells as possible, while holding healthy cell destruction to a minimum. Cancer patients require substantial physical and emotional support to help them deal with the stresses of both the disease and the treatment.

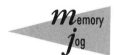

The effective treatment of cancer with chemotherapy and radiation therapy is inhibited by the fact that in order to kill malignant cells, healthy cells are also destroyed.

Reasoning Exercises: Cell Division

Patty Daniels is a 25-year-old, white female, pregnant with her first child. She is being seen in the obstetrical clinic for her first prenatal visit.

1. Patty tells the nurse, "I drank a glass of wine at a party before I found out that I was pregnant. I'm worried that I might have hurt the baby." Based on an understanding of alcohol use in pregnancy, which of the following responses is the most appropriate?
   A. "We don't really know how much alcohol is too much during pregnancy. Don't drink anymore and try not to worry about it."
   B. "As long as your drinking is moderate, I wouldn't worry about it. There were plenty of healthy babies born to drinking mothers before they ever discovered fetal alcohol syndrome."
   C. "An occasional drink shouldn't hurt the baby. Research has

shown that the risk to the fetus increases as the amount and frequency of alcohol consumption increases."

D. "I can understand why you're so upset, but an occasional drink shouldn't hurt the baby."

The correct response is **C.** This patient needs two things from the nurse: information about alcohol use in pregnancy and reassurance about the potential risk to her own baby. Alcohol is a known teratogenic substance, but it is unclear how much alcohol it takes, and at what point in development, to adversely affect the fetus. Research has shown that the incidence of fetal alcohol syndrome and related disorders increases as the amount and frequency of alcohol consumption increase. An occasional drink should not harm the fetus. **C** is the correct response because it is the only answer that offers reassurance and accurate information without catastrophizing the situation.

2. The nurse explains to Patty that good prenatal nutrition is essential for the healthy growth and development of her baby. Which of the following nutritional factors has the most significant impact on the eventual outcome of her pregnancy?

A. The severity of first trimester nausea or vomiting and its interference with adequate nutritional intake

B. The ready availability of the essential minerals (*e.g.,* calcium, iron) necessary for proper tissue and organ formation

C. The availability of appropriate nutrients at critical points in fetal development

D. The percentage of protein intake, as compared with that of other nutrient groups

The correct response is **C.** Growth and development in a fetus occur as a result of an increase in both the number of cells (*i.e.,* cell division) and in cell size. This requires an adequate supply of appropriate nutrients, available to the fetus when needed. When dietary deficiencies interfere with cell growth, it is possible to reverse the process by eliminating the deficiency. However, if dietary deficiencies interfere with cell division, they may result in permanent defects that will have a permanent effect on the fetus.

Situation Update

Patty is now 41 weeks gestation. A nonstress test performed in her physician's office was nonreactive. She has been admitted to the Labor and Delivery Unit to undergo a contraction stress test.

3. The contraction stress test (CST) is frequently used in the management of postdate pregnancies. The main reason that a CST is performed is which of the following?

   A. To determine whether or not the fetus is ready to be delivered

   B. To determine whether or not the placenta is adequately oxygenating the fetus

   C. To determine whether or not the fetus can tolerate normal labor, prior to elective induction

   D. To determine whether or not the uterus will be able to contract efficiently enough to establish an adequate labor pattern

The correct response is **B.** The CST identifies the fetus at risk for intrauterine asphyxia, by monitoring the fetal heart rate in response to uterine contractions. Labor is normally an asphyxiating condition. If the fetal-placental unit is healthy, there is enough O_2 reserve to support the fetus during the stress of the contraction. In postdate pregnancies, the placenta begins to degenerate so that there is less O_2 reserve available.

4. During the CST, the baseline fetal heart rate was 130 to 140 beats/min. Which of the following findings gives the best indication that Patty's fetus may not be able to tolerate labor?

   A. A series of late decelerations with a drop in fetal heart rate to 116 beats/min

   B. A single variable deceleration with a drop in fetal heart rate to 90 beats/min

   C. A series of early decelerations with a drop in fetal heart rate to 116 beats/min

   D. A single late deceleration with a drop in fetal heart rate to 90 beats/min

The correct response is **A.** Early decelerations result from fetal head compression and do not indicate fetal distress. Variable decelerations result from umbilical cord compression and may or may not indicate distress. A single, isolated variable deceleration is probably not ominous. Late decelerations result from uteroplacental insufficiency and indicate fetal distress. A persistent run of late decelerations is more ominous than a single, isolated one.

5. Based on the results of the contraction stress test, the decision is made to deliver Patty's baby by cesarean section. Which of the following observations at birth indicate that the infant may have experienced intrauterine stress-asphyxia at some point earlier in the pregnancy?

A. One-min Apgar = 5; 5-min Apgar = 8
B. Thick, bright green meconium present in the amniotic fluid
C. Vigorous stimulation required to initiate respiration
D. Yellowish-brown, stained amniotic fluid, infant's skin stained similarly

Meconium-stained amniotic fluid is a classic sign of fetal asphyxia or distress. Fresh meconium is bright green in color, but it turns a yellowish-brown color as it ages. The correct response is **D,** because yellowish-brown, stained amniotic fluid and infant skin indicate that the fetus passed meconium at some point earlier in the pregnancy.

MOBILITY

MARIAN B. SIDES

16

THE HUMAN BODY FUNCTIONS BEST WHEN IT CAN MOVE ABOUT FREELY IN ITS ENVIRONMENT

Illustration of Principle

Mobility is a quality of the human body that enables man to move about freely and interact with the world around him. This freedom to move about ranges from no movement (comatose) to excessive movement (hyperactivity). Optimal mobility assumes that the body will strike a comfortable balance between these two extremes.

The ability to move freely and purposefully in the environment enables one to satisfy basic human needs, move away from danger, and move toward pleasant events.

When the body is able to maintain balance through movement, nursing intervention is minimal. As immobility increases and autonomy decreases, the nurse plays a more active role in providing care.

PRINCIPLE

A DECREASE IN THE QUANTITY AND QUALITY OF MOBILITY REDUCES SELF-CONTROL AND THREATENS SELF-IMAGE

Illustration of Principle

The freedom to control motor activity is very important to one's self-image. The freedom of self-worth is directly related to independence and autonomy.

185

For example, the patient with upper extremity burns may not be able to perform the basic activities of daily living. Although this limitation is focused and temporary, the need to rely on others is threatening. The patient who has a debilitating rheumatoid arthritis and is bedridden feels an even greater threat to his independence and self-worth because this limitation is generalized and progressive.

In planning care for this type of patient, the nurse must be sensitive to the psychological impact of these limitations and promote independent functioning whenever possible.

PRINCIPLE

THE EXTENT AND DURATION OF IMMOBILIZATION DETERMINES THE KIND OF INTERVENTION REQUIRED

Illustration of Principle

Mobility takes on characteristic features related to extent and duration when illness occurs. These features help shape and give direction to nursing intervention. For example, the patient who has a hip spica cast or a Stryker frame requires greater assistance for a longer period of time than the patient who has a cast following a surgical reduction of a limb fracture. The nurse must be sensitive to the extent and duration of immobility that limits the individual's freedom to function independently.

The manner in which the immobilization is imposed upon the patient is also important in determining appropriate nursing response. For example, the patient who is recovering from a myocardial infarction may be ordered to bedrest to conserve energy. Patient compliance in this case requires self-discipline and an understanding of the relationship between bedrest and recovery. He must be willing to cooperate and follow this protocol. After all, the patient knows he *can* move about but *must* not.

The patient in traction for a fractured femur is immobilized by the mechanical treatment protocol (traction) as well as his functional disability (fracture). In this case the patient knows he can't move about *now* but will be able to later.

The patient with lower extremity amputations is limited primarily by his own functional disability rather than by some external medical protocol. This patient has permanent restrictions on his mobility. He is not mobile now and will not be later.

Each of the above limitations creates a different set of circumstances to which the patient must adjust. It is important to understand the threat imposed by each type of immobility. The nurse must carefully assess the patient's understanding of his limitations and the way in which he is coping, and she must provide the necessary intervention, including safe physical care, emotional support, and adequate health teaching.

In establishing your plan of care, ask yourself these questions:

1. How long *has* he been immobilized?
2. How long *will* he be immobilized?
3. To what extent is he immobilized?
4. How is he coping with this limitation?

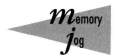

PRINCIPLE

A DECREASE IN MOBILITY INCREASES THE RISK FOR COMPLICATIONS IN MAJOR BODY PROCESSES

Illustration of Principle

Situational immobilization of a body part such as a cast to the arm or a brace to the knee imposes little threat to the normal body functions. However, patients who are subjected to prolonged and extensive immobilization are at risk for many complications and hazards of immobility. The impact of immobility on major body processes and the selected nursing management of deviations from normalcy are discussed in the sections to follow.

Musculoskeletal Processes

The bones and muscles of the body provide a structural framework that enables it to perform purposeful and independent activities. In turn, the constant motion of the body keeps the musculoskeletal processes in good working order and helps maintain structural integrity. When movement is curtailed, rapid and progressive deterioration in bony structure and muscle mass occurs. Prolonged immobilization is accompanied by an increase in the loss of calcium from the bones. The incidence of fractures may increase in bones unable to support body weight. Debilitating changes in joint structure result from immobilization of body parts. These changes are manifested in a loss of flexibility in the joint and gradual decrease in range of motion. The joint eventually becomes stiffer, and contractures result.

Immobilization causes a deterioration in musculoskeletal strength and a loss of joint mobility.

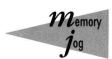

The initial step in managing the actual or potential health hazards caused by immobility is to make an accurate assessment of your patient's mobility status. The nurse must know the processes causing immobilization, limits imposed by medical treatment regimen, and the health status prior to immobilization. These assessment data are a necessary baseline for establishment of your patient-care goals.

The intervention behaviors of the nurse are directed at supporting the normal functions of the body and maintaining strength, endurance, and flexibility of the musculoskeletal system. All nursing actions are directed at providing a safe environment and preventing injury and complications.

Exercise

A planned exercise program should be executed to maintain and recover muscle strength and joint mobility. The amount and type of exercise used will depend upon the patient's physical limitations and medical restrictions. Range-of-motion exercises, transfer activities, and ambulation will help maintain joint mobility and reduce loss of calcium from the bone.

The nurse should encourage the patient to perform independently all activities that are permitted by his limitations in order to achieve an optional level of mobility. In other words, the nurse should not perform activities that the patient can do for himself.

Diet

The nurse should monitor the patient's dietary intake of calcium when mobility is curtailed. Calcium intake of 800 mg per day will produce adequate calcium levels and will reduce skeletal mineral loss. A healthy, balanced diet is necessary also to counter muscle weakness and fatigue. Hypercalcemia can occur from overingestion of calcium. Your patient will complain of anorexia, nausea, weakness, headaches, pain, or cramping.

Positioning

Good body alignment is essential to optimal musculoskeletal functioning and joint mobility. It is also essential to prevent complications. The nurse should be highly sensitive to the need to establish proper positioning, appropriate body supports, and change in position as frequently as necessary.

Comfort

Changes in musculoskeletal processes are often accompanied by joint pain, inflammation, edema, or surgical discomfort. The nurse should respond to alternatives in comfort by taking appropriate measures for pain control, particularly before exercise and activity. These measures may include administering pain medication, changing positions, or providing support to extremities and body parts or making heat or cold applications.

Your patient's progress must be monitored and evaluated in an ongoing manner to determine the effectiveness of your interventions. The initial assessment data are used to determine the extent to which your goals are achieved.

> How well does your patient perform range-of-motion exercises in comparison with his initial performance? What changes in muscular strength, endurance, and joint mobility indicate that you were successful in your nursing interventions?

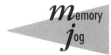

The success of your exercise program, for example, can be evaluated by observing skeletal strength and muscle tone by means of normal activities of daily living. Evidence can be evaluated by observing how long a patient can perform a particular task before becoming fatigued. The patient himself is frequently a good evaluator of progress.

Respiratory Processes

Normal ventilation is necessary to keep the lungs expanded and to prevent respiratory infection in the immobilized patient.

A decrease in physical activity reduces the stimuli for breathing and decreases movement of air in and out of lungs. When a person is supine, respiratory secretions collect in the lungs and create ideal media for bacterial growth. Atelectasis or collapse of alveoli can result from a decrease in ventilation.

> The patient who is immobilized is at risk for development of respiratory infection and collapse of the alveoli.

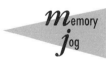

The first responsibility of the nurse in caring for the immobilized patient is to conduct a thorough assessment of the quality of his breathing. The goal of nursing care is to reduce pulmonary secretions and increase pulmonary ventilation. Interventions aimed at this goal will prevent infection and alveolar collapse. These interventions include deep breathing and coughing exercises, frequent change in position, and room humidification. Suctioning and hyperventilation may be necessary to assist the patient who is unable to perform these exercises.

What are the key indicators that adequate ventilation is being accomplished? What is the respiratory pattern? Blood–gas values? How do the lungs sound? How does your patient look?

Circulatory Processes

The heart must work harder when the body is in a flat, supine position to redistribute blood from the legs to other parts of the systemic circulation. As noted earlier, muscular strength decreases with immobilization, thus further reducing the effectiveness of the peripheral pumping action and increasing the stress on the heart. Likewise, the pumping action that occurs in the blood vessels in the extremities markedly slows when the body is moving. Venous thrombosis can begin to form almost immediately after immobilization in patients whose health is compromised. Individuals at risk include the elderly, persons with cardiovascular problems, the obese, and those who are severely ill.

Physical immobilization reduces the pumping action of the heart and slows the emptying of vessels. The longer the duration of immobilization, the greater the risk of venous thrombosis.

The nurse should monitor carefully the cardiovascular status of all patients who are immobilized. The primary goal is to maintain circulatory status and prevent complications. Mobilization of the extremities with range-of-motion exercise should be accomplished as indicated. Vital signs should be monitored, and the nurse should assess the patient for clinical signs of venous thrombosis. Common signs are edema in the extremities, pain, tenderness, and erythema. Intolerance of postural changes may be accompanied by a decrease in blood pressure, an increase in pulse rate, dizziness, and blurred vision. A sudden change from supine to upright position should be avoided. The nurse should assist patients in sitting up for the first time after surgery and after long periods of immobilization to avoid hypostatic problems.

Pulmonary emboli can occur in patients who are immobilized with cardiovascular problems or other conditions that compromise the pumping action of the heart. Dyspnea is the most common obvious symptom. The nurse must constantly evaluate the patient's tolerance of immobility and his response to efforts to increase mobility.

Ask yourself these questions: Are vital signs within your patient's normal limits? Can he change position from supine to upright without difficulty? Are the feet swollen? Is there pain or tenderness in the calves? Are there any other signs of poor blood flow? How does your patient feel?

Immobilization contributes to problems in elimination. Alterations in gastrointestinal and urinary functions are discussed in Chapter 11. Problems related to neurological processes are also precipitated by immobility. These issues are addressed in Chapter 16.

Patients who are immobilized are at great risk for skin breakdown. Ischemic changes in the skin and muscles result from prolonged pressure on body parts and bony prominences. A turning schedule or pattern of movement should be established. Meticulous skin care and a well-balanced diet are essential preventive measures.

The ultimate goal of nursing intervention is to assist the patient to return to an optimal level of wellness and to minimize the untoward effects imposed by the restriction on movement (see Fig. 16-1). Pathological changes in each body system should be anticipated. Efforts should be directed at maintaining functional capacity and preventing deterioration of body processes.

For each of the physiological processes identified under hazards of immobility, ask yourself these questions: What can I do for this individual that will make the most difference in his health status? What can I do to prevent pneumonia, to prevent constipation, to prevent decubiti formation, to prevent thrombi formation and muscular weakness? If these problems have already developed, then what can I do to correct them and help the patient to regain normalcy or to accept the limitations?

Memory jog

Most interventions that support the normal functioning of body processes can be performed independently by the nurse. If these opportunities are recognized and acted upon in a timely manner, the nurse can expedite the patient's return to wellness. Astute decision-making and nursing judgment must be carefully exercised in selecting intervention measures so that actions are appropriate and relevant to each situation. For example, skin massage may be appropriate to prevent skin breakdown and promote circulation, but leg massage may be contraindicated for patients who are on prolonged bedrest. Nursing intervention must, therefore, clearly and sensibly relate to the underlying patient care problems.

M aintain functional capacity

O ptimize return to normalcy

B uild ego strength

I ndividualize care

L isten to your patient

I ntervene only when necessary

T each good therapeutic care

"Y es," I can do it, attitude!

Memory jog

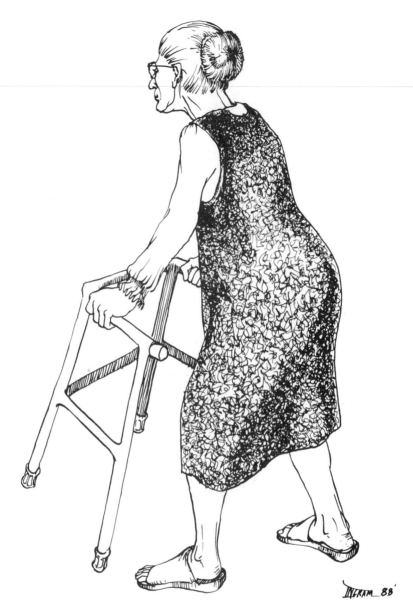

FIGURE 16-1. MAXIMIZING POTENTIAL FOR MOVEMENT.

Reasoning Exercises: Mobility

Mrs. Sonja Felice, 82 years old, suffered a fractured ankle and bruised ribs falling down a staircase in her daughter's home. Two days after the accident, Mrs. Felice is progressing well in the hospital.

1. Which of the following assessment data related to circulation is most significant for Mrs. Felice at this time?

    A. Ankle edema and muscular weakness

    B. Rapid pulse, decreased blood pressure

    C. Sudden dizziness when sitting up

    D. Dyspnea and anxiety

The intended reponse is *B*. Although each of the responses may appropriately pertain to the patient's status post-fracture, the question calls for data related to *circulation,* the key word in this question. A rapid pulse and decreased blood pressure could signal internal bleeding following the trauma from the patient's fall and is thus the most significant data relating to circulation.

2. When planning for Mrs. Felice, your goal is to maintain normal circulation. This can best be accomplished by

    A. Dangling feet twice a day

    B. Active range-of-motion exercise

    C. Deep breathing and periodic hyperventilation

    D. Application of elastic stockings to legs

The intended response is *D*. Again, the focus of the question is on *circulation,* the key word in the stem. Dangling the patient's feet (*A*) will cause venous blood to pool in the lower extremities, thus actually impeding normal circulation. Range-of-motion exercises are aimed at improving and maintaining *joint* movement and would have little effect on blood flow (*B*). Response *C* is incorrect, since deep-breathing exercises are used to improve *pulmonary* function, not circulatory function.

3. Radiographic studies indicate that Mrs. Felice has greater than 50% demineralization of bone. You recognize that this suggests which of the following bone abnormalities:

    A. Osteoporosis

    B. Osteomyelitis

    C. Osteochondritis

    D. Osteomalacia

The intended response is *A*. Demineralization of bone occurs in osteoporosis, often as a result of advanced age and immobility. The presence of osteoporotic changes likely contributed greatly to the patient's development of fracture, since demineralized (decalcified) bone is very porous and fragile.

4. Mrs. Felice does not want to turn and deep breathe because it is uncomfortable and sometimes painful. Which of the following responses would be most effective?

   A. Mrs. Felice, if you don't breathe deeply and turn, you will develop pneumonia.

   B. You'll become very weak, Mrs. Felice, and it will be very difficult for you to walk.

   C. I know it must be uncomfortable, Mrs. Felice. Let me hold your chest while you take a deep breath and cough.

   D. I know it hurts, Mrs. Felice, but breathing and turning are the best thing for you.

The intended response is *C,* because this response recognizes and validates the patient's discomfort while also addressing nursing action to *reduce* the discomfort with deep breathing. Response *A* utilizes a rational approach, connecting the failure to deep breathe with pneumonia—an approach that is most often totally unsuccessful in correcting negative behaviors. Responses *B* and *D* likewise utilize rational approaches and do not offer a strategy to diminish the pain that comes with deep breathing.

COMMUNICATION

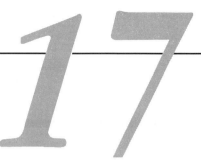

NANCY B. CAILLES

17

PRINCIPLE

MAN IS A SOCIAL BEING WHO IS IN CONSTANT COMMUNICATION WITH OTHERS IN HIS ENVIRONMENT

Illustration of Principle

Man, in general, is a creature who both seeks and receives pleasure from socialization with others—through speech, action, expression—even through tools of communication such as painting, poetry, or song. Man is constantly engaged in a process of communication, even when he is not consciously aware of it. For example, an individual who removes himself from the crowd at a large party and remains in a quiet corner of the room sipping a drink is not actively speaking with others at the party, but he *is* communicating! His separation from the group communicates his message of "I wish to be alone for awhile" or "I don't feel comfortable in this large group." Man, then, communicates in a variety of ways, both verbal and nonverbal. A smile shared with a familiar face, a handshake with an old friend, or an embrace with a beloved family member communicates a message as effectively and clearly as the spoken word.

Illness presents an *increased* need for man to communicate, because illness causes new situations with new needs, problems, and concerns. At the same time, however, illness may alter the individual's ability to communicate effectively, thus calling upon health-care givers to implement measures that facilitate the patient's expression and communication. For example, a patient who has undergone surgery for tracheostomy has a definite *increased* need to communicate with his health-care provider; at the same time, he has a *decreased* ability to communicate by virtue of his surgical experience.

Nurses, then, must become critically aware of their essential roles as com-

195

municators—of receivers and transmitters of thoughts, feelings, desires, and fears. The establishment of effective helping relationships depends heavily on the nurse's ability and willingness to be an open listener and communicator, ready to hear the patient's communicated messages and accept the value of that message to the patient.

PRINCIPLE

VERBAL COMMUNICATION INVOLVES THE RELAYING OF IDEAS, THOUGHTS, EMOTIONS, AND DRIVES THROUGH CONTENT, SPEED, VOLUME, PITCH, AND PATTERN OF SPEECH

Illustration of Principle

The process of communication between human beings involves more than just the transmission and receipt of a spoken message; the elements of *how* the message is sent, and thus, received, influence communication as much as *what* is being said. Because nursing is a service involving constant interactions with individuals, both requiring and providing health care, understanding the elements of the communication process is critical to the provision of holistic and comprehensive nursing care.

The elements of verbal communication are as follows:

Speech Content

Content comprises what is being said or discussed, the topic of the conversation, the message idea. The nurse, in order to fully appreciate speech content, must practice being an attentive *listener,* so that the message that is intended can be fully appreciated or accepted. The nurse should take note that the spoken message is congruent with other elements of verbal communication, such as pitch or volume. For example, if the patient verbally denies any pain or discomfort and states, "I'm fine, really," but at the same time is clenching his teeth and has an unusual pitch in his speech, the nurse may need to reevaluate the patient's denial of pain.

In conversations with patients and staff as well, the nurse should use astute listening skills to keep focused on the speech content, rather than attempt to formulate responses. No pat answer to a spoken message exists; if unsure about what to respond to a message, the nurse does best to simply repeat what has been said to encourage the patient or other individual to express himself more fully.

Consider this example:

Patient: "I've been in the hospital for over 2 weeks now. I don't think I'll ever get better."

The nurse caring for this client may be unsure of the true meaning of the patient's statement and may feel ill at ease with providing a sense of reassurance that may not be warranted. The best response would be one that *encourages the patient to express himself more fully,* so that the nurse can gather more information and thus understand the patient's statements.

An example of an effective response might then be, "You seem concerned about getting better."

Speech Pitch or Tone

Speech pitch is the intonation or pitch in voice with which a verbal message is communicated. Clearly, all of us can appreciate that a certain tone or pitch in voice can definitely change the meaning of a spoken message. A complimentary message such as "Your new hairstyle is so different!" can be quickly changed to a negative, disapproving message with a tone of sarcasm added to the verbal message. Tone or pitch then reflects an attitude, opinion, or emotion about the speech content that cannot be ignored if one is to fully comprehend and appreciate the communicated message. Nurses should not only concentrate on picking up the tone of the messages received from patients but must also focus on avoiding sending messages with tones of disapproval, doubt, shock, or disgust back to patients and others.

Consider this example:

Nurse #1:   "Do you really think the biopsy will show a malignancy?"

Nurse #2:   "Do you *really* think the biopsy will show a malignancy?"

With the addition of the underlined word "really" in the second message, a new tone is established in the nurse's statement to the patient, one that may indicate doubt or disapproval to the receiver of that message.

Speed and Volume of Speech

Speed and volume are listed in unison, since they tend to work together in speech. When an individual is feeling very saddened, is experiencing grief or loss, has undergone a difficult period of adjustment or of failure, or is embarrassed about what is being said, the volume and speed with which that individual speaks tend to decrease. Few students, for example, would announce loudly to their colleagues, "Look! I've failed an important exam!" That difficult message would much more likely be communicated in a slow, hesitating manner and in a soft or low volume. Likewise, when an individual is feeling intense emotion such as anger or fright, or when he is experiencing joy, elation, or significant accomplishment, he is most likely to communicate with increased volume and speed. Consider a group of fans at a football game cheering on their team with especially loud volume or a married couple engaged in a heated argument that has escalated from quiet, slower speech to a feverish pitch of loud interchanges between the two.

Thus, the nurse must be attuned to changes in volume and speech as well as pitch to pick up unspoken messages that patients or colleagues may be expressing. Likewise, the nurse would do well to alter her own volume and speech to better coincide with the person with whom she is communicating. In the example of a patient speaking in a soft voice to the nurse and saying, "I think that I may have made a mess in the bed," the nurse should note the softness of the volume and comprehend that the patient is not only expressing a need for assistance—but is also expressing a sense of possible embarrassment over losing control of his elimination.

Speech Pattern

Speech pattern involves the rhythm with which we speak and words that are interspaced in communicated messages that alter that rhythm. Common interspaced words that affect speech patterns include "uh," "er," "you know," and "like." Changes in speech pattern, like changes in pitch, volume, and speed, may indicate a feeling tone or emotion that the patient is expressing. For example, persons who are unused to public speaking and feel ill at ease in front of a group or audience tend to stammer a bit with their words and will use the words "uh" and "er" a great deal in their speech. This change in speech pattern highlights the speaker's sense of anxiety and discomfort in public speaking. Consider these examples. What feeling tone might be expressed?

A 15-year-old male patient explains his purpose for seeking medical attention to the admitting clinic nurse.

> *Patient:* "I think . . . uh . . . that I . . . you know . . . I . . . uh . . . have . . . like I might have V.D."

Here the speech pattern clearly indicates the patient's discomfort over his medical problem and may also indicate his anxiety over discussing it openly with the nurse.

An 18-year-old college freshman tells her classmate how she fared on her first class examination.

> *Student:* "Well, I mean, I did okay, I guess, I mean, I didn't flunk, or anything like that, you know, I mean, you know, it was an okay grade, you know, I guess I did all right."

An astute listener could pick up, in this situation, that the student is avoiding the discussion of her test score with her classmate by never really answering the classmate directly, but rather, by using multiple speech patterns, is expressing her own insecurity about her test performance.

When the nurse becomes aware of changes in speech pattern, the nurse should focus on listening attentively and allowing the patient added time to complete his thoughts and formulate those thoughts into messages. Avoid hurrying the patient or attempting to complete his sentences for him, since these actions will likely impair the communication process.

Patient: "I need my . . . uh . . . you know . . . that thing . . . that blue thing . . . uh . . ."

Nurse: "You need your bedpan? Your blanket? Your towel? What do you need? Your robe?"

In the above example, the nurse frustrates the communication between herself and the patient by attempting to finish the patient's sentence and hurry his thoughts. It would be more appropriate to encourage the patient to think for a few seconds or so and allow him to identify what it is he needs, rather than interrupt his speech and risk blocking his communication.

PRINCIPLE

MESSAGES MAY BE COMMUNICATED WITHOUT THE USE OF WORDS BY *NONVERBAL* COMMUNICATION. NONVERBAL COMMUNICATION INVOLVES THE POSTURES, MOVEMENTS, EXPRESSIONS, MANNERISMS, AND GESTURES OF THE HUMAN BODY THAT RELAY MESSAGES AND MEANINGS

Illustration of Principle

Nonverbal communication, sometimes referred to as "body language," is an unspoken expression of thoughts, feelings, and drives that is as much a useful tool in the communication process as verbal or spoken messages. Consider the behavior of an expectant father in a waiting room. The nurse might note pacing, hand wringing, or inability to sit in a chair for more than a few minutes. The individual may flip through various magazines without really reading or comprehending even a single paragraph. He may drink one cup of coffee after another or smoke excessively. All of these behaviors reflect his mental and emotional states, and are thus valuable tools of communication. Consider also the behavior of young children when they see a department store Santa Claus, the facial expression of a young bride and groom as they exchange marital vows at the altar, or the body posture of a row of students sitting through a long and tedious lecture on an uninteresting topic. It is obvious that nonverbal communication can be a useful tool of human expression.

The nurse must learn to be a keen observer of nonverbal cues that convey a message in order to completely comprehend and appreciate a patient's conveyed message. Focusing on *all* aspects of a patient's communication style will help the nurse to better understand the patient and anticipate his needs.

Golden Rules of Effective Communication

1. Always choose responses that allow or encourage the patient to express himself more fully.

Since man has the inherent need to express himself and illness often increases that basic need, responses by the nurse that facilitate greater expression for the patient are most often the most satisfactory in a helping relationship. Reflecting or restating what the patient has previously said helps the patient to focus and clarify the ideas or feelings he is endeavoring to express. The nurse may also encourage expression directly. Such responses might include these examples:

"Tell me more of what you have been feeling."

"Go on."

"Can you share more of that experience with me?"

It is evident that the above responses communicate to the patient the nurse's interest and concern as well as her openness to the patient and his ideas and feelings.

2. Listen for the "feeling tone" of the patient's communicated message.

Remember that feelings and emotions are often not directly stated, but rather, are expressed by the intonation, speed, or volume of the speech. The nurse ought to be attentive for such signals in the communication process that will assist her in better understanding the real message being conveyed to her by the patient. Consider the example. What feeling tone is being expressed?

"I just can't go on like this! Sometimes I think I can't do *anything* right!"

Here the patient is clearly expressing feelings of frustration, helplessness, and even hopelessness. The nurse could facilitate further expression of these feelings by responding in the following manner:

"You seem frustrated. Can you tell me a bit more about your situation?"

By focusing on the feeling tone of what has been said by the patient, the nurse helps draw the patient's feeling out in the open, to be better understood and thus more effectively managed.

3. Encourage hope in the patient, but avoid providing false reassurances.

It is well documented that all patients need and benefit from a sense of hope—no matter how critically, chronically, or terminally ill. However, the nurse must be careful not to provide the patient with a false sense of comfort or reassurance, since this may cause the patient to experience increased anxieties when the reality of the situation does not reflect the reassurance provided. Thus, the nurse must exercise caution when expressing personal beliefs about the patient's situation, prognosis, or outcome.

Examples of falsely reassuring responses include the following:

"I'm sure everything will turn out okay with your surgery."

"I know you've done everything you could."

"Your physician is very experienced with this disease. I'm confident you'll be well in no time."

No human being can ever safely predict the future or fully understand the present, and responses to patients such as those listed above attempt to achieve those unreachable goals. Such responses may, in fact, backfire in the future, when the falsely reassured patient does not in reality experience what the nurse blithely promises.

4. Avoid responses that catastrophize the patient's situation.

Patients facing illness, surgery, or medical interventions may view their situations with reservations based upon fear, anxiety, or lack of understanding. Nurses could easily escalate the patient's sense of discomfort by catastrophizing, that is, creating an even worse scenario than the patient himself has visualized.

Consider this example:

Patient: "I didn't know what to do! I couldn't get my breath, and I felt like I was choking!"

Nurse: "You must have been terrified! What a frightening experience you've had!"

Even though it is appropriate for the nurse to reflect to the patient that she appreciates the patient's sense of fear in the above situation, she makes the patient's situation sound much worse than how the patient perceives it, or how it was in reality. Telling the patient that he "must have been terrified" is an example of catastrophizing, and the nurse here, rather than supporting the patient, may cause the patient to have even greater concern, worry, or fear about the situation he encountered.

5. When unsure about what the patient is saying, either verbally or nonverbally, clarify!

Effective communication is dependent upon the perception and understanding or comprehension of the relayed message. If the nurse is unsure about what is being said, or if she questions her comprehension of the patient's true meaning in the message, it is appropriate and necessary to ask for clarification. This rule may also apply if the patient's speech is impaired and difficult to understand; if the patient uses colloquialisms or slang; or if the patient speaks in dialect. Asking for clarification of what has been conveyed expresses to the patient the nurse's interest in him and her need to fully appreciate the thoughts and feelings being expressed. Consider this example:

Patient: "Nurse, I need to pass water. Get me that bottle, would you?"

The patient is using a different term for urination than the nurse might be familiar with by stating "I need to pass water." Likewise, he refers to the urinal as a "bottle." The nurse, if unsure of the patient's meaning, should clarify his statements so that effective and helpful communication may take place.

6. Avoid negating feelings that are being expressed.

Patients, as stated previously, will have unique perceptions of their illnesses, treatment, care, and progress that may or may not be rooted in fact. The nurse should utilize responses to patients that will aid them in clarifying and expressing their feelings and avoid responses that negate or diminish the patient's feelings or concerns. Nurses are most prone to use statements that diminish patient's feelings when the patients are expressing negative emotions, since the caring nurse does not wish the patient to endure psychic unrest or pain. However, the patient needs to express any negative emotions just as much as positive ones, and negating or diminishing thus does not serve the patient in a helping way.

Consider this example:

Patient: "I hate being in the hospital! I don't like being so dependent on others."

Nurse: "It's not really that bad, is it?"

In this situation, the nurse intended to reduce some of the patient's negative perception of his hospitalization, but in her response, she instead diminished the patient's perception, and thus feelings, as being unwarranted and exaggerated. This response would likely frustrate the patient and may well block any further communication of his true feelings.

A more effective response by the nurse in the situation would be

Nurse: "It sounds as though you're having a difficult time being hospitalized."

With this response, the nurse calls for further clarification of the issues and concerns of this patient and likewise expresses her interest in the patient's state of well being.

7. Avoid confronting the patient until the situation is fully known and understood.

When a patient's behavior is inappropriate and requires limitations or restriction, such as an acting-out patient in the psychiatric setting, confrontation of the patient may be necessary. The nurse confronting the patient should identify calmly and concisely the inappropriate behavior that the patient has engaged in; how that behavior has influenced himself, others, or the environment; and finally, what steps should be taken to alter the situation and decrease or halt the behavior labeled inappropriate. The nurse must be cautious with the use of confrontation, however, and should be sure to examine all the facts of the situation before making a decision to confront. The use of direct confrontation with patients may escalate their feelings of self-doubt or insecurity, because this exchange between patient and nurse is, by nature, often anxiety-provoking.

8. Extend "communication courtesy" to patients.

Simple measures of communication courtesy can go a long way to enhance the communication process between individuals. If the patient senses that the nurse is truly interested and attentive, he is obviously much more likely to feel comfortable in expressing himself. Therefore, to create an atmosphere more conducive to communication, the nurse should observe some basic rules of communication courtesy:

Don't interrupt the patient when he is speaking.

Don't rush the patient to complete his message or attempt to complete his sentences for him.

Maintain good eye contact with the patient.

Maintain a comfortable distance from the patient.

Use touch with the patient as appropriate.

These measures will serve the nurse to facilitate communication with her patients, and thus, foster the helping relationship.

Reasoning Exercises: Communication

Amy Stevens is a 17-year-old student admitted for evaluation of lower abdominal pain. She tells the nurse, "I wish my friends would come to visit me. I don't like being here alone."

1. Which of the following would be the most appropriate response of the nurse?
    A. "You sound very lonely. Shall I stay with you for awhile?"
    B. "I'm sure your friends will come to see you soon."
    C. "It's a little too early for visiting hours. You'll have to wait until this afternoon."
    D. "It's hard to be alone. Would you like me to stay with you?"

The intended response is **D,** since this response acknowledges the patient's feelings and offers support. Response **A** tends to catastrophize the patient's situation by saying "you must be very lonely." Response **B** provides false reassurance, because the nurse has no real way of knowing if in fact friends will come to visit Amy. Finally, **C** is incorrect because it provides only a factual response and does not attend to the feeling tone of Amy's remarks.

Samuel Davidson is a 68-year-old being treated for metastatic prostate carcinoma. He says, "You may as well give up on me, Nurse. I'll never get better."

2. The nurse would appropriately respond:
   A. "But you really are improving. Try to keep a positive attitude."
   B. "I won't give up on you, Mr. Davidson. I know you'll get better."
   C. "I'm not sure what you are saying. You feel you're not improving?"
   D. "Recovering from cancer takes a while. Be patient."

The intended response is **C,** since the nurse is clarifying the patient's intended message and at once is offering to listen to him further, thus facilitating his expression of his concerns and feelings. Response **A** denies the patient's feeling tone of despair and frustration, offering what may be false reassurance. Response **B** mimics response **A** in its offering of reassurance that the patient will "get better." Finally, response **D** focuses on facts and realities, without addressing the feeling tone of what the patient is expressing verbally.

Joyce Lisle is a patient on a medical-surgical unit who has undergone biopsy for abnormal uterine bleeding. Joyce questions the nurse about the procedure and then says, "Do you think I have cancer?"

3. The nurse should respond to Joyce's question with which of the following statements?
   A. "It's impossible to know for sure until your biopsy report is complete."
   B. "Often biopsies are negative."
   C. "I can understand how you must feel. I'd be frightened, too."
   D. "I really can't say. Are you concerned about what the biopsy will show?"

The intended response is **D,** since it is honest and at the same time, encourages further expression by the patient. Response **A** is a factual statement, yet it does not respond to the patient's unspoken sense of concern over the biopsy results. **B** may be a correct statement, but it does not address the patient's unique situation, and may be false reassurance. Response **C** both assumes that the nurse *does* have an understanding of this patient's unique perceptions and experiences as well as catastrophizes by focusing on the issue of fear by stating "I'd be frightened too." This response sends the message to the patient that she *should* be frightened about the results of the biopsy, which is clearly an undesired effect in this situation.

INTERPERSONAL RELATIONSHIPS

ANN SHEERER FILIPSKI

PRINCIPLE

MAN IS A SOCIAL BEING EVER IN INTERACTION WITH OTHERS IN THE ENVIRONMENT

Illustration of Principle

From the moment of birth until one's death, man is in contact with the environment and those within it. As an initially dependent being, the physical and emotional needs of each infant must be met by others. These contacts provide the means for the developing infant's continued survival and growth. Additionally, although early interactions may seem unidirectional (the caretaker gives, the infant receives), they rapidly become *progressively more reciprocal* in nature. For example, the caretaker gives warmth and reassurance; the infant experiences pleasure and smiles. The caretaker feels capable and gratified; the infant comes to know "I am pleasing." Thus, a pattern is established, and the developing self of the child comes to have certain expectations of, needs for, and capacities to affect other humans.

> Human interaction is reciprocal in nature.

Memory jog

Over time and with repeated interactions, humans develop relationships. The nature of a relationship is influenced by both the present and past events and experiences of each individual involved. Thus, no two relationships are ever exactly alike.

205

Relationships are also of varying degrees of depth. Our contacts with another may be brief or limited in scope. Even though they may be repeated, little personal exposure results, and such a relationship would likely be considered superficial or social in nature. In contrast, with increasing levels of personal exposure or shared experience, a friendship may result. In this case, it is also likely that the relationship meets a larger number of needs for each individual or is more mutually gratifying. Intimate or deep relationships are those in which extensive exposure of aspects of the "self" of each person occurs. Further, the quality or quantity of shared experience also continues to increase.

> Relationships vary in degrees of depth. There is often an inverse relationship between depth of interaction and the number of relationships of that type a given individual has.

The obvious means of sharing past and present experiences or revealing aspects of the self is through *communication.* This tool is essential in establishing and maintaining a relationship.

PRINCIPLE

BEHAVIOR OCCURS IN THE INTERPERSONAL CONTEXT

Illustration of Principle

Behavior, or how one "acts," communicates much about an individual to the larger world. It reveals much about one's psychological or *inner world,* how one perceives, thinks, feels, or actualizes intentions. In addition to these internal influences upon the individual, behavior is also shaped by *external* factors. These external influences are all related to aspects of the social or interpersonal area. How one interprets cues in a given setting or environment or experiences others' expectations of them, or what one's culture dictates, all influences behavior and the responses of others to a given behavior.

> There is a constant dynamic interplay between one's social or relationship experiences and one's inner emotional state.

Principle

Illustration of Principle

Our individual needs and wants influence our relationships with others. Because of our early infantile experiences in which others met our physical and emotional needs, this pattern can feel comfortable, and at times we may wish to have it continue. However, with further growth and development and the capacity to gratify many of our own needs, autonomy is also experienced as pleasurable. Thus, from early childhood into old age, a constant individual balance between independence and dependence in relationships is sought. What makes relationship issues so complex is the fact that at any given time, two individuals struggle with this balance internally and interpersonally. If both individuals are particularly needy or dependent at a given time, can their needs be met within the context of their relationship? Or if both are highly independent and struggling to maintain their autonomy, what happens to the aspects of self-exposure and quantity of shared experience?

Obviously, some of this potential difficulty is alleviated with the large number of relationships that most individuals have concurrently. This allows for many potential sources of need gratification.

A further factor affecting relations with others is the nature of one's *interactional skills,* particularly observation and communication. One needs a means of collecting and sharing information or negotiating issues of responsibility if a relationship is to develop and progress. How else are decisions to be made about the respective needs of individuals and if or how they can be met?

Lastly, the *social context* can also influence an interpersonal relationship. Do married couples behave the same way publicly in the United States and India? Do two persons relate in the same way if when introduced, they are labeled as coworkers rather than one as supervisor and the other as subordinate?

> The ability to utilize external cues and interpersonal feedback can profoundly influence the nature and course of a relationship.

Predictable chronologic phases occur as any relationship develops. Generally early, initial contacts between two people allow for some sharing of information and personal exposure. If a level of trust can be established here, then the sharing process is likely to continue in a mutually agreed upon manner. It is at this working level or phase that the potential for increased growth and mutual gratification can best be achieved. Lastly, termination occurs in all relationships; sometimes because of imposed external circumstances and in others based upon the decision of those involved. Ideally, the successful completion of this process fosters the growth and further development of each participant.

> Human relationships progress through initial, working, and termination phases.

The *therapeutic nurse-patient relationship* constitutes a specialized form of interpersonal relationship. How does this relationship differ from others? First, its formation often occurs under somewhat unusual circumstances. In the initial phase, the focus of information sharing is often upon the patient's experience, past and present. Relatively little information about the nurse of a personal nature is shared with the patient. Further, the focus of the relationship is often to meet specific needs of the patient that he is presently unable to meet himself. The patient is *not* expected to meet the nurse's needs.

There is also the expectation that the relationship itself is to be enabling. In other words, in addition to meeting identified health needs of the patient, the experience of a therapeutic relationship and interactions is to be validating and growth-producing. And by definition, the nurse–patient relationship is goal-oriented and limited in scope and duration. The nurse is expected to be cognizant of these issues and evaluate the status of the relationship in an ongoing fashion.

> The therapeutic relationship between nurse and patient can be utilized as a tool in fostering growth and facilitating change.

PRINCIPLE

PREREQUISITES TO SATISFYING INTERPERSONAL RELATIONSHIPS ARE BASIC TRUST AND A SENSE OF SELF AS SEPARATE FROM, BUT RELATED TO, OTHERS

Illustration of Principle

In order to form mature and mutually rewarding relationships with others, an individual must trust that the interpersonal world is basically a safe and good place. He or she must have had past relationships that were more good than bad or more gratifying than disappointing. Otherwise, uncertainty and anxiety will color any contacts with others and leave little energy available to the self for adequate functioning or adaptation to changing circumstances, let alone the risk taking that relationships require.

It is only through the prolonged process of psychological growth and development that one begins to formulate an understanding of one's self. This includes a sense of what is unique to the individual (likes, dislikes, interests, capabilities, strengths, and weaknesses) and what is shared in common with others. One also needs to know what can be given to others as well as obtained from them. If achieved, the quality of relationships increases.

Past delay or arrest in emotional development and subsequent alteration or impairment in the self will become visible in patient behavior. This includes the nature of one's interpersonal relationships. Conversely, one's experiences in the interpersonal sphere and relationships can continue to influence internal psychic development throughout the life span.

Thus, the nurse has obvious tools available in meeting the emotional health needs of patients. First, assessment of the nature of a given individual's relationships and the observation of how the patient relates to the nurse provide some possible clues about past experiences and unmet needs. Observation of behavior also gives clues about the nature of the patient's perceptions, thoughts, feelings, and actions. Difficulties in any of these areas are then amenable to nursing intervention.

Evaluation of the patient's responses to nursing interventions may demonstrate that change has occurred. And through more therapeutic and gratifying interactions and relationships with the nurse and others, it is hoped that further individual growth can take place.

> How one behaves influences how others respond to us and our relationships. Our relationships influence how we behave.

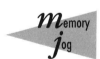

Recall that the nurse-patient relationship is often based upon and developed around our ability to meet the patient's needs he cannot meet alone. Like other relationships, to be satisfying, the nurse-patient relationship must also be based upon trust. Trust is the cornerstone in the nurse-patient relationship. Without it, little can be accomplished. Interestingly, *how* we meet the needs of patients can do much to build or destroy that trust.

Further, the self of both patient and nurse enter into the therapeutic relationship. In many instances, the self of the patient is either deficient (particularly in psychiatric settings) or temporarily threatened and vulnerable (*e.g.,* the mastectomy patient who experiences a change in body image). The self of the nurse is often used as a tool in aiding patients. Thus, the nurse must be knowledgeable about the patient *and* herself. She will therefore be assessing both selves in an ongoing fashion by a review of behavior and introspection.

> The nurse must demonstrate self-awareness and an ability to examine her own behavior.

PRINCIPLE

THE QUALITY AND QUANTITY OF ONE'S INTERPERSONAL NETWORK MAY AUGMENT OR DIMINISH THE ABILITY TO COPE WITH STRESS

Illustration of Principle

As a social being, clearly man is more than a biologic organism. Other humans provide us with a vast number of possibilities for gratification of needs. Even if not dependent upon others for help in meeting survival and safety needs, man's need to belong or become self-actualized, as articulated by Maslow, is highly dependent upon experiences with others.

Research tells us that relationships—their absence or presence—influences our chances of survival, not just in the sense of physical safety but in coping with stress and adversity. Those who experience the loss of a significant relationship are subsequently at greater risk of illness, injury, and death for some period of time. Statistics tell us those who are married live longer. Thus, the availability of others and our contacts with them serve to aid us in making the adaptations required in life.

How are others beneficial to us? They provide comfort and nurturance. They validate us as individuals and our experiences. They allow us to give. We can bond together to achieve a common purpose or share a sorrow.

Without others and relationships, we often behave differently. Do you always dress the same way? Does the priority placed on comfort when selecting clothing vary if you plan to stay home alone or are expecting company? Probably. Similarly, our inner experience may well change also if our contacts or relationships with others are disrupted. The phenomenon of winter "cabin fever" illustrates what even a brief change in contacts with others can do to our emotional state.

> The quality of an individual's relationships has impact on emotional health. Conversely, the state of one's emotional health influences the nature of relationships.

Reasoning Exercise: Interpersonal Relations

Rose McGrath is a 68-year-old retired teacher admitted to psychiatry for treatment of depression.

1. Ms. McGrath isolates herself in her room for much of the day. She is quiet and somewhat disheveled in appearance. When approached by the nurse during her first hospital day she makes no eye contact. In attempting to address issues of grooming and hygiene, the nurse might best say:
   A. Here are your linens. Now go clean up before lunch.
   B. You look a mess. Let's do something about that right now.
   C. I think you'll feel better after you have a chance to bathe and dress. I'll help you.
   D. Why haven't you gotten dressed? It's after 10 o'clock.

The intended response is **C.** The nurse is offering her assistance to the client in a respectful way. This response is most likely to engender beginning trust.

2. The nurse learns that Ms. McGrath's husband died 6 months ago. Each of the following factors would tend to place her at high risk for depression *except:*
   A. She expressed anger and feelings of abandonment following his death.
   B. She was unable to cry or attend her husband's funeral.
   C. She has also lost a parent and a brother during the past year.
   D. She cared for Mr. McGrath during his lengthy illness and rarely socialized with others.

The intended response is **A.** Each of the other factors suggests the progressive decline in close relationships or contacts with others, or a block in the normal grieving process completion. The number and quality of relationships and adequate resolution of loss are factors in alleviating stress.

3. Which of the following responses by the patient when the nurse arrives 10 minutes late for a planned "talk" suggests that trust has been established?
   A. Oh, you're here. What were we going to do again?
   B. I didn't think I'd ever see you again, nurse.

    C. I thought you'd come as soon as you could.

    D. Who are you? I forgot your name.

The intended response is **C**. The patient is expressing confidence in the nurse and also the belief that she is important enough for the nurse to honor their commitment.

4. Which of the following descriptions of Ms. McGrath's behavior in relationships would the nurse consider most typical?

    A. She has many friends and many very close friends.

    B. She finds it easiest to be on the receiving end.

    C. She finds it easiest to express angry feelings.

    D. She finds it easiest to give to others.

The intended response is **D**. Characteristically, because of low self-esteem the depressed patient feels unworthy of others' attention and has difficulty expressing negative feelings. Additionally, because of this limited willingness to share a range of feelings and expectation of little from others, relationships at the deep levels are fewer in number.

5. As the time for Ms. McGrath's discharge approaches, she and the nurse begin to discuss the termination process. Which of the following statements by Ms. McGrath would increase the nurse's confidence that their relationship has been helpful?

    A. How will I ever manage? No one out there will want to bother with me like you have.

    B. Nothing is going to be different. I'll come back to see you, and you can come and see me.

    C. Oh nurse, you've been so wonderful. I'll be lost without you.

    D. I feel so much better now. Help me figure out how I've done it so I can stay out of here.

The intended response is **D**. As part of the termination process it is helpful for both nurse and patient to review the course of the relationship and to identify the work accomplished and future goals. Additionally, a therapeutic relationship is to be validating and enabling, not one creating unnecessary dependence or artificial independence.

PERSONAL INTEGRITY 19

ANN SHEERER FILIPSKI

PRINCIPLE

A SENSE OF SELF BEGINS TO DEVELOP EARLY IN LIFE AND IS DEPENDENT UPON NURTURANCE AND EXTERNAL VALIDATION

Illustration of Principle

Each person begins life in unique circumstances. With an innate set of individual characteristics as determined by genetic material and the influences and events within the prenatal and birth environment, each human being must then begin the complex and lifelong task of continued growth and development. Despite individual differences in makeup and life situations, there is a logical and orderly progression to human development that has been observed by personality theorists like Freud, Erikson, and Sullivan.

> Theories of human personality recognize the progression through "stages" of development that are dependent upon the physical maturation of the individual and the response of the surrounding environment.

Memory Jog

Because of the relative immaturity of their physiological and psychological apparatuses, all infants and young children must rely upon the external environment and those within it to meet their needs. Just as the maturing body's physical survival and growth are dependent upon the provision of food and shelter, the maturing self or "emotional body" must be provided with nurturance and external validation.

213

Early psychological needs are met in many seemingly simple ways. Physical contact with the world can produce varied sensations for the infant, some pleasant and some not so pleasant. Witness the different responses by most children to a cold, wet diaper versus being held and rocked by a familiar adult. Being protected from environmental threats or disruptions in a comfortable state and consistent contacts with caring others lead to a sense of the world and those within it as safe, reliable, and pleasing. Further, contacts and interactions with the larger world and other beings provide the developing individual with many opportunities to both validate experience and learn more about oneself.

Ideally, over time the individual can gain an awareness of his physical being (or body image), a sense of identity (both real and desired), a means of developing and preserving self-esteem (coping mechanisms), and the ability to examine oneself and behavior (self-awareness). The foundation for this multifaceted, dynamic sense of self is firmly rooted in the individual's early experiences, but it continues to mature and be subject to alteration throughout life.

> The aspects of the person to be integrated into the "self" include body image, identity, self-esteem, and self-awareness.

By virtue of their contacts with patients in many varied settings and states of health, the nurse is in a unique position to assess for potential or actual alterations in the sense of self, formulate appropriate nursing diagnosis, and intervene in a manner designed to facilitate further growth and development. These efforts must be guided by an awareness of the "normal" process of human development. Further, the nurse must recognize that even when the patient's physical being is the priority or focus of attention, *no* nursing contact or intervention is without impact upon the patient's self.

> Each nursing action has an impact upon the patient's self and potential for fostering integration of the personality.

Principle

THE SELF IS THE VEHICLE IN WHICH ONE FUNCTIONS IN THE LARGER WORLD

Illustration of Principle

The self of any individual is dynamic and multifaceted. Aspects of the self are made known or communicated to others by behavior. How a person conducts oneself or acts is utilized as a tool in understanding or gaining knowledge about that person. We recognize that behavior has meaning and because man is complex, an action is influenced by a multiplicity of factors.

Internal influences upon behavior include the individual's perceptions, thoughts, feelings, and actions. External influences include such things as the environment and setting, cultural norms, and the expectations of others. Thus, any attempt to understand an individual's behavior must consider both the self (or unique attributes of the person) and the context of the larger external environment.

> Behavior is complex, meaningful, and multidetermined.

Memory jog

Most observers tend to evaluate other's behavior strictly from their own perspectives. The nurse, however, is responsible for expanding this narrow focus. An awareness of both the internal and external influences upon the patient's behavior must be included in the use of nursing process.

Any given behavior may be the end result of unique or altered internal influences. For example, patients with sensory impairments may have altered perceptions about a given situation. Those who are intellectually limited because of handicaps or physical immaturity will likely respond differently to varied patient education efforts. An impulsive patient may handle frustrating situations in characteristic and often counterproductive ways. With knowledge of the unique internal influences upon a patient's behavior the nurse is better prepared to intervene therapeutically.

The nurse must also be aware of many external influences upon patient behavior. For example, the setting in which one finds oneself may well influence individual response to the statement "Undress, please." Or the behavioral response to being served rare roast beef may vary if one is a vegetarian, a Hindu, or a cattle rancher in the Midwest. And lastly, the expectations of others may also influence how one behaves. The patient giving his own insulin injection for the first time may respond very differently to "I'll help if you need me," versus "I don't know if you can manage."

> Sensory stimuli → perceptions
> Perceptions (interpreted and labeled) → thoughts
> Thoughts and evoked memories → feelings
> Feelings experienced and acted upon →
> *Behavior*

Memory jog

Armed with the knowledge of patient behavior and the various influences upon it, the nurse can then direct her interventions toward the individual or the environment. The overriding goal is always to foster the patient's ability to function as effectively as possible.

EACH INDIVIDUAL MUST DEVELOP MEANS OF MAINTAINING THE INTEGRITY OF THE SELF IN ALTERING CIRCUMSTANCES

Illustration of Principle

All living organisms must be able to adapt to the changing circumstances in life. Thus, within man both physiological and psychological means are available to help maintain "normal" homeostatic balance.

For example, exposed to infectious agents within the environment, man has certain protective mechanisms that automatically assist him in maintaining a healthy body. Certain physical and chemical barriers, the inflammatory process, and the immune system all act to sustain physical integrity. Similarly, in interaction with the external environment, man has *psychological* mechanisms available to help him sustain emotional health. Mechanisms such as denial, repression, sublimation, and compensation are utilized to safeguard the self. They help to preserve self-esteem while allowing for some modification in one's sense of identity and desired self-image when faced with environmental limitations or the demand for change. Like the physiological mechanisms mentioned earlier, these defense mechanisms are also somewhat "automatic." Frequently used in normal everyday life, they may be called upon to maintain the integrity of the self long before the individual is even aware of any personal threat. They are vital to man's emotional health and ability to sustain himself.

Memory Jog

> During normal maturation, the individual develops a collection of defense mechanisms or coping skills that aid in maintaining the health of the self.

Successful adaptation for the individual in a physical sense means the protective mechanisms have maintained an acceptable level of homeostasis and bodily integrity. The state of health may be disrupted, however, if the bodily threat is so severe as to be overwhelming, the protective mechanisms are themselves deficient or impaired, or the prolonged use of the normal mechanisms leads to exhaustion and further vulnerability or insult.

Psychologically, successful adaptation allows the individual to preserve personal integrity without undue distress for himself or others. If the defense mechanisms are inadequate in number or quality, the external assaults or environmental stresses are too severe, or the use of the defenses themselves jeopardize the individual or others, then emotional health is disrupted.

> Successful adaptation allows the individual to meet the demands of the environment without undue distress or disruption for himself or others.

The focus of nursing attention is always related to the variables of patient, environment, and health. Thus, in any situation, the nurse will be seeking to maximize the state of the patient's self.

This may be accomplished through the use of any or all of the following interventions:

▷ Assisting the patient in recognizing and responding to changing environmental circumstances

▷ Supporting the patient's use of effective, adaptive coping or defense mechanisms

▷ Identifying alterations in health or deficits in the patient's ability to act autonomously or maintain personal integrity and means to remedy these

▷ Lending the assistance of the self of the nurse in the patient's efforts to acquire new or more effective defense mechanisms and continued psychological growth and development

PRINCIPLE

THREAT TO THE INDIVIDUAL RESULTS IN FEAR OR ANXIETY

Illustration of Principle

The experiences of fear and anxiety are universal. Both responses serve protective functions in that they alert the individual to potential threats and disruptions in one's normal, steady state. *Fear* is generally considered object-specific. This means that a readily identifiable threat exists (often to one's physical well-being) in the environment. As a result, the individual experiences distress (fear) and responds with a "flight, fight, or fright" reaction. Both the threat and the subsequent response would be understood or viewed as predictable by most individuals. For example, if while crossing the street one were suddenly to see a speeding car approach, both fear for one's safety and attempts to run from the path of the vehicle would be common reactions.

> Fear is a response to the presence of an immediate environmental threat to the individual's survival or physical well-being.

In contrast, *anxiety* is a more subjective experience. The anxious person feels uncertain and ill at ease or may even experience an acute sense of panic and impending doom. Often with anxiety, the individual may be uncertain or unclear about the source of his or her distress. Even if identified, the "threat" is often highly individualized and may be unrealistic. The experience is generally precipitated by an assault to one's sense of self or other aspects of personal integrity.

Anxiety is a sense of vague uneasiness and discomfort experienced in response to the presence of subjectively determined threats to the self.

PRINCIPLE

ANXIETY ELICITS THE USE OF DEFENSE MECHANISMS AND COPING STRATEGIES IN ATTEMPTS TO PRESERVE THE INTEGRITY OF THE SELF

Illustration of Principle

The experience of anxiety serves to alert the individual faced with actual or potential threats. Although some patients may be able to describe or label their internal, subjective experience as "anxiety," more often the nurse infers its presence from her observation of them. Anxiety produces physiological, emotional, and cognitive manifestations in all individuals, and these manifestations are closely related to the severity of the distress experienced. Further, these same manifestations may produce behavioral change.

LEVELS OF ANXIETY	MANIFESTATIONS
Mild—common event in everyday life. Use of defense mechanisms prevents significant impairment in ability to function.	Physiological ↑ Pulse and respirations Mild GI symptoms—*i.e.*, "butterflies" Dry mouth ↑ Diaphoresis—*i.e.*, "sweaty palms" ↑ Muscle tension
	Emotional Some sense of tension—"nervous" *(continued)*

LEVELS OF ANXIETY	MANIFESTATIONS
	Mild lability—giggling or nervous laughter, more easily irritated or tearful
	Cognitive Able to focus attention ↑ Awareness of environment
Moderate—present when faced with excessive or repeated demands for change or threats to the self. May see exaggeration of normal defensive operations or some impairment in ability to function.	Physiological Tachycardia and tachypnea Nausea, anorexia, constipation, or diarrhea Excessive perspiration Restlessness, excessive motor activity, painful muscle tension Urinary frequency or retention
	Emotional Labile mood—irritability, anger, hostility or tearfulness, withdrawal, apathy
	Cognitive ↓ Concentration and attention ↑ Distractibility ↑ Preoccupied ↓ Recall ↑ May see distortions in perceptions or judgment and decision-making
Severe or Panic State—Present when the threat to the self is overwhelming; defensive operations have been inadequate, disruptive, or failed. *Marked* impairment in ability to function results.	Physiological Autonomic nervous system symptoms remain and may become the focus of patient's attention or concern. Frank somatic symptoms such as fainting, chest pains, shortness of breath may be reported or observed. Marked psychomotor agitation or assaultive

(continued)

LEVELS OF ANXIETY	MANIFESTATIONS
	behavior may be seen.
	Hypervigilance
	Emotional
	Unstable mood and poor
	affective regulation or control
	Terror, rage, or aggression
	Inappropriate affect
	Cognitive
	Poor reality testing
	Internally focused and
	preoccupied
	Difficulties with attention
	Impaired judgment
	Faulty decision-making

The use of defense mechanisms to safeguard the self is generally an adaptive mechanism. Their use allows the individual to function effectively in the face of new or unusual circumstances. Sometimes, however, the mechanisms are inadequate, and the anxiety no longer serves merely as a signal of potential threat. It may become so pronounced as to impair functioning and lead to disruption in the experience of the self.

Memory Jog

> The presence of anxiety can be inferred from observation of patient behavior.

The role of the nurse with the anxious patient is as varied as the manifestations and severity of anxiety. Thus, the importance of accurate assessment is clear as is the need to select interventions that will be effective and appropriate to the level of anxiety.

In general, patients need assistance in containing the manifestations of anxiety and in preserving the self, particularly with increasing levels of distress or impairment. As anxiety increases, nursing interventions utilize verbal or cognitive modes of a less sophisticated nature. And conversely, with less disruption at mild levels of anxiety, it is more appropriate to assist the patient in identifying the presence of anxiety and its manifestations, gaining insight as to its causes or precipitants, and developing means to manage it more effectively or adapt to changes.

> Factors to be considered in determining nursing interventions for patients experiencing anxiety include the level of current distress, nature of defense mechanisms, and the integrity of the self.

Reasoning Exercises: Personal Integrity

Margaret Jones, the evening charge nurse, is contacted by the emergency room. She is informed of a new admission, "John Doe," a young adult male. Described as "uncooperative" and "suspicious," he provided no information to the examining physician and was brought to the hospital by the police.

1. Which of the following information obtained during the nursing assessment would be most suggestive of psychopathology?

    A. John seems to be hard of hearing.

    B. John lives in an urban, high-crime area.

    C. John has a history of violent behavior.

    D. John does not understand or speak English.

The intended response is **C.** Each of the other options provides a possible explanation for John's reported "uncooperative" and "suspicious" behavior. Without knowledge of them, others might view his actions as very maladaptive.

2. Additional history is obtained from John's family and past medical records. He has been diagnosed as suffering from schizophrenia, paranoid type. Emotional arrest in such patients is most likely to have occurred during what stage of development?

    A. Autonomy versus shame and doubt

    B. Intimacy versus isolation

    C. Generativity versus stagnation

    D. Trust versus mistrust

The intended response is **D.** The nature of this disorder's symptoms and the defenses utilized to protect the self suggest very early emotional trauma has left the patient with difficulty in establishing trusting relationships with others.

3. John tells the nurse, "You know I'm the last Czar of Russia don't you? The KGB and CIA are both looking for me!" The nurse must

recognize that these statements likely reflect all of the following *except:*

A. Delusional beliefs

B. Use of defense mechanisms

C. Impaired self-concept

D. Sense of entitlement

The intended response is D. Delusions of persecution or grandeur are common features in this subtype of schizophrenia. Both reflect attempts to defend against underlying feelings of isolation and low self-esteem. Thus, the client provides himself with a delusional explanation—his differentness is *special* in some way. It allows the fear and anxiety to be externalized to an environmental source.

4. John remains aloof and distant, seeming to avoid contacts with other patients or unit staff. In order to establish a relationship it will be most helpful if the nurse

   A. Approaches him directly and converses about topics like unit events or daily activities

   B. Encourages him to participate in cooperative activities with other patients

   C. Provides warm and supportive contact, allowing John to select the focus of conversation

   D. Asks John to discuss his obvious discomfort in the presence of others to gain insight

The intended response is A. Other options presently are likely to be interpreted as threatening by John and would thus serve to *increase* his anxiety. With increased anxiety, his abilities to test reality are likely to decrease, leading to further impairment in functioning.

5. John becomes tense and anxious following a visit from his mother. He begins pacing in the hallway and when approached, begins to shout angrily and threatens to "get you all!" All of the following would be reasonable, immediate approaches to this behavior *except:*

   A. Speak calmly to John in a nonthreatening but direct manner.

   B. Ask John to explore why he's become so uncomfortable following his mother's visit.

   C. Mobilize additional personnel to aid in physical management if needed.

   D. Clear the hallway of other patients and minimize distracting activity.

The intended response is **B.** John's loss of control and other behavior suggest anxiety of severe proportions. Thus, ambiguous or highly verbal approaches are likely to be *unsuccessful* because the patient's ability to sustain attention or think clearly is markedly compromised.

6. Nurse Jones has spent considerable time with John. Which of the following questions might indicate that he has progressed in gaining insight and is willing to enter the working phase of a therapeutic relationship?

    A. You know I don't want to talk; why do you bother me?

    B. Who do you work for—the FBI or CIA?

    C. I've been in the hospital before. How can I keep from coming back here all the time?

    D. Oh you again! What do you want—more things to write in my chart?

The intended response is **C.** This response suggests that some level of trust has been developed, and the patient is willing to utilize the self of the nurse in his efforts to develop new coping skills that are more effective.

20 GROWTH AND DEVELOPMENT

Cynthia Smego

PRINCIPLE

BIOLOGICAL GROWTH IS VERY RAPID DURING THE FIRST 12 MONTHS OF LIFE. MOTOR DEVELOPMENT FOLLOWS SPECIFIC PATTERNS
(CEPHALOCAUDAL PROXIMALDISTAL)

Illustration of Principle

Overall increase in the size of the body and continual maturation of body systems during infancy are remarkable. During each of the first 6 months of life, an infant will gain approximately 1½ pounds, thereby doubling his body weight by 6 months. Weight gain decreases somewhat during the second 6 months. Yet, by 12 months of age, he will have tripled his body weight. Increases in length or height will be primarily confined to the trunk.

The most remarkable developmental changes are related to the nervous system as evidenced by the progressive fine and gross motor developments that occur during this stage.

PRINCIPLE

INFANTS MUST DEVELOP A SENSE OF TRUST. THIS IS ESTABLISHED THROUGH THE RELATIONSHIP WITH THE PRIMARY CAREGIVER(S)

Illustration of Principle

A consistent, loving, protective, and responsive primary caregiver is essential for the development of trust. Yet, the infant also has a strong role to play and

225

TABLE 20-1. GROSS MOTOR DEVELOPMENT (EACH MILESTONE ADDS TO THE DEVELOPMENT OF POSTURE, BALANCE, AND FUTURE LOCOMOTION.)

Newborn	Maintains head control for short periods
4 months	Lifts head and upper body to bear weight on forearms Can roll onto his side
5 months	Can roll from front to back with ease
6 months	Lifts head and upper body to bear weight on hands Can roll from back to abdomen from prone position
7 months	Adds to the upright position mastered at 6 months by being able to bear weight with one hand while exploring with the other Can sit alone now, often leaning forward onto hands for support
8 months	Has mastered skill of sitting alone Will begin to actively explore his surroundings Will use both hands now (falls over frequently)
9 months	Can pull self up on furniture
10 months	Will be able to achieve sitting position from prone position by himself Crawls well When standing with support, will try to step with one foot
11 months	Will walk along furniture
12 months	Can walk while holding hands with caregiver

must be loving and responsive to the caregiver as well. Each must provide the other with positive feedback for the relationship to develop. Through a complex process of displaying his needs and having them met in a gratifying way, the infant develops a sense of trust in his primary caregiver, (usually parent), and in his environment.

Very early on, the infant will begin to make associations between his needs and actions that lead to the fulfillment of those needs. As the infant grows and develops, he will make increasingly more complex associations between needs and their fulfillment. For example, when the newborn infant feels uncomfortable because he is hungry, he will cry. Crying will bring a nipple to his mouth. He will soon associate hunger and crying with the satisfaction gained from sucking. Later, he will recognize that when he cries, he not only gets the nipple, but he will hear his mother's voice. Her voice will soon be associated with the comfort and security he feels in her arms. As this process continues to be reinforced, he will soon begin to accept and trust that this cycle will occur whenever he expresses his needs. Although this is a simple example, it illustrates a process that will be built upon throughout the first 12 months.

TABLE 20-2. FINE MOTOR DEVELOPMENT (DEVELOPING INCREASED DEXTERITY, LEARNING TO USE HANDS AND FINGERS TO EXPLORE SELF AND ENVIRONMENT)

Newborn	Is not aware of own hands or fingers; unless by accident, they reach his mouth Grasp is reflexive
1 to 5 months	Discovers hands, fingers, feet and plays with them Will replace primitive, reflexive grasp with purposeful, voluntary grasp by 5 months Purposeful grasp at 5 months is usually two-handed
6 months	Level of skill with hands is greatly increased Can hold items easily (bottles, cookies, toys) Can only handle one object at a time Actively uses hands for exploration
7 months	Will be able to transfer objects between hands Likes to bang objects Learns to use fingers for increased exploration
10 months	Pincher grasp is established
11 to 12 months	Likes to manipulate objects Enjoys putting things into larger objects (the beginning understanding of the concept of object permanence)

PRINCIPLE

INFANTS LEARN THROUGH PARTICIPATION WITH THEIR PRIMARY CAREGIVER AND BY ACTIVELY EXPLORING THEMSELVES AND THEIR ENVIRONMENT

Illustration of Principle

Cognitive development during the first 24 months is referred to as the sensorimotor phase. The first four stages take place from birth to 12 months. During this phase, the infant will learn that he is separate from other objects and beings within the environment, the groundwork for the concept of object permanence will be laid, and he will begin to equate symbols with mental images (*i.e.,* "bye-bye" means someone is leaving).

During the first few months of life, the infant learns through the use of reflexes. Through repetition, the infant will begin to recognize the development of patterns. Recognition of these patterns sets the stage for the replacement of voluntary actions for the reflex behavior. From 1 to 4 months, reflexes become deliberate efforts to gain a desired response. Until approximately 8 months, he will continue to test his new abilities in a variety of ways. As a result of his experiments, he will begin to develop a sense of causality. Intentions will become more deliberate as he begins to see himself as separate from his environment and from his parents.

Expanding upon the example given in Principle 2, one can see how patterns developed from reflexive behavior will be tried and tested until a sense of cause and effect is developed. Once again, when a newborn is hungry, he cries and is given a nipple. Soon, an association is made between the nipple and the comfort of the satisfaction of a need. As this process is repeated time and again, the infant will begin to recognize the development of a consistent pattern. When he begins to add the element of the loving caregiver to this pattern, he will begin to test the reflex in order to gain the comfort of his mother even in the absence of hunger. At this point, reflexive behavior is replaced by voluntary actions. In other words, actions become deliberate—he cries, his mother comes.

The groundwork for the development of object permanence is held during infancy. The infant begins to first recognize that the removal of something from sight doesn't necessarily mean that it is gone forever by his interaction with parents. This is best illustrated by reviewing the attachment and separation process. The process of attachment begins at birth and continues throughout the first year. The infant will develop a sense of attachment and separation by progressing through *overlapping* stages.

1. From birth until approximately 2 months of age, the infant will respond to anyone and everyone.

2. From 8 to 12 weeks, infants will respond primarily to parents. Although the infant enjoys the comfort of mother, most others are perceived as equally comforting and loving. At this stage, because the primary caregiver is always readily available to meet his every need, the infant does not perceive himself as separate.

3. At 6 months of age, infants will show a definite preference for mother. Between 4 to 8 months, an infant will begin to have an awareness of himself as separate from mother. This is the point at which anxiety will be evident whenever mother and baby are separated. Infants begin to learn about object permanence as a result of sight; they will protest desperately, believing that if mom is out of sight, mom is gone forever. Yet, when she reappears and anxiety subsides, the infant's concept of her predictability and permanence will be reinforced.

4. By about 7 months, the infant will begin to show preference to other familiar family members or consistent caregivers. During this stage, he will begin to recognize the differences between the familiar and unfamiliar. Protest and anxiety will begin to be displayed when confronted with strangers.

SPECIAL NEEDS AND PROBLEMS

1. Love, comfort, and security (trust)
2. Adequate nutrition for growth
3. Prevention of injury
   a. Foreign object aspiration
   b. Suffocation
   c. Falls
   d. Poisoning
   e. Burns
4. Immunization administration

NURSING CONSIDERATIONS

1. Emotional support to family
2. Education and guidance
3. Maintenance of infant-parent trust relationship

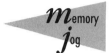

PRINCIPLE

BIOLOGICAL GROWTH IS SLOWER AND STEADIER DURING THE TODDLER YEARS AS COMPARED WITH THE MONTHS OF INFANCY.
BODY ORGANS ACHIEVE MORE MATURE FUNCTIONING. IMPROVED MOTOR SKILLS CREATE MANY NEW OPPORTUNITIES FOR THE TODDLER

Illustration of Principle

Overall growth is much slower at this time. By 2½ years of age, most toddlers will have quadrupled their birth weight. Increases in height are also less dramatic. Most of their height increase will be a result of increase in the length of their legs. Toddlers will gain approximately 3 inches in height each year. Growth of the head is also slower and steadier. The anterior fontanel will close between 12 and 18 months. Chest circumference will continue to increase and will surpass head circumference.

Most body systems are relatively mature by the end of the toddler years. One of the most obvious body system changes is related to the gastrointestinal system. Most children can successfully achieve voluntary control over elimination between 18 and 24 months.

Studies made at this time in both fine and gross motor development can be seen in all that the toddler does.

Increased fine motor control is evidenced by increased dexterity. Toddlers can hold and release (throw) arms at will, open doors, pick up tiny objects and examine them closely, and put their little fingers into the most impossible places.

Increased gross motor control is evident by the rapid progress made in locomotion. From 15 months to 2 years, the toddler progresses rapidly from walking with ease to running fairly well. By 2 years of age, most toddlers will have mastered the stairs, one foot at a time. The 2½ year old can jump and stand on one foot for brief periods of time. By the age of 3 years, the toddler can stand on tip toe, climb stairs by alternating feet, and stand on one foot at a time with ease.

PRINCIPLE

COGNITIVE DEVELOPMENT AT THIS STAGE IS PRIMARILY RELATED TO LANGUAGE DEVELOPMENT, PRIMITIVE REASONING, AND TRIAL AND ERROR EXPERIMENTATION

Illustration of Principle

Much of the language development is accomplished through liptation and imitation. For example, as parents continue to use the word "up" every time they pick up their child, the toddler soon learns to say "up" whenever he wants to be held. Much to the dismay of many parents, the egocentric toddler also enjoys the selective use of the words that he has mastered. "No" and "mine" are two perfect examples. From 12 to 24 months, toddlers usually have developed a vocabulary of approximately 300 words. By 2 years of age, the toddler is able to group words into simple sentences to convey a meaning, such as "Me outside" or "Grandma go bye-bye." More remarkable, though, than their vocabulary is their level of comprehension. They are able to understand much more than what they can say.

An illustration can be made by picturing the toddler who has wandered away from mother, momentarily, to explore the kitchen cabinets alone. Upon hearing the familiar rattle of the pots and pans, Mom yells, "Hey, what are you doing in there?" from the other room. The toddler will instantly stop and think to himself, "Who, me? I'm just checking out the cabinets. Are you yelling at me or just asking? Okay, just a minute. Here I come." Certainly these sentences are more complex than he's capable of, but they illustrate the complexity of his level of comprehension.

The level of reasoning of the toddler is quite primitive. It is described as transductional. He makes generalizations and applies them loosely. For example, he reasons that if one sweater is scratchy, therefore, all sweaters are scratchy. So, whenever his parents try to dress him in a sweater, he will protest violently. Another example of such reasoning can be illustrated by examining the typical mealtime behavior of the toddler. After crying for one-half hour for something to eat, the toddler is finally served dinner. With four things to choose from on his plate, he'll try the most appealing item first. If it happens to be something that he doesn't like, he'll immediately assume that everything will taste just as bad and refuse despite all efforts from his parents. This is transductional thinking—making generalizations from particular to particular.

The toddler's approach to learning and discovery is one of trial and error. The memory of the toddler is very short, and he will frequently have to learn the same lesson over and over again. Because he has a high level of understanding of the concept of object permanence, the toddler will now know that if something is missing, it may be located in any number of possible hiding places. He will set out, using a trial and error approach, until he locates the missing item.

PRINCIPLE

THE TODDLER MUST DEVELOP A SENSE OF AUTONOMY

Illustration of Principle

The activities of the toddler are directed toward the exploration of and control over the environment. The daily mission of the toddler is to explore and learn as much as he possibly can. This is certainly evidenced by the fact that toddlers are into everything—almost always at once. They play in the water of the toilet, rummage through closets, put their fingers into the darnedest places, and are almost always creating a mess. That is how they learn, and of course it is also how they frequently get themselves into a hundred jams. All of this activity is also helping them to learn to be less dependent upon their parents. As they venture out into their world, they become less concerned about separation from their parents, yet they still need visual and verbal reassurance of their parents' closeness. For example, a 2 year old can play alone with his toys for extended periods of time. As long as the parent is still there each time he looks up, he is content.

Usually at this stage, they are very fearful of strangers, particularly when their parents are present.

During the toddler years, independence must be balanced with appropriate guidance. Limit setting by parents should be constructive and encourage self-control, reasonable autonomy, and independence. Discipline may be necessary. If so, it should be carried out in an appropriate, consistent, and timely fashion.

SPECIAL NEEDS AND PROBLEMS

1. Temper tantrums
2. Negativism
3. Sibling rivalry
4. Toilet training
5. Dental hygiene
6. Prevention of injury
   a. Drowning
   b. Burns
   c. Poisoning
   d. Falls
   e. Aspiration

NURSING CONSIDERATIONS

1. Helping parents to learn to "set limits"
2. Accident prevention

PRINCIPLE

RATE OF PHYSICAL GROWTH STABILIZES. MOTOR SKILLS ARE REFINED

Illustration of Principle

The preschooler is characteristically more slender, stands more erect, and is more graceful than the toddler. Average weight gain is approximately 5 pounds per year. As with the toddler, the preschooler adds 2.5 to 3 inches per year to his height with most of it occurring in the legs rather than the trunk.

Advances in motor development are chiefly related to continued refinement of all skills.

PRINCIPLE

THE PRESCHOOLER LEARNS THROUGH A MORE ADVANCED EXPLORATION OF THE ENVIRONMENT. THESE ARE THE "WHY" YEARS THROUGH WHICH THEY DEVELOP A SENSE OF INITIATIVE

Illustration of Principle

The preschooler is best described as an inquisitive, creative, aggressive, foolhardy ball of energy. These characteristics can easily be seen whenever preschoolers are seen at "work"—exploring! To them, the world is full of wonder and magic. The environment offers many new and wonderful experiences and opportunities for discovery, and the preschooler intends to see and experience them all. He develops a sense of himself and his world through this exploration and a seemingly endless string of questions. *Why* is the key word of their vocabulary.

As the preschooler sets out on his own to conquer the world, he learns many lessons. Because he doesn't know his own limits, the preschooler will often get into more mischief than he can handle. He begins to develop a sense of good versus bad, right versus wrong. These principles are the foundation of the development of a sense of conscience. He will constantly test the limits set by his parents in order to determine what is good or bad behavior. At this stage, the child remains quite self-centered and will worry about the consequences of his actions only in reference to himself. He has little use for the concerns of others except for his parents. He fears the disapproval of his parents and will usually do things or not do them in order to stay in their good graces. Children of this age group strive to be cooperative and responsible members of the family.

PRINCIPLE
THINKING IS PRELOGICAL AND MAGICAL

Illustration of Principle

Conceptual thinking can be described as prelogical in that the preschooler is unable to perceive parts in terms of the whole. They only understand what they can see. For example, if two glasses of different sizes contain the same amount of juice, the preschooler will believe that the larger glass has more. To him, bigger means more. By the same token, a small, fat candy bar will never be as satisfactory as a large, thin one.

Children at this age have a very poor sense of body boundaries. For example, they wholeheartedly believe that if they have a cut or have an injection that the "hole" must be covered in order to prevent anything from escaping from their bodies. Boundaries are a critical necessity for the injured preschooler.

The preschooler can only understand time in relation to events. For example, when separated from his parents, the preschooler is calmed much more easily with the comment, "Your mother will be home after Mr. Rogers," and not from "She'll be here at 2 PM."

Because the preschooler depends upon his parents for answers to his questions, this is a time when parental fears can be easily transferred to the child, for example fear of the dark, fear of the cellar. In order to control fears, the child will often use magical thinking in an attempt to control fears or to solve mysteries. The preschooler believes that thinking or wishing for something will make the event occur. The preschooler will create "special friends" to take the blame for his actions. Only a preschooler can see the monster in the closet or under the bed. Children of this age delight in the magic of Santa.

SPECIAL NEEDS AND PROBLEMS

1. Consistency in limit setting

2. Sleep disturbances (nightmares)

3. Prevention of injury, falls, or poisoning

4. Communicable diseases

5. Child abuse or neglect

NURSING CONSIDERATIONS

1. Protection of body image

2. Helping parents prepare for day school or preschool

3. Concrete answers to questions

PRINCIPLE

THROUGHOUT THE SCHOOL YEARS, PHYSICAL GROWTH REMAINS SLOW AND STEADY

Illustration of Principle

From the ages of 6 to 12 years, physical growth will proceed at a slow yet steady pace. Children will gain approximately 2 inches per year in height and will have doubled their weight over the 6-year period. Toward the end of the school-age years, girls will begin to surpass boys in height and weight. Shedding of the primary teeth occurs at this time.

Characteristically, school-age children appear leaner and taller with improved posture as compared with the preschooler. They become more graceful as their coordination and motor skills improve.

PRINCIPLE

DURING THIS DEVELOPMENTAL STAGE, CHILDREN MUST DEVELOP A SENSE OF INDUSTRY

Illustration of Principle

Throughout the school-age years, children will be struggling with developing a sense of industry. Failure to do so will result in feelings of inadequacy or inferiority. The developmental tasks of the child in this age group are met through the challenges and conflicts encountered at school and through the development of peer group relationships. With each new experience, the child will be developing a sense of self-worth (self-esteem and body image), evaluating family and social values, and learning to cope with a variety of failures and successes.

Principle

THROUGH FORMAL EDUCATION, CHILDREN WILL ACHIEVE A SENSE OF PERSONAL COMPETENCE BY GAINING KNOWLEDGE AND TECHNICAL SKILLS

Illustration of Principle

The entrance into school marks a period of significant change for children. They are entering a new world. They leave the security and freedom of the home and family environment and enter a system that is very structured, one with new rules and regulations. They must learn to respect and obey an adult other than their parents. Teachers exert a great deal of influence over children. Hero worship is typical during this stage.

During this developmental stage, children are very active and eager intellectually. They enjoy new experiences and delight in the acquisition of new abilities and skills. They are excited to discover the answers to the many unanswered questions of the previous developmental stage.

Piaget describes this developmental stage as one of *concrete operations,* which is the process of using thoughts to experience work and to describe actions or events. In other words, children learn to "think" through a process and can perform it in their minds rather than having to act out the actual activity. This skill will become refined with increased use throughout the school years.

For example, a 4-year-old child could find his way to the park six blocks from home after having been there several times. Simply stated, he has learned the way—he can act it out. Yet an 8 year old could think of going to the park, and in his mind he could find his way. Furthermore, when asked the way to that same park, he could easily give directions; he can mentally perform the task.

Principle

CHILDREN ARE FACED WITH MAKING THEIR FIRST TRUE COMMITMENT TO RELATIONSHIPS OUTSIDE THE HOME. PEER GROUP VERSUS FAMILY VALUES ARE OFTEN A SOURCE OF CONFLICT

Illustration of Principle

Throughout the years 6 to 12, children will seek independence from their parents by increasing their identification with the peer group. The peer group exerts a tremendous amount of influence over the daily activities of the school-aged child. During these years, children are in the process of laying the groundwork for the development of self-esteem and self-worth. This is accomplished as they integrate family and peer group values. Quite often, they are faced with a conflict of standards. It is not always easy or desirable to defy their parents in order to conform to the pressures of the group. As a result, children are faced with the task of self- and social evaluation.

These are the wonderful years of best friends, blood buddies, secret places, clubs of exclusive memberships and rigid group rules. Peer relations dictate how the group members walk, talk, and dress. Roles are frequently assumed according to group standards.

Children will often modify their behavior and beliefs in order to conform to peer group values and pressures. Yet, when in serious conflict with the values taught by parents, family values will almost always prevail.

SPECIAL CONCERNS AND PROBLEMS

1. Dishonest behavior
    a. Cheating
    b. Lying
    c. Stealing
2. Latch-key children
3. Need for sexual exploration
4. Injury prevention (often sports-related)
5. Dental hygiene
6. Skin disorders
7. Behavioral disorders (attention deficient disorder—ADD)
8. Learning disabilities

NURSING CONSIDERATIONS

1. Reinforce positive body image perceptions
2. Support educational needs while hospitalized

PRINCIPLE

PHYSICAL GROWTH AND BODILY CHANGES ARE DRAMATIC AND VISIBLE DURING ADOLESCENCE

Illustration of Principle

The physical changes that occur in adolescence are caused by hormones. Sexual maturation is also closely associated with a dramatic increase in physical growth. The "growth spurt" occurs over a relatively short period of time—2 to 3 years. During adolescence, children will achieve the remainder of their linear growth, and body systems will reach full maturity. The onset of puberty is variable for both sexes and is widened by the development of secondary sex characteristics.

Girls—Puberty can begin at any point between the ages of 8 and 14 years. Once puberty begins, all physical changes are usually completed within approximately 3 years. The onset of menstruation usually occurs about 2 to 2½ years after the onset of puberty.

Boys—Puberty begins later for boys than for girls, usually with its onset between 10 and 16 years of age. Major developmental changes for boys are related to increases in height and musculature, maturation of the gonads, and the development of secondary sex characteristics.

PRINCIPLE
THE TASK OF ADOLESCENTS IS TO DEVELOP A SENSE OF IDENTITY

Illustration of Principle

As a result of the onset and rapid development of physical growth and sexual maturation, adolescents must face many new and unfamiliar feelings about themselves and their bodies. This is a time when children are confronted with an increased sensitivity for peer approval and acceptance.

The adolescent will strive for a sense of self and separation from the family. This is a complex process that involves first an intense need for peer identity, which leads ultimately to the development of self-identity.

PRINCIPLE
COGNITIVE GROWTH AT THIS STAGE IS RELATED TO THE DEVELOPMENT OF ABSTRACT THINKING. THIS IS THE PERIOD OF FORMAL OPERATIONS

Illustration of Principle

Piaget's fourth stage of cognitive development is the period of *formal operations.* During this stage, adolescents will develop the capacity for abstract thinking. They will become capable of scientific reasoning and formal logic. They can begin to direct their thoughts to the future, to the possibilities that lie ahead of them. By utilizing these new abilities and thought processes, they can begin to plan the future and see themselves and others—the world—in a much more realistic fashion.

PRINCIPLE

CONCERNS RELATED TO BODY IMAGE ARE OF PARAMOUNT CONCERN TO THE ADOLESCENT

Illustration of Principle

As a result of the rapid growth and sexual development of their bodies, adolescents typically suffer from difficulties in adjusting to their new appearances. Depending upon their personal perceptions and the perceptions of their peers, adolescents may attempt to hide their bodies or, on the other hand, may flaunt them. Peer acceptance of their appearance is very important to adolescents. They are constantly comparing themselves with others. They will make judgments about themselves, about what is normal based on peer standards and norms. This process will eventually influence their perceptions of personal body, perceptions that they will maintain throughout the remainder of their lives.

Memory jog

SPECIAL PROBLEMS OR CONCERNS

1. Protection from injury (motor vehicles, firearms)
2. Substance abuse (smoking, alcohol, drugs)
3. Sports-related injury
4. Acne
5. Alterations in maturation
   a. Short stature, tall stature
   b. Precocious puberty
   c. Dysmenorrhea
6. Adolescent pregnancy
7. Sexually transmitted diseases

NURSING CONSIDERATIONS

1. Nutrition guidance
2. Sexual counseling
3. Personal hygiene
4. Contraception

CONCEPT: SOCIAL DEVELOPMENT IN CHILDHOOD

Social development throughout childhood is closely linked to interaction with people (peers, parents, family) and through play activities.

PRINCIPLE

PLAY IS THE WORK OF A CHILD

Illustration of Principle

Infant

Infant play activities are primarily centered around his body. The infant finds pleasure through these play activities that are the major source of sensory stimulation for infants. A great deal of intrapersonal contact during play is of the greatest importance to infants, more than the quality of the toy. For example, paper to crumple is just as stimulating as a colorful rattle; likewise, wooden spoons and plastic bowls are very entertaining.

Toddler

The toddler requires a higher level of intrapersonal interaction during play. The toddler is capable of parallel play or playing beside another child. One of the most characteristic elements of toddler play is the toddler's use of vivid imagination. They can paint the house for hours with a brush and a pail of water, and they can "keep house" as well as any parent. For the toddler, falling is a very important means of play. They enjoy radios, television, and reading stories.

Preschooler

Preschoolers particularly enjoy "associative play." Most characteristic of the preschooler, though, is imitative play. They enjoy dress up, playing house, doctor kits, or any activity in which they can pretend or act out adult roles. Preschoolers have a difficult time separating reality from fantasy. This is particularly evident when their imaginary friends stay for dinner after the play activity has ended. The development of imaginary friends or playmates is normal and quite useful for the child of this age. They can keep a child company when no one else has time, suffer many misfortunes, and take the blame without protest when called upon.

School-Aged Child

Play at this stage is a total reflection of the child's developmental growth. It is more organized, intelligent, and creative. Play in peer groups of the same sex is most particular of children of this developmental age group. "Team play" teaches the child many lessons: taking turns, respect for rules, support of team goals, team success or failure, nature of competition.

Adolescent

Play activities are primarily related to peer group activities, which may be organized school activities, sports, or just "hanging out" in groups. Adolescents enjoy games and activities that test their intellectual abilities as well as their physical abilities.

Reasoning Exercises: Growth and Development

Mrs. Owens brings Patrick, aged 2 months, to the clinic for a well child visit and to receive his first immunizations. The nurse weighs Patrick and performs a physical examination. He weighs 12 pounds. His birth weight was 8 pounds, 6 ounces. His vital signs are within normal limits. By physical examination, Patrick appears to be very healthy and well cared for.

1. After the nurse weighs Patrick, Mrs. Owens states, "Patrick seems to be so fat. He's much bigger than my sister's little girl was at 2 months." The nurse should respond by explaining that

   A. Not all babies grow at the same pace.

   B. Girls tend to be smaller than boys.

   C. His weight is within normal limits.

   D. Supplementation with water will help slow down his weight gain.

The nurse would understand that normal weight gain for infants is approximately 1½ pounds per month until approximately 6 months of age. Patrick has increased his weight by approximately 4 pounds, which is within the normal limits. Therefore, **C** is the correct response.

2. The nurse should recognize which of the following to be true of Patrick's fine motor development at this age?

   A. Until the establishment of the pincer grasp he will be unable to hold things.

   B. The 2 month old's grasp is primarily reflexive.

   C. At 2 months he should be able to grasp an object by holding it with two hands.

   D. He will not be able to hold a rattle until 3 months of age.

The correct response is **B**. The nurse should recognize that the 2 month old's grasp is purely reflexive. An infant may hold something in his hands for short periods of time, but only because something happened to come into contact with his open hand. The way in which an infant holds onto the blankets and sheets is a good example of the reflexive grasp of the 2 month old.

3. The nurse should encourage Mrs. Owens to focus on play activities that will stimulate the senses. All the following toys would be appropriate for Patrick except which of the following?

   A. Unbreakable mirrors

   B. Nursery mobiles

   C. Music boxes

   D. Squeaky animals

Although Patrick will find the noise made by the squeaky animal interesting, it will not offer much stimulation unless someone is there to play with him. Therefore, **D** is the correct response. Each of the other responses are appropriate choices for a 2 month old, providing sensory stimulation. At 2 months of age the infant can interact independently with the mirror, mobile, and the music box.

Kelly Jones, aged 3 years, is brought to the emergency room by her mother following an accidental ingestion of acetaminophen. When questioned, Mrs. Jones states that she believes that Kelly ingested approximately 20 tablets. She further states that she believes that the ingestion occurred within the last hour.

1. Immediately upon arrival in the emergency room the nurse should

   A. Assess vital signs

   B. Administer O_2

   C. Start IV fluids

   D. Perform an arterial puncture for blood gases

A is the correct response. The establishment of baseline vital signs should always be done first. Although hyperventilation and resultant respiratory alkalosis is the most obvious clinical manifestation, acetaminophen does not exert its peak effect until 2 to 4 hours following ingestion. Performing an arterial puncture for blood-gas analysis will be important, but it is not the first thing that the nurse should do. There is no indication at this time for the administration of O_2 or IV fluids.

2. The nurse should understand that acute overdose of acetaminophen most severely affects which of the following body organs?

   A. Lungs

   B. Brain

   C. Liver

   D. Kidneys

Damage to the liver is not done by the drug itself, but by the metabolites that are toxic to the liver. With large amounts of metabolites, the liver is unable to produce enough fluthathione to negate its toxic effects, and liver necrosis will result. The correct response is **C**.

3. In order to help Mrs. Jones plan to child proof her home, the nurse should understand which of the following about the preschool-aged child?

    A. Preschoolers are not very obedient; they will often play with things that they are told not to touch.

    B. Preschoolers take pills only to get attention of their parents.

    C. Preschoolers are very inquisitive and often explore things that they should not.

    D. Preschoolers will only take poisons or pills if they are left unattended.

C is the correct response. The preschool aged child's task is to explore as many objects and situations as possible on a daily basis. Many accidental ingestions have occurred while the parent is right in the room with the child. Because the preschooler is inquisitive and seems to always get into everything under the sun, sometimes all at once, it is important that the nurse help the parent to focus on childproofing the home in order to prevent accidents from occurring.

4. Which of the following instructions given by the nurse would be most helpful to Mrs. Jones?

    A. Post the telephone number of the poison control center by the telephone.

    B. Never leave a preschool child unattended.

    C. Preschoolers usually learn from their experiences; therefore, the child is not likely to ingest poison again.

    D. Place "danger" label on all dangerous substances, and teach the child to recognize the label and not touch those substances.

D is the correct response. The child at this age will easily learn to avoid items that are labeled, indicating the items are or substances are dangerous. "Mr. Yuck" labels are an example of one such label. It would be most helpful for the nurse to help Mrs. Jones to focus on strategies that will help prevent ingestion in the future.

21

SURGICAL INTERVENTION

NANCY B. CAILLES

PRINCIPLE

THE PRIMARY GOAL FOR THE IMMEDIATE POSTOPERATIVE PATIENT IS TO ESTABLISH BALANCE

Illustration of Principle

Surgical intervention presents a major insult to the normal functioning of the body's systems.

Critical assessment of the immediate postoperative patient includes

▷ Patency of airway
▷ Vital signs—values and qualities
▷ Adequacy of peripheral circulation
▷ Regulation of core body temperature
▷ Fluid status and regulation
▷ Level of consciousness and orientation

Nursing Management

Optimally, all data gathered from these assessment criteria would indicate a return to normal state, evidencing a reestablishment of physiological balance. Since surgical patients are cooled to reduce risk for bleeding, the nurse should note a steady increase in body temperature to normal or slightly elevated levels. Recovering patients should show an increase in level of consciousness and awareness, becoming able to correctly orient themselves to the postsurgical environment. Respirations should become spontaneous, unlabored, and adequate as the effects of anesthesia dissipate.

243

Assessment data that indicate a movement *away* from normal parameters should alert the nurse to possible postoperative complications. Accelerating respiratory rates may indicate inadequate oxygenation; precipitious falls in arterial blood pressure may signal fluid loss or hemorrhage. The nurse should remain alert for any such indications and take appropriate action to ensure the postoperative well-being and safety of the patient.

PRINCIPLE

SURGICAL INTERVENTION INHERENTLY PLACES THE PATIENT AT RISK FOR INFECTION

Illustration of Principle

Since most surgical procedures involve the opening of skin layers, the body's first line of defense against the invasion of microorganisms and contaminants is compromised, placing the surgical patient at risk for the development of infection. Additionally, surgical intervention compromises defense against infection in the following ways:

▷ Surgery may involve the opening of sterile body cavities, such as the lung, bladder, uterus, or peritoneum.

▷ Surgery places an additional stress on the body, possibly decreasing its resistance to infection.

▷ Postoperative convalescence may influence risk for infection secondary to anorexia associated with discomfort or anesthesia, bedrest with decreased circulation, or contamination of the wound associated with handling during dressing changes and irrigations.

Nursing Management

Because of these risks, the nurse must have an ongoing awareness of the patient's immune status following surgery, focusing on signs of developing infection:

▷ Elevated body temperature

▷ Elevated white blood cell count

▷ Increase in severity of pain at the surgical site

▷ Increase in swelling, redness, or tenderness at the surgical site

▷ Change in wound drainage from the expected (sanguinous, serosanguinous) to purulent

The nurse should assess the patient's operative site routinely for evidence of the progress of healing. Wounds healing in the expected manner should have the following characteristics:

▷ Wound edges in close approximation (first intention healing)

▷ Sutures or staples intact, with no evidence of pulling or gaping of the wound edges

▷ Absence of redness, swelling, or tenderness at wound site

▷ Absence of foul odor or purulent drainage from surgical wound

The nurse should plan interventions aimed at preventing or containing postoperative infection, such as careful handling of dressing materials, use of sterile technique in wound care, and observance of isolation restrictions for wound drainage should they apply. The most valuable method for infection management, however, is the simplest—*thorough handwashing* before and after contact with the patient.

> Since surgery involves the opening of skin layers, the body is at risk for infection from invading microorganisms. The nurse should conscientiously utilize handwashing before and after contact with the patient to reduce the risk for the development of postoperative infection.

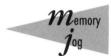

Memory Jog

PRINCIPLE

THE STRESS OF SURGICAL INTERVENTION INCREASES THE BODY'S NUTRITIONAL NEEDS TO EFFECT HEALING

Illustration of Principle

Nutritional factors play a significant role in timely and complete postoperative healing. Typically, the recovering patient requires the following:

▷ Increased protein for tissue repair

▷ Increased carbohydrate to be used by the body for energy, thus sparing the protein for tissue repair

▷ Increased fluids as allowed to flush out residual anesthesia and reduce risk for postoperative fluid and electrolyte imbalance

▷ Increased vitamin C for tissue healing

Nursing Management

The nurse should assess the readiness for oral intake of foods and fluids, guided by physician order and the patient's ability to swallow and retain intake following surgery. Mild, transient anorexia can be expected in the early recovery period and can be managed by offering the patient small, frequent feedings rather than full meals. Oral fluids should be encouraged as early as possible and permitted. If the patient enjoyed a healthy nutritional status prior to surgery, a general (regular) postoperative diet will provide ample amounts of the above nutritional requirements to promote healing. However, if the patient was in a poor nutritional state preoperatively as evidenced by significant weight loss, poor skin turgor and repair, and pale coloring then additional nutritional snacks and supplements are indicated. Hyperalimentation (parenteral nutrition) is indicated as a therapy to counteract serious malnutrition that could compromise healing during the recovery period.

*M*emory
*J*og

> Postoperative patients should have ample sources of protein, carbohydrate, fluids, and vitamin C to promote effective and timely healing in the recovery period.

PRINCIPLE

PROCESSES OR MEASURES THAT SLOW OR HALT PERISTALSIS DECREASE THE BODY'S ABILITY TO METABOLIZE AND ABSORB FOODS

Illustration of Principle

This principle is readily applied to the surgical patient because general anesthesia markedly decreases or halts the process of peristalsis in the gastrointestinal tract, thus negatively influencing the body's ability to metabolize, absorb, transport, or eliminate foods. For this reason, patients who have undergone surgery with general anesthesia, patients who have experienced prolonged surgeries, or clients who have had abdominal surgery should be assessed carefully for readiness for and tolerance to oral intake.

Nursing Management

In view of this effect of anesthesia and surgery, the nurse caring for the postoperative patient should include as a *routine* assessment the activity of peristalsis by the auscultation of bowel sounds. Absence of bowel sounds is common after surgery and is an indication that the patient is *not* ready for oral intake. This patient should remain NPO until peristaltic activity is noted, and then may be advanced to ice chips and clear fluids gradually. Presence of bowel sound activity in all four quadrants indicates a readiness for oral intake.

Typically, oral fluids for postoperative patients are advanced from clear fluids such as ice chips, water, or juices to more complex foods and fluids steadily as oral tolerance is verified. Patients who experience severe nausea or vomiting with oral intake should be reversed back to NPO status until oral tolerance is assured.

Providing complex foods to a patient with inadequate peristalsis places him at risk for a number of complications, including constipation, fecal impaction, bowel obstruction, and paralytic ileus. It is evident from this list of possible complications that postoperative diet is an important consideration for the nurse.

It is important to note that continuous use of narcotic analgesia for pain management in the postoperative phase may precipitate constipation, with abdominal firmness and bloating, abdominal fullness and discomfort, and decreased or absent passing of flatus and stool. Because narcotics significantly reduce peristaltic activity in much the same way as general anesthesia does, the nurse caring for the postsurgical patient receiving narcotic pain medications should monitor elimination patterns and subsequent readiness and tolerance of oral intake.

> Since perioperative anesthesia can slow or halt peristalsis, the nurse must check for the presence of active bowel sounds before allowing the postoperative patient foods or fluids.

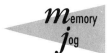

PRINCIPLE

POSTOPERATIVE PAIN DECREASES WITH EACH SUCCESSIVE DAY AFTER SURGERY

Illustration of Principle

Unlike the chronic pain associated with arthritis or advanced malignancy, postoperative pain diminishes in its intensity and frequency with each successive day following surgery. Typically, the patient will experience his most severe or acute pain on the first postoperative day, with diminution of pain as recovery progresses. In light of this principle, postoperative pain management is typically initiated with medication of greater strength and duration, such as narcotic analgesia. Intravenous or intramuscular routes are most often selected to enhance pain management. Analgesia is then slowly tapered with each successive day, and the patient will likely be placed on oral analgesia of less potency as his recovery progresses.

Nursing Management

Prior to administering pain medication, the nurse should assess the patient's pain for the following characteristics:

▷ Location (helpful to ask patient to *point* to source of pain)

▷ Type (dull, aching, sharp, stabbing, burning)

▷ Severity (on a scale of 1 to 10, with 10 being most severe)

▷ Frequency (how often pain recurs following medication)

▷ Success of previous management (pain relief with previous medication)

Following administration of medication, the nurse should observe for relief of pain as well as any side-effects of the medication, such as drowsiness, lethargy, disorientation, hypotension, and so on. The nurse can enhance pain relief with medication by using measures to calm and reassure the patient, since anxiety will exacerbate the pain experience. The patient should receive instruction on measures that will decrease postoperative pain, such as splinting the abdomen for coughing and movement after abdominal surgery or laying the patient in the lateral position to facilitate expulsion of flatus.

It is evident, then, that if the patient's pain does *not* seem to be decreasing with each successive postoperative day, the possibility of physiological or psychologic factors that could exacerbate pain should be explored. For example, if the patient continues to complain of acute pain in his fourth and fifth days postappendectomy, the possibility of a physiological problem such as peritonitis or a psychological problem such as anxiety should be ruled out to determine the cause of the continued pain.

> Postoperative pain is an expected occurrence that should decrease as each postoperative day passes. Nurses should anticipate using stronger, typically narcotic analgesia the first few days, tapering the strength and frequency of medication as pain subsides.

PRINCIPLE

THE PROCESS OF SURGICAL INTERVENTION POTENTIATES CHANGES IN BOTH BODY IMAGE AND ROLE PERCEPTION OF THE SURGICAL PATIENT

Illustration of Principle

Depending on the type and involvement of surgery, a patient may be faced with significant changes in his perceptions about his physical appearance, his attractiveness and desirability, and his concept of gender roles and work roles in employment as well as in a family structure. A patient with bowel obstruction facing the surgical creation of a temporary colostomy is confronted with changes in his body image and potential anxiety over his physical appearance and attractiveness. A male patient undergoing prostate surgery may feel ill at ease about exposure of his genitals to a predominantly female nursing staff. A middle-aged female could easily fear hysterectomy surgery, not only for the physical changes this surgery will cause, but also for the interruption in daily living that the postoperative convalescence will bring about. Finally, even minor surgery such as removal of a mole may cause anxiety for the patient if there is a question about a possible malignancy of that mole tissue.

Nursing Management

The nurse caring for the surgical patient should routinely include in a preoperative assessment questions that will provide information about the patient's background, work and family roles, and perceptions of self. The nurse should anticipate typical questions the patient may have, and plan to address any concerns that most surgical patients have when facing upcoming surgery, knowledge specifically correlating to the type of surgery. For example, most surgical patients will have questions about the length of their postoperative recovery period, what if any restrictions they will have after surgery, any dietary modifications they may need to make, or how postoperative pain will be managed. The nurse caring for the patient undergoing a total abdominal hysterectomy, then, should share with the patient preoperatively that the expected hospitalization will be approximately 4 to 6 days following surgery, during which time her diet will be advanced slowly as tolerated. The patient may expect some limitations on her physical activity (heavy housework, stair climbing) and on sexual intercourse for a period of 4 to 6 weeks postoperatively. Pain will be managed with narcotic injections and then with oral analgesics.

Preparation of the patient in such a manner helps to decrease preoperative fears and anxieties, which should then make the recovery period less difficult and more predictable. Likewise, providing the patient with answers to questions will reduce the unknowns of the surgical experience and will foster greater understanding and cooperation between patient and nurse.

PRINCIPLE

THE IDEAL MANAGEMENT OF THE UNKNOWNS IN THE SURGICAL EXPERIENCE IS THE PROVISION OF ADEQUATE
AND TIMELY PREOPERATIVE PATIENT TEACHING

Illustration of Principle

As discussed in the illustration of the previous principle, informational preparation of the patient undergoing surgery is a critical nursing intervention. The patient facing surgery will undergo a number of changes in normal day-to-day functioning that will be foreign or unknown to him. For example, the patient may have concerns about exposure of his body in the surgical suite or may fear that he will expose himself emotionally because of loss of inhibitions under anesthesia's influence. Patients may cling to erroneous old wives' tales about medical interventions that could cause them unnecessary anxiety. If the patient believes that receiving a blood transfusion means that the individual is critically ill or close to death, for example, he may unnecessarily fear administration of blood products before, during, or after surgery. Informational instruction pertinent to the type of surgery and explained in simple, concise terms will help dispel misconceptions and thus reduce the patient's preoperative anxiety over the "unknowns" that he faces related to the surgical procedure.

It is presumptuous and foolhardy for the nurse to believe that patients are medically aware and enlightened and that they thus understand the general concepts and procedures involved in their surgeries. For example, if the nurse tells the patient that he will be held *NPO* prior to his surgery, there is an underlying belief that the patient will have an appreciation of the meaning of that abbreviation and its application to preoperative management. Because all patients are unique and have different levels of education and awareness, the nurse is wisest to evaluate the patient's level of knowledge, rather than assume that he possesses a set level of knowledge, no matter how simple the principles, concepts, or procedures involved.

Some predictable unknowns that can be managed effectively through adequate and timely preoperative teaching include the following:

▷ The need for turning, coughing, and deep breathing after surgery to mobilize lung secretions and prevent pneumonia

▷ The role of early ambulation in preventing complications associated with immobility (*e.g.* venous stasis, thrombus)

▷ The purpose of NPO and diet advancement orders

▷ The purpose and function of tubes or drains postoperatively (Penrose drain, Jackson-Pratt, IV tubing, endotracheal tube)

▷ Methods of pain management, including medication, positioning, transcutaneous nerve stimulator units

Memory jog

> Timely and appropriate preoperative teaching is a valuable way to reduce postoperative anxieties and complications.

Reasoning Exercises: Surgical Intervention

Louise Eubanks is scheduled for a biopsy with possible mastectomy of her right breast after a lump in the upper outer quadrant was noted by her physician and outlined on mammography.

1. During the admission procedures, Louise asks the nurse, "Will I have a lot of pain with this type of surgery?" The most appropriate response of the nurse would be

A. "You seem worried about your upcoming surgery."

B. "Your physician will order medications to control any pain you experience following your surgery."

C. "All patients react differently to surgery—it's impossible to tell what pain you might experience after the procedure."

D. "The nurses will make sure that you don't have any pain following your surgery."

The intended response is **B**, since it provides the most accurate information about pain and pain management following surgery. Response **A** focuses on the patient's concerns and possible fears but supplies no information about postoperative pain management. Response **C** is incorrect, because postoperative pain *is* predictable and expected. Response **D** may offer the patient false reassurance, because it isn't always possible to eliminate a postoperative patient's pain completely. Much as we nurses would like our patients to be pain-free, this goal is clearly unrealistic.

2. The night prior to surgery, the nurse enters the room to find Louise alone quietly weeping. The most appropriate initial response of the nurse would be to

A. Leave the room quietly and close the patient's door

B. Apologize for disturbing the patient and return to the room later

C. Sit with the patient silently and use therapeutic touch

D. Ask the patient if there is a family member the patient would like to be with

The intended response is **C**, since sitting with the patient and using touch therapeutically conveys the nurse's interest and concern for the patient, which will help to reduce the patient's preoperative fears and anxieties. Responses **A** and **B** convey a message of avoidance of the patient and offer no support to the patient. Response **D** is ineffective because the nurse is not offering self, but rather a family member to support the patient.

Louise undergoes a modified radical mastectomy with complete removal of her right breast and some axillary lymph nodes following confirmation of breast malignancy.

3. The nurse preparing a care plan for Louise should include all of the following nursing diagnoses *except:*

A. Self-care deficit related to use of the upper right extremity

B. Disturbance in self-concept and body image

C. Fluid volume deficit related to lymphatic surgery

D. Alteration in comfort related to surgical procedure

The intended response is **C**, since the lymphatic surgery would lead to a fluid volume *excess,* with resultant edema of the upper right extremity. (Remember—this is an *except* question.) Response **A** is appropriate for this patient because the surgery will result in a temporary impairment of the patient's ability to use her upper right extremity freely. Response **B** is appropriate to the patient because the surgical procedure is a disfiguring one, with resultant changes in body image and self-concept. Finally, response **D** is appropriate to the patient, because pain and discomfort are expected outcomes of surgery.

4. On her second postoperative day, Louise complains of severe pain in her upper right surgical and shoulder areas. Which of the following analgesic medications would the nurse most likely administer to Louise?

   A. Morphine grains i I.M.

   B. Demerol 75 mg I.M.

   C. Percodan tablets ii P.O.

   D. Tylenol #3 1 tablet P.O.

The intended response is **B**, since narcotic analgesia administered per I.M. route is most indicated for postoperative pain on the second post-surgical day. Although response **A** also offers a narcotic analgesic with an I.M. route, the dosage is *much too high* (1 grain = 60 mg). Responses **C** and **D** are incorrect, because the oral route of analgesia would be much less effective for pain management for a second day postoperative patient.

5. The nurse caring for Louise on her second postsurgical day should reinforce teaching for the patient to do all of the following *except*

   A. Turn, cough, and deep-breathe several times each shift

   B. Maintain a semi-Fowler's position when in bed

   C. Elevate the affected arm on pillows

   D. Expect a scant amount of clear serous drainage in the surgical Hemovac

The intended response is **D**, since the drainage in the surgical Hemovac would likely be sanguinous (deep red) or serosanguinous (reddish-pink) and not clear serous. If the patient was expecting a clear drainage, the presence of a deep red drainage in her Hemovac drain would likely cause her undue alarm and concern. Responses **A, B,** and **C** are appropriate interventions to prevent postoperative complications. Response **A** serves to decrease risk of stasis pneumonia, response **B** to enhance ventilation capacity and lung expansion, and response **C** to reduce postoperative edema in the affected extremity.

PHARMACOLOGIC INTERVENTION AND MEDICATION DOSAGE CALCULATION

NANCY B. CAILLES

PRINCIPLE

THE FIRST STEP TO CALCULATING A PRESCRIBED MEDICATION DOSAGE IS TO COMMUNICATE

Illustration of Principle

When we think about the process of *communication*, we think about the use of language in order to relay a message. Indeed, the process of calculating correct dosages of medication requires that same process, that is, the use of language. The languages utilized in medication administration are the three systems of weights and measures utilized in medical practice in the United States, each system having unique words, symbols, and abbreviations to describe the same ideas, just as three different languages would. For example, fluid measurements of medications can be communicated in terms of drams, teaspoons, or milliliters, and can be symbolized as ʒ, tsp, or mL. In order to administer the correct dose of a prescribed medication, the nurse must be "fluent" in the three systems of weights and measures or measurement languages, so that "translation" of words and symbols used in each of the three different systems will be done correctly.

Three systems of weights and measures currently used in medical practice in the United States are the English system, apothecary system, and metric system.

English System

The system of weights and measures that is probably most familiar to the American nurse is the English system, since it is this system used in America to measure most food products, liquids, gasoline, ingredients for recipes.

Key measures of the English system include the following:

Volume

teaspoon (tsp)

tablespoon (tbsp)

cup (c)

ounce (oz)

pint (pt)

quart (qt)

gallon (gal)

Weight

teaspoon (tsp)

tablespoon (tbsp)

cup (c)

ounce (oz)

pound (lb)

Amounts of medication are expressed in whole numbers and fractions, such as "2 tsp" or "½ tbsp".

The second system of weights and measures is the

Apothecary System

Utilized in ancient times for the distribution of medicinal potions and treatments, its measures are foreign to Americans and are now used exclusively in medical and pharmaceutical practice.

Key measures of the apothecarcy system include the following:

Volume

drop

minim (m.)

dram ($\mathfrak{z}$)

ounce ($\mathfrak{z}$)

Weight

grain (gr)

Amounts of medication are expressed in terms of the Roman numeral system, either in small case or in upper case. For example, *gr X* means 10 grains and $\mathfrak{z}$ *ii* means 2 drams. Fractions of whole numbers are expressed as such, that is, "gr ⅙" or "one sixth of a grain."

Metric System

The third and final system is also the simplest and most exact system of measurement, the metric system. This system is based on the number 10 and its multiples. For example, the prefix *milli* in milligram expresses *one-thousandth gram.* Fractions of whole numbers are expressed in terms of *decimals* in the tenths and hundredths. In this system, very small quantities of medications can be measured much more accurately than in the other two systems, because decimals are far more precise than are fraction dosages used in the English and apothecary systems. It is the exactness, then, of the metric system that makes it the system most ideal and valuable for medical practice.

Key measures of the metric system include

Volume
liter (L)
milliliter (mL)
cubic centimeter (cc)

Weight
gram (g)
milligram (mg)
kilogram (kg)

Amounts of medication are expressed in whole numbers or decimals of whole numbers, such as "1000 mL", "1.5 cc" or "0.5 mg."

The first step in calculating the correct dosage of a medication, then, is to identify which system, or "language," is being used in the medication order compared with the medication label—to communicate between the order and label.

Consider the example below:

Order: ASA gr X Q4° PRN for temp 100°F

Label: ASA 350 mg = 1 tablet

In the example above, the nurse notes that the physician's order reads "Aspirin 10 grains for temperatures greater than 100°F." The medication label, however, indicates that the medication weight is measured in terms of milligrams.

In this first step, then, the nurse *communicates* between order and label and notes that the order is written in the apothecary system, but the medication is distributed according to the label in the metric system.

PRINCIPLE

MEDICATION CALCULATIONS CANNOT BE COMPLETED WHEN UNLIKE SYSTEMS OF MEASURES ARE BEING UTILIZED. THE NURSE MUST **CONVERT** THE UNITS OF MEASURE UTILIZED IN THE MEDICATION **ORDER** TO THE UNITS UTILIZED ON THE MEDICATION **LABEL**

Illustration of Principle

Remembering that the systems of measurement are like three different languages, the nurse must be able to translate the meanings of words and symbols used in one system to another system, so that both the order and the label are "speaking the same language."

Consider the sample below:

Order: Morphine sulfate gr 1/6 IM STAT

Label: Morphine sulfate 10 mg = 1.0 cc

Since the order is written in the apothecary system and the label in the metric system, the nurse, prior to dosage calculation, must convert or translate the units of measure in the order to the units of measure on the label.

Since 60 mg = 1 gr; the conversion is

gr 1/6 $\times$ 60 = 10 mg

Our medication order in this example *now* reads:

morphine sulfate 10 mg IM STAT

PRINCIPLE

THE LAST STEP IN DETERMINING THE CORRECT DOSAGE OF A MEDICATION IS TO **CALCULATE**

Illustration of Principle

Once the nurse has communicated between the medication order and label and has performed any necessary conversions, the calculation of the medication dosage is possible.

Therefore, the calculation of correct dosage is as simple as the 3 C's—*Communicate, Convert, Calculate.*

Completing the example from above:

Since morphine sulfate gr 1/6 = 10 mg as desired dose in metric, the dose calculation can be completed by utilizing this simple formula:

$$\frac{\text{Amount of med ordered}}{\text{Amount of med available}} \times \text{Unit} = \text{Med Dose}$$

$$\frac{10 \text{ mg}}{10 \text{ mg}} \times 1 \text{ cc} = 1 \times 1 = \textit{1 cc}$$

Since the NCLEX examination requires mathematical conversions from one system of measurement to another by memory and without assistance from charts or conversion tables, we recommend that candidates for the examination learn the following conversion equivalents.

Volume

1 mL = 1 cc = 15 M = 15 drops

1 dram = 5 cc = 1 tsp

1 ounce = 30 cc = 2 tbsp

Weight

1 gr = 60 mg

1 g = 1000 mg

1 kg = 2/2 lb

Reasoning Exercises

Try to recall the equivalencies for these conversions below.

1. 1 L = _____ mL
2. 2 drams = _____ mL
3. 30 mL = _____ tbsp
4. 10 gr = _____ mg
5. 1 tsp = _____ 3
6. 30 M = _____ ml
7. gr 1/6 = _____ mg
8. 1 gm = _____ mg
9. 45 drops = _____ mL
10. 10 kg = _____ lb

The correct responses for the above conversions are

1. 1000
2. 10
3. 2
4. 600
5. 1
6. 2
7. 10
8. 1000
9. 3
10. 22

PRINCIPLE

FLOW RATES OF IV FLUIDS MAY BE EXPRESSED IN TERMS OF **MILLILITERS PER HOUR** OR **DROPS PER MINUTE**

Illustration of Principle

The mathematical calculations required to determine flow rates for IV fluids are relatively simple, utilizing this formula:

$$\frac{\text{Total amount of IV fluid to infuse in milliliters}}{\text{Total time of infusion in hours}}$$

Consider the example below:

Order

$$\text{1000 cc of D5W to infuse in 8 hr}$$

Since the nurse is aware that cubic centimeters is an equal measure for milliliters, the flow rate of milliliters per hour is easily calculated using the formula above.

$$\frac{1000 \text{ mL}}{8 \text{ hr}} = 125 \text{ mL/hr flow rate}$$

In order to calculate the drops per minute, another factor must be added to the mathematical formula above, the *drop factor,* that is, the number of drops per milliliter that the IV tubing delivers.

Thus, in order to determine the drops per minute in the IV fluid order above, the formula the nurse would utilize is

$$\frac{\begin{array}{c}\text{Total amount of IV fluid}\\ \text{in milliliters}\end{array}}{\begin{array}{c}\text{Total time of infusion}\\ \text{in minutes}\end{array}} \times \text{Drop Factor} = \text{drops per minute}$$

From the example above, the calculation of drops per minute would be performed as follows:

$$\frac{1000 \text{ mL}}{8 \times 60 = 480 \text{ min}} \times \text{Drop Factor} = 10 \text{ drops/mL}$$

$$\frac{1000 \text{ mL}}{480 \text{ min}} \times 10 = 2.08 \times 10 = 20 \text{ drops/min}$$

In the example above, the number 8 in the hundredths decimal place is dropped, since it is too small a measure to have meaning.

PRINCIPLE

WHEN A SET DOSAGE OF MEDICATION IS ADDED TO IV FLUIDS, THE FLOW RATE SHOULD BE CALCULATED IN TERMS OF AMOUNT OF MEDICATION INFUSED RATHER THAN AMOUNT OF IV FLUIDS INFUSED

Illustration of Principle

A physician may order a client to receive a set concentration or dosage of medication by IV drip route, and this requires that the nurse focus attention on the amount of medication infusing per hour or per minute, rather than the amount of IV fluids infusing.

Consider the example below:

The physician has ordered a client to receive a total dosage of 20,000 units of Heparin in 500 cc of IV fluid. The client is to receive 1000 units/hr. The drop factor is 10 drops per milliliter. How many drops per minute will the client receive?

First, the total time of infusion must be determined in order to calculate drops/minute.

If the client is to receive a total dosage of 20,000 units at 1000 units/hour, the IV infusion is then to run for 20 hours. Thus, the total time of infusion is *20 hours,* or 1200 minutes.

Now, the IV infusion calculation formula may be utilized:

$$\frac{500 \text{ cc}}{1200 \text{ min}} \times 10 = .41 \times 10 = 4.1 \text{ or 4 drops/min}$$

Reasoning Exercises: Pharmacologic Intervention and Medication Dosage Calculation

Try to apply the principles for medication and IV fluid calculations in the reasoning exercises below.

1. The physician has ordered the patient to receive gr 1/150 preoperatively. The label indicates that atropine 0.4 mg = 1 cc. How many cc should the nurse administer?

    A. 0.5 cc

    B. 0.8 cc

C. 1.0 cc

D. 1.2 cc

The correct response is **C.**

Since the medication order is in the apothecary system and the label is in the metric system, a conversion of order to label is necessary in this situation.

$$\text{gr } 1/150 \times 60 = 0.4 \text{ mg}$$

Next, the calculation formula is utilized:

$$\frac{0.4 \text{ mg}}{0.4 \text{ mg}} \times 1 \text{ cc} = 1 \times 1 = \textit{1 cc}$$

2. Mr. Davis is to receive phenobarbital gr i ss P.O. The label reads phenobarbital 100 mg = 10 mL. How many mL should the nurse administer?

A. 5 mL

B. 7 mL

C. 9 mL

D. 11 mL

The correct response is **C.**

Again, a conversion from the apothecary system to the metric system is required before a calculation of dosage can be completed.

gr i ss = gr 1½, since the symbol "ss" stands for "half"
in the apothecary system.

$$\text{gr } 1\frac{1}{2} \times 60 = 90 \text{ mg}$$

Next, the calculation formula is utilized:

$$\frac{90 \text{ mg}}{100 \text{ mg}} \times 10 \text{ mL} = 0.9 \times 10 \text{ mL} = \textit{9.0 mL}$$

3. If a multidose vial of heparin contains 20,000 units in 10 cc, how many cc should the nurse administer to a patient who requires a 5000-unit dose?

A. 2.0 cc

B. 2.5 cc

C. 3.0 cc

D. 3.5 cc

The correct response is **B.**

Since both the order and the label are written in the same system (units), no conversion is required in this situation. The calculation formula can be immediately utilized:

$$\frac{5000 \text{ units}}{20{,}000 \text{ units}} \times 10 = .25 \times 10 = \textit{2.5 cc}$$

4. One liter of IV fluid is to infuse in 8 hours. The drop factor of the IV equipment is 10 drops/mL. How many drops per minute will the IV infuse?

A. 16 drops/min

B. 19 drops/min

C. 21 drops/min

D. 23 drops/min

The correct response is **C.**

No conversion is necessary with IV infusion rate problems. The formula for IV rate calculations may be used:

$$\frac{\text{Total amount of IV fluid to infuse in mL}}{\text{Total time to infuse in minutes}} \times \text{Drop Factor}$$

Since 1 liter = 1000 mL, the formula is implemented in the following way:

$$\frac{1000 \text{ mL}}{480 \text{ min}} \times 10 - 2.08 \times 10 = 20.8 \text{ or } \textit{21 drops/min}$$

5. The physician orders 1 gr of lidocaine in 500 cc 5% D/W to infuse at 4 mg/min per pump. How many cc/hr should the patient receive?

A. 80 cc/hr

B. 100 cc/hr

C. 120 cc/hr

D. 140 cc/hr

The correct response is **C.**

Determine the total amount of time in which the IV with lidocaine is to infuse.

Step One

$$\frac{100 \text{ mg } (1 \text{ g})}{4 \text{ mg/min}} \quad 250 \text{ min total infusion time}$$

Determine the rate of flow of lidocaine per hour in cc.

Step Two

$$\frac{500 \text{ cc (total amount of fluid)}}{250 \text{ min}} = 2 \text{ cc/min or } 120 \text{ cc/hr}$$

NUTRITION*

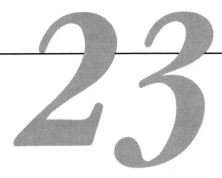

DIANE M. BLACK

PRINCIPLE

CARBOHYDRATES ARE THE HUMAN BODY'S FUEL SOURCE

Illustration of Principle

Much as a car needs gasoline to run, the human body needs carbohydrates to carry out its functions. Carbohydrates are needed for the following functions:

Energy source

Cellular nutrition

Maintenance of body temperature

Sparing usage of protein and fats

Promotion of lower GI functioning

Maintenance of blood glucose levels

When a car increases its speed, its gasoline requirements are greatly increased. Likewise, the human body needs carbohydrates in increased amounts in the presence of fever, hyperthyroidism, excessive exercise, and pregnancy. When the body does not receive an adequate supply of carbohydrates, it must utilize other sources, such as protein and fats, resulting in loss of weight.

* The categories of proteins, fats, carbohydrates, and vitamins are discussed in this chapter. Minerals are discussed in other chapters.

263

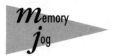

Carbohydrates are the most readily usable form of energy for body metabolism.

Sugars, starches, and fiber are the main forms in which carbohydrates occur in food. Sugars and starches are the main sources of energy for the body. Food sources of starches are plant foods, vegetables, breads, cereals, and grains; for example:

Potatoes

Macaroni

Rice

Food sources of sugars are fruits; for example:

Honey

Molasses

Grapefruit

Apples

Fiber, another plant component that is a carbohydrate, does not furnish energy but is needed for lower GI functioning.

Carbohydrate deficiency is manifested clinically as loss of weight, with protein sources being utilized for energy as fats are broken down to produce a state of ketosis. Prolonged carbohydrate deficiencies can lead to liver damage. Decreased fiber in the diet can lead to constipation and diverticulosis and may increase the occurrence of hemorrhoids, varicose veins, and hiatal hernias by increasing pressure in the colon.

Clients that present with carbohydrate deficiency may be anorexic or bulimic.

Clinical manifestations of overconsumption of carbohydrates are the opposite of those of carbohydrate deficiency. Excessive intake of starches and sugars can lead to obesity and dental caries.

Other clients at risk of impaired carbohydrate metabolism are clients with diabetes mellitus, in which carbohydrates are not metabolized because of a deficiency in insulin production by the pancreas.

PRINCIPLE

PROTEINS ARE THE BUILDING BLOCKS OF THE BODY, WHICH BREAK DOWN INTO AMINO ACIDS

Illustration of Principle

Proteins are the fundamental portion of the cell, much as a brick is the fundamental block of the building. The body is constantly under construction, with

new cell and tissue production. Therefore, the body requires protein throughout the lifespan, and particularly during periods of rapid growth (*e.g.,* pregnancy [baby under construction]; infancy to young adulthood).

Proteins are present in the human body in a number of forms and perform
various functions. One type of protein is an enzyme. Enzymes are proteins that
break down other proteins. Another type of protein, albumin, helps maintain
fluid balance in the body. Antibodies are proteins, as are hormones such as
thyroid and insulin. Proteins known as lipoproteins act as transport mechanisms. One important protein is collagen, which helps develop scar tissue.

> Proteins are the major nutrient for cellular and tissue growth and repair.

It is important to remember that when increased proteins are needed for
tissue repair, increased carbohydrates are required to meet the body's energy
needs and thus spare the protein for tissue repair.

Protein sources containing essential amino acids are those foods of high
biological value, such as eggs, milk and dairy products, meat, fish, and poultry.

The client who lacks protein in the diet in sufficient amounts will appear
weak and apathetic, with poor fat stores under the skin. The skin may appear
patchy and scaly, the hair loses its color, and wounds fail to heal.

Proteins are lost in the drainage of open wounds and in urine. Increased
protein intake is needed to promote tissue growth and repair when damage or
injury occurs in the body (*i.e.,* decubitus ulcers, surgery, preeclampsia). Protein is also needed when bodies are in states of catabolism, such as in clients
with anorexia, cachexia, or malnutrition (kwashiorkor and marasmus).

On the other hand, protein is not needed when the by-products of protein
metabolism (nitrogen) cannot be excreted or utilized, as in renal failure (urea
cannot be excreted) and cirrhosis of the liver (nitrogen binds with hydrogen
to form ammonia, leading to hepatic encephalopathy).

PRINCIPLE

FATS ARE THE BODY'S FUEL AND ENERGY STORAGE SYSTEMS AND ITS "CUSHIONS OF LIFE."

Illustration of Principle

Much like a gas station, which stores gasoline until it is pumped into cars, fats
are the repository of fuel for the human body. Excess carbohydrates are turned
into fats and stored for later use. Fats are also protein-sparing, which reduces
the need to use protein for energy. Fat has several other functions, such as
maintaining body temperature by acting as insulation, cushioning vital organs,
and facilitating absorption of fat-soluble vitamins A, D, E, and K.

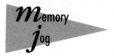

Fats are stored forms of energy that need carbohydrates for complete oxidation.

Fats are also classified as lipids. Those that are liquid are considered oils, while those that are solid are considered fats, which break down into triglycerides and fatty acids. Fatty acids are classified as saturated or unsaturated. Saturated fatty acids tend to be solid at room temperature (*i.e.,* a steak left on a table will begin to show white patches of fat as it reaches room temperature). Thus, animals are the greatest source of saturated fat.

The following are examples of saturated fats:

Beef

Pork

Poultry

Milk and milk products

Butter

Ice cream

Egg yolk

Unsaturated fats do not solidify at room temperature; thereby, vegetable oils are largely unsaturated fats. Examples of unsaturated fats are:

Safflower oil

Corn oil

Soybean oil

Essential fatty acids are needed by the body for normal nutrition but cannot be synthesized.

Cholesterol is a fat-soluble substance that is synthesized and stored in the liver. It is found in the blood and serves as a transporter of fat and a producer of vitamin D and hormones. Sources of cholesterol are egg yolk and animal brain. Other sources include butter, cream, cheese, and organ meats (heart, kidney, liver).

If there is inadequate fat in the body, there is no fuel for energy, no cushion, and no insulation. For example, a premature infant cannot regulate body temperature or meet the body's energy demands. Consequently, the infant is put under a radiant heater for thermoregulation and given high-calorie nutrition intravenously to meet energy demands.

On the other hand, too much intake of fat in the form of triglycerides and cholesterol can lead to obesity and various problems, such as atherosclerosis leading to myocardial infarction, cerebrovascular accident, peripheral vascular disease, or rupture of an artery.

Other clients at risk with intake of fats would include those with gallbladder dysfunction or pancreatitis. Bile is produced in the liver and stored in the gallbladder. Bile aids in emulsifying fats or breaking down fats into small particles for digestion and absorption. Thus if the common bile duct is blocked or liver disease is present, the client must restrict the intake of fat. If such a client eats fat digestion is blocked, but the client's hunger is satiated. Fat is then excreted as fatty acids along with vitamins A, D, E, and K. Therefore, this type of client needs supplementary intake of fat-soluble vitamins with increased intake of carbohydrates.

PRINCIPLE

VITAMINS ARE NUTRIENTS NECESSARY FOR LIFE AND GROWTH PROCESSES. VITAMINS FACILITATE THE USE OF ENERGY NUTRIENTS, THE REGULATION OF SOME BODY FUNCTIONS, AND THE MAINTENANCE OF BODY STRUCTURES. VITAMINS ARE CLASSIFIED AS EITHER FAT-SOLUBLE OR WATER-SOLUBLE.

Illustration of Principle

The fat-soluble vitamins are vitamins A, D, E, and K. These vitamins are soluble in fats and are absorbed from the intestinal tract in much the same way as fats.

> Bile is needed to emulsify fats; therefore, bile is necessary for absorption of fat-soluble vitamins.

These vitamins are stored in the body, mostly in the liver. Each vitamin has its own food sources, function, and symptoms of deficiency.

Vitamin A aids in the adaption of vision to dim light, maintenance of skin and mucous membranes, and formation of bones and teeth. Food sources high in vitamin A include yellow carotene foods and green leafy vegetables. Other sources are fish liver oil and animal liver. A deficiency of vitamin A can lead to night blindness and lowered resistance to infection.

Vitamin D aids in the absorption and mobilization of calcium for the development and maintenance of bones and teeth.

> Vitamin D is called the "sunshine vitamin."

Fortified milk is a food source high in vitamin D. A diet deficient in this vitamin will parallel a deficiency of calcium, leading to rickets and osteomalacia.

The functions of vitamin E are to protect vitamin A from oxidation in the intestines and guard the red blood cells from hemolysis. Vitamin E also increases the structural integrity of the cell membrane. Food sources include whole grains, nuts, and salad oils. A deficiency can lead to increased hemolysis of red blood cells.

Vitamin K, the blood-clotting vitamin, is needed for the formation of prothrombin. Food sources include green leafy vegetables. Vitamin K can also be synthesized by intestinal bacteria. A deficiency of this vitamin can lead to hemorrhage from lack of prothrombin.

Vitamin K injections are routinely given to newborns to enhance pro-thrombin production and prevent hemorrhagic disorders.

Clients who develop problems with fat absorption will also develop problems with fat-soluble vitamin depletion. Cholelithiasis with blocked ducts inhibits bile use, continued intake of mineral oil prevents absorption of nutrients, and celiac diseases prevent fat absorption. Clients that develop steatorrheic stools will eventually manifest signs and symptoms of fat-soluble vitamin deficiencies.

Any interference with fat absorption in the GI tract will also interfere in the absorption of fat-soluble vitamins.

Illustration of Principle

Water-soluble vitamins are the B and C complex vitamins. These vitamins are soluble in water and absorbed in the small intestines. Once the body has attained maximum saturation, the excess is excreted in the urine.

Vitamin C, also known as ascorbic acid, has a significant role in the formation of collagen. It also functions in the metabolism of amino acids, the absorption of iron, and the conversion of folatin to folinic acid.

Vitamin C is needed in increased amounts during growth phases and in tissue healing.

Vitamin C is found in citrus fruits such as strawberries, orange juice, and grapefruit. Dark green leafy vegetables are also high in vitamin C.

A deficiency of ascorbic acid can result in scurvy, a disease characterized by easy bruising, sore mouth and gums, and joint tenderness due to disruption of cartilage.

TABLE 23-1. VITAMIN B COMPLEX

Vitamin	Food Sources	Deficiency
Thiamine	Dry yeast, wheat germ, pork, enriched bread	Beriberi (nervous system manifestations)
Riboflavin	Organ meats, green leafy vegetables,	Cheilosis (scaly skin, cracked lips)
Niacin	Meat, poultry, fish, enriched products	Pellagra (dermatitis)
B_6 (pyridoxine)	Organ meats, legumes, nuts	CNS abnormalities
Pantothenic acid	Organ meats, eggs, yeast	
B_{12}	Organ meats, milk, fish	Pernicious anemia (lack of intrinsic factor)
Folacin	Green leafy vegetables	Macrocytic anemia
Biotin	Organ meats, peanuts	Anemia

Alcoholism, prolonged fasting (anorexia), and gastric carcinoma predispose clients to water-soluble vitamin deficiencies.

Vitamin B complex includes 12 fractions, the major ones being thiamine, riboflavin, niacin, B_{12}, folacin, pantothenic acid, and biotin. The major function of these vitamins is to aid in metabolism to provide energy.

Reasoning Exercises: Nutrition

Dianne, a 28-year-old female, is admitted to the hospital with a diagnosis of anorexia nervosa. She is 5'6" tall and weighs 90 pounds. She appears weak and lethargic, with very poor skin turgor.

1. Dianne is placed on a high-protein, high-carbohydrate diet. The primary function of carbohydrates in the body is to
   A. Develop a cushion around vital organs
   B. Break down and transport proteins
   C. Supply energy to the body
   D. Maintain fluid balance

   The intended response is **C**, since carbohydrates break down into sugars, which furnish the body with energy. **A** refers to a function of fats. **B** and **D** refer to functions of proteins.

2. Which of the following meals would be most appropriate for Dianne on a high-protein, high-carbohydrate diet?
   A. Liver and onions, roll, lettuce salad, ½ cup fruit cocktail, 1 glass of milk

B. Hamburger on a bun, brussel sprouts, ½ orange, can of soda pop

C. Bagel and cream cheese, olives, mineral water

D. Tortilla, peas, cooked noodles, instant chocolate pudding, herbal tea

The intended response is **A,** since it contains sources of protein, primarily liver and milk. Small amounts of protein are in the roll and fruit. High amounts of carbohydrates are found in the onions, roll, lettuce, and fruit. **B** is incorrect. There is a high amount of protein only in the hamburger, with a small amount in the bun. The bun, brussel sprouts, and orange contain carbohydrates. **B** does not have as high an amount of protein and carbohydrates as **A. C** is incorrect, since this meal is high in fats and carbohydrates. **D** is incorrect because it is high only in carbohydrates.

3. Dianne refuses to eat and continues to lose weight. She is placed on hyperalimentation. Proteins are given in the form of

A. Complex proteins

B. Amino acids

C. Triglycerides

D. Monosaccharides

The intended response is **B,** since proteins break down into amino acids. **A** is incorrect. Complex proteins cannot be given directly in an intravenous solution. **C** is incorrect because fats break down into triglycerides. **D** is incorrect, since monosaccharides are sugars.

4. Dianne's urine is tested for sugar every 6 hours while she is on intravenous hyperalimentation. The rationale for this nursing strategy is

A. Spilling of sugar is an adverse effect leading to increase of the IV flow rate.

B. Diabetes mellitus often develops when a client is started on hyperalimentation.

C. Osmotic diuresis and electrolyte imbalances can occur.

D. Glycosuria may develop if hyperalimentation is infused faster than it can be metabolized.

The intended response is **D.** Intravenous hyperalimentation solution is hypertonic, usually consisting of a 10% dextrose solution. If the pancreas cannot produce enough insulin for metabolism of the glucose, sugar is spilled in the urine, and insulin must be given intravenously or subcutaneously. **A** is incorrect because this would only add to increased serum glucose levels and further sugar spillage and physiologic problems. **B** is incorrect because diabetes does not develop but a state of hyperglycemia may occur. Although osmotic diuresis and electrolyte imbalances may occur with intravenous hyperalimentation, they bear no relationship to urine tests for sugar; therefore, **C** is incorrect.

5. Dianne is given a daily dose of multivitamins. The rationale for treatment is to
    A. Enhance carbohydrate, protein, and fat metabolism
    B. Supplement the diet with nutrients needed for health maintenance and growth
    C. Help build fat deposits in muscles for support of the skeleton
    D. Build stronger bones and teeth

The intended response is **B.** Vitamins are nutrients in the diet that help maintain homeostasis. **A** is incorrect because it refers only to water-soluble vitamins. **C** is erroneous. **D** is incorrect because it addresses only one vitamin function rather than the functions of all vitamins.

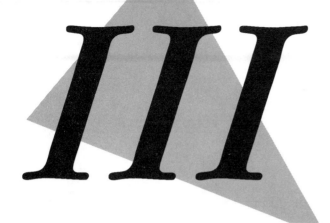

COMPREHENSIVE
REASONING
EXERCISES

ADULT HEALTH EXAM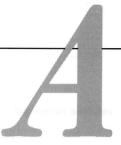

Bob Parker is a 63-year-old mailman brought to the hospital by ambulance. Physical examination reveals right hemiplegia. Admitting diagnosis is cerebral vascular accident, cerebral hemorrhage.

1. The nurse assessing Mr. Parker should check for signs of increased intracranial pressure, which would include
   A. Tachycardia, bradypnea, hypertension
   B. Bradycardia, bradypnea, hypertension
   C. Bradycardia, tachypnea, hypotension
   D. Tachycardia, bradypnea, hypotension

2. A goal of care for Mr. Parker is to reduce intracranial pressure. Which of the following interventions should be included in Mr. Parker's care plan?
   A. Administer sedative medications at set intervals
   B. Cough and deep breathe every 2 hours
   C. Encourage him to use Valsalva's maneuver
   D. Elevate the head of the bed 30 degrees

3. Mr. Parker demonstrates flaccid paralysis of his right extremities. Which of the following nursing actions would help most to prevent the development of joint ankylosis?
   A. Elevate the extremities on pillows
   B. Place the extremities in soft splints
   C. Perform PROM several times each shift
   D. Position extremities using rolled washcloths and towels

275

4. Mr. Parker is diagnosed as having a neurogenic bladder. Which of the following actions would be most appropriate in preventing urinary retention?

   A. Straight catheter every 8 hours

   B. Offer the bedpan every 4 hours

   C. Run warm water over the patient's hands

   D. Utilize the credé method

5. Which of the following would be a realistic discharge goal for Mr. Parker?

   A. He will feed himself independently a general diet.

   B. He will perform self-ADL, including bathing and dressing.

   C. He will resume premorbid bowel and bladder elimination patterns.

   D. He will ambulate short distances with assistance using a tripod cane.

Chet Allen is a 29-year-old health club instructor admitted to the emergency room with loss of pain sensation and weakness of lower extremities for 2 days. A preliminary diagnosis of Guillain-Barré is made.

6. Chet is placed on the neurologic unit to observe the progression of his disease. The nursing diagnosis of greatest priority would be which of the following?

   A. Safety impaired, related to paralysis

   B. Knowledge deficit, related to disease process

   C. Coping ineffective, related to fear of the unknown

   D. Gas exchange impaired, related to progressive weakness

7. Chet requires intubation and is placed on mechanical ventilation. The physician orders suctioning every 1 hour. The proper order for suctioning would be

   A. Mouth, nose, endotracheal tube

   B. Nose, mouth, endotracheal tube

   C. Endotracheal tube, nose, mouth

   D. Endotracheal tube, mouth, nose

8. Which of the following is the most valid indicator that Chet no longer requires mechanical ventilation?

   A. Chet is assisting ventilation at regular intervals.

   B. Chet's arterial pH value is WNL at a reduced FIO_2.

   C. Chet's respiratory rate averages 32 breaths/min during weaning.

   D. Chet frequently attempts to extubate himself.

Wayne Derrick is a 31-year-old policeman admitted with complaints of fatigue, difficulty with fine finger movements, and weakness in his legs. It has been determined that Wayne has amyotropic lateral sclerosis.

9. The nursing diagnosis of greatest priority as Wayne's disease progresses would be which of these?
   A. Alteration in nutrition
   B. Impaired physical mobility
   C. Impairment in skin integrity
   D. Ineffective gas exchange

10. Which of the following would help to prevent the most serious complication of Wayne's disease?
    A. Encourage him to turn, cough, and deep breathe
    B. Educate Wayne and his family about the disease process
    C. Encourage him to eat foods rich in iron
    D. Instruct him to increase intake of fresh fruit juices

Clara Evers is admitted for management of fecal impaction after several days of constipation. Radiographic studies indicate the presence of a large bowel obstruction. Presently Clara's abdomen is firm and distended, and she has experienced three bouts of nausea and emesis.

11. The physician has ordered the insertion of a Salem Sump nasogastric tube connected to intermittent low suction. The nurse preparing equipment for this procedure should procure which of the following solutions for irrigation?
    A. Distilled water
    B. Sterile water
    C. Normal saline
    D. Dextrose

12. As the nurse is inserting the Salem Sump tube, Clara suddenly begins to cough and gasp. The nurse should
    A. Stop the insertion, allow the patient to rest, then continue inserting the tube
    B. Encourage the patient to take deep breaths through her mouth while the tube is being inserted
    C. Instruct the patient to take a few sips of water and swallow as the tube is being inserted
    D. Remove the inserted tube, allow the patient to rest, and then attempt to reinsert

13. Which of the following colors of gastric drainate in the Salem sump tube would indicate the need for the nurse to perform a Hemoccult test?

    A. Clear

    B. Green

    C. Pale yellow

    D. Dark brown

14. Because Clara is NPO with intermittent suction of gastric content, the nurse should *especially* monitor which of the following serum electrolyte levels?

    A. Calcium

    B. Potassium

    C. Sodium

    D. Magnesium

15. Following 3 days of medical therapy, abdominal x-ray shows reduction of the fecal impaction. Clara has begun to pass frequent, watery stools. Which of the following nursing actions would be of *greatest* priority for Clara at this time?

    A. Provide frequent skin and perianal care

    B. Monitor her intake of IV fluids

    C. Assess her skin turgor and moisture of mucous membranes

    D. Turn and reposition her every 2 hours

16. In preparing Clara for discharge, the nurse provides teaching to the patient on bowel management and prevention of constipation. Which of the following statements should the nurse include in her teaching plan?

    A. "It's important for you to have a regular bowel movement once each day."

    B. "Take a laxative tablet or enema daily to prevent constipation."

    C. "Drink oral fluids often, and get regular exercise."

    D. "Avoid foods high in bulk, like breads and vegetables, since these are constipating."

Lenny Langford is a 17-year-old student admitted with complaint of severe right flank pain radiating to the scrotum. A diagnosis of epididymo-orchitis and supermetic cord torsion is reached by CT scan. A unilateral orchiectomy is performed.

17. Lenny's orchitis is traced to a chlamydial infection. Which of the following statements in a client's health history would support a diagnosis of chlamydial infection?

A. Lenny has been sexually active since age 14.

B. Lenny has been experiencing nausea, vomiting, and malaise for several days prior to the onset of his pain.

C. Lenny has noticed bloody urine for the past 2 days.

D. Lenny has noticed three fluid-filled blisters on his penis.

18. Postoperatively, Lenny is to wear a scrotal support. The *principal* reason for a scrotal support to the operative site is to

A. Reduce swelling

B. Reduce postoperative pain

C. Reduce hematoma formation

D. Decrease risk of hemorrhage

19. Which of the following statements by Lenny *best* indicates that patient teaching to prevent reinfection has been effective?

A. "As soon as I notice any changes in my penis or pain, I'll call my doctor."

B. "I know I won't get the infection again if I take all of the antibiotics the doctor ordered."

C. "I will need to be more careful about choosing my sexual partners."

D. "I will wear a condom during sexual activity."

20. Prior to his discharge, Lenny should be instructed to follow all of the following *except*

A. Avoid sexual activity for 4 to 6 weeks after surgery

B. Avoid heavy lifting or straining

C. Report any changes from his normal urinary function to his physician

D. Apply warm compresses to the scrotal area for discomfort

Mr. Jay is admitted to a neurological unit for evaluation after having suffered a grand mal seizure at home.

21. Which of these signs of seizure did Mr. Jay likely experience *first?*

A. Subtle, unusual sensory illusion (aura)

B. Loud moan or shrill cry

C. Slight tremors of the facial muscles

D. Blurring and dimming of vision

22. Mr. Jay is placed on seizure precautions during his hospitalization. The nurse should include all of the following interventions for seizure precautions *except*

A. Place a padded tongue blade at the patient's bedside

B. Apply soft padding to the patient's side rails

C. Maintain the patient's side rails in the up position at all times

D. Maintain an O_2 administration set at the patient's bedside

23. Mr. Jay experiences another seizure during this hospitalization. Which of the following data about Mr. Jay would cause the nurse the *greatest* concern?

A. BP 180/110

B. Pulse 120

C. Pupils dilated, unreactive to light

D. Respirations snoring and labored

24. Following the seizure, the nurse caring for Mr. Jay should implement which of the following actions *first*?

A. Insert an airway into the patient's mouth

B. Take a complete set of vital signs

C. Prepare an administration of Valium 10 mg IV

D. Turn the patient onto his left side

25. The nurse should carefully observe Mr. Jay's respirations. During which phase of grand mal seizure is the patient most likely to demonstrate apnea?

A. Preictal phase

B. Clonic phase

C. Tonic phase

D. Postictal phase

26. Following a series of tests, Mr. Jay is diagnosed with idiopathic seizure disorder. He is placed on Dilantin (phenytoin) 100 mg three times a day in preparation for discharge. The nurse teaching Mr. Jay about this medication should include which of the following?

A. "Since this medication causes drowsiness, you may not drive a car without supervision."

B. "You should avoid alcohol while on this medication."

C. "This medication may cause your urine to become very dark."

D. "Any changes in your vision should be reported to your physician immediately."

27. The day of discharge, Mrs. Jay tells the nurse, "I'm afraid to take my husband home. If he has another seizure, I won't know what to do!" Which of the following instructions to Mrs. Jay would be *most* helpful?

A. "Keep the phone numbers of the fire department ambulance service posted near every house telephone."

B. "Keep a padded tongue blade in an accessible place on each floor of your house."

C. "During a seizure, turn him on his side and stay with him."

D. "After the seizure, open his mouth wide and check his breathing."

Mary C. is a 54-year-old housewife admitted for complaint of chest pain diagnosed as stable angina pectoris. The frequency and intensity of her angina attacks have increased since her husband's sudden death 4 months ago, but her recent ECG shows no significant abnormalities. Following coronary angiography, she is diagnosed with coronary artery disease (CAD).

28. Which of the following statements by Mrs. C. in her health history would not correlate with a diagnosis of stable angina pectoris?

    A. "The nitro tablet takes the pain away in a few minutes."

    B. "I feel pressure in my chest, and it moves down my left arm."

    C. "The pain comes on even when I'm lying still and resting."

    D. "I sweat a lot during an attack, and my hands get all clammy."

29. Which of the following elements of Mrs. C.'s life style would *most* influence her predisposition to CAD and angina?

    A. Mary C. had onset of her menopause at age 47.

    B. Mary C. has a history of heart disease in maternal and paternal family tree.

    C. Mary C. smokes approximately one pack of cigarettes each day, increasing her smoking under stress.

    D. Mary C. has been eating very irregularly since the death of her spouse.

30. Mrs. C.'s anginal pain would likely be managed by any of the following medications *except*

    A. Nitroglycerin

    B. Inderal

    C. Procardia

    D. Digoxin

31. The nurse teaching Mrs. C. about management of anginal pain with nitrate medication should include which of the following directions to the client in her teaching plan?

    A. "Place your nitro tab under your tongue when your chest pain begins."

B. "If chest pain persists, you may take another tablet every 30 minutes after the first dose."

C. "The medication will probably cause your skin to become cool, pale, and clammy."

D. "If the medication causes you to have a headache or to feel dizzy, discontinue use and notify your physician immediately."

32. Mrs. C.'s physician has placed her on a low salt, low fat, low cholesterol diet. Which of the following menus should the nurse encourage in her diet teaching plan?

A. Poached eggs, ham slice, unbuttered toast with jam, coffee

B. Beef bouillon soup with croutons, cold cuts and fruit plate, tea

C. Fresh lettuce salad with lemon and oil dressing, broiled chicken, skim milk

D. Macaroni and cheese casserole, fresh fruit salad, buttered croissant

Stanley Keeler has undergone radical neck surgery with placement of a tracheostomy tube.

33. Which of the following should the nurse consider of *greatest* priority during Stanley's first 24 hours postoperatively?

A. Monitor temperature for signs of infection

B. Assess for patency of tracheostomy airway

C. Observe quality, rate, and rhythm of respirations

D. Monitor blood pressure for indication of bleeding

34. Which of the following steps should Stanley's nurse take *first* when preparing to perform trach care?

A. Wash hands thoroughly

B. Open all necessary kits and dressings

C. Apply sterile gloves

D. Pour cleansing solutions into sterile containers

35. The nurse preparing for trach care should place Stanley in which of these positions?

A. Sims'

B. Side-lying

C. Semi-Fowler's

D. Supine

36. The nurse suctioning Stanley's trach should take which of the following steps *first?*
    A. Suction secretions from inner cannula
    B. Instruct Stanley to cough and deep breathe
    C. Hyperoxygenate Stanley per O_2 cuff or Ambu bag
    D. Remove soiled dressings from around the trach tube

37. Stanley's family is learning about trach care in preparation for Stanley's discharge from the hospital. Which of the following elements of teaching should be considered *most* important for Stanley's family?
    A. Method of cleansing the inner cannula
    B. Use of the obturator
    C. Suctioning
    D. CPR

38. Stanley's nurse should teach his family all of the following signs of respiratory distress *except*
    A. Decreased pulse rate
    B. Restlessness
    C. Nostril flaring
    D. Dusky skin color

Jim Cooper is a 29-year-old business executive admitted to the acute medical unit with diagnosis of cocaine toxicity. Mr. Cooper's spouse acknowledges Jim's history of cocaine use in the admission history and assessment.

39. Of the following symptoms associated with cocaine toxicity, which should Mr. Cooper's nurse consider the *most* serious?
    A. Hypertension
    B. Hyperthermia
    C. Cardiac arrhythmia
    D. Convulsions

40. Jim's vital signs are apical rate 160, respirations 38, BP 198/102. The nurse should employ all the following interventions *except*
    A. Connect Jim to continuous ECG heart monitor to assess for irregular rhythm
    B. Administer O_2 per nasal cannula at 5 L/min to increase oxygenation
    C. Place Jim in high Fowler's position to facilitate respirations
    D. Initiate IV fluids for possible medication administration as ordered

41. Jim's physician has written the following orders. Which should the nurse caring for Jim implement *first*?

   A. Insert oral airway

   B. Insert Foley catheter and attach to gravity drainage

   C. Place patient on hypothermia blanket with rectal probe

   D. Initiate seizure precautions

42. Jim is becoming extremely agitated and combative. Which of the following nursing interventions would be the *most* appropriate?

   A. Place Jim in a private, secluded room

   B. Disallow any visitation by family or friends

   C. Place Jim in soft restraints and Posey vest

   D. Place Jim in a large, open, quiet area and remain in constant attendance

43. Which of the following findings would indicate a positive change in Jim's states of hyperthermia and dehydration?

   A. Apical rate is 126.

   B. BP is 96/60.

   C. Hourly urine output is 75 cc.

   D. CVP reading is 1.

Mr. Fountain is seen at a public health clinic with complaint of recurrent cough and low-grade fever. As part of his physical examination, Mr. Fountain receives a Mantoux skin test.

44. The nurse administering the Mantoux skin test should inform Mr. Fountain about all of the following *except*

   A. "If this test shows a positive reaction, a lung biopsy will be scheduled."

   B. "If the skin around the test site becomes reddened or puffy, the test is likely positive."

   C. "A positive reaction of this test indicates that you have been exposed to tuberculosis."

   D. "You will need to come back to the clinic in 2 days to have the test site checked by the nurse."

45. Mr. Fountain's Mantoux is found positive, and follow-up testing confirms diagnosis of tuberculosis. Which of the following tests would provide the *most* definitive diagnosis of TB?

   A. Blood cultures

   B. Sputum culture

    C. Chest X-ray

    D. Lung nuclear scan

46. Mr. Fountain is admitted to the respiratory unit and placed in isolation. Which of the following nursing actions would be appropriate for Mr. Fountain?

    A. Wear gown, mask, and gloves whenever coming into contact with the patient

    B. Instruct the patient to cover his mouth when he coughs and wash his hands often

    C. Provide disposable equipment, dishes, and silverware for patient use

    D. Spray disinfectant on used tissues before disposal

47. Mr. Fountain asks if members of his immediate family could have "caught" tuberculosis from him. Which response reflects a correct understanding of transmission of TB?

    A. "This disease is not very contagious. I'm sure they will not develop TB."

    B. "If anyone in your family begins to develop symptoms of the disease, we will recommend that a skin test be done."

    C. "The members of your family may possibly develop the disease. They should have chest x-rays performed every 6 months."

    D. "TB is contagious. It's best to have the members of your family receive skin testing as soon as possible."

48. Mr. Fountain is placed on isoniazid (INH) and rifampin therapy. After several days on these medications, he tells the nurse, "I'm feeling one hundred per cent better now. I don't think I'll be needing the medication too much longer." Which response of the nurse is most appropriate?

    A. "You will need to continue taking the medications until all your symptoms disappear."

    B. "You will remain on the medication until your Mantoux skin tests return negative for the disease."

    C. "Normally, the medication is required for 1 or 2 months, even if the symptoms have disappeared."

    D. "You will need to remain on medication for a long period of time, to prevent recurrence of your disease and infection of others."

49. The nurse preparing Mr. Fountain for discharge should alert the patient to symptoms that would indicate recurrence of tuberculosis, including all of the following *except*

    A. Persistent cough

    B. Fever

    C. Hematemesis

    D. Hemoptysis

50. Which of the following statements by Mr. Fountain indicates the *best* understanding of follow-up care upon discharge?

    A. "I'll try to eat regular, well-balanced meals when I go home."

    B. "I'll return to my doctor at the clinic each year for an examination."

    C. "I plan to stay out of smoke-filled rooms when I return to my job at the factory."

    D. "I'll be sure to take the medications the doctor prescribed for me."

Ella Stevens is a 66-year-old housewife who suffers from deficient production of antidiuretic hormone (ADH) from the pituitary gland.

51. The nurse caring for Ella explains that she is suffering from which of the following endocrine disorders?

    A. Diabetes insipidus

    B. Diabetes mellitus

    C. Cushing's syndrome

    D. Graves' disease

52. Ella would have which of the following symptoms secondary to her ADH deficiency?

    A. Peripheral edema

    B. Polydipsia

    C. Anuria

    D. Taut skin turgor

53. In light of Ella's ADH deficiency, the nurse would expect her serum electrolyte values to show which of the following imbalances?

    A. Hypokalemia

    B. Hyponatremia

    C. Hypocalcemia

    D. Hypochloridemia

54. The nurse caring for Ella should employ all of the following measures *except*

    A. Administer vasopressin tannate as ordered

    B. Limit oral intake of fluids to 1000 cc/day

    C. Measure intake and output

    D. Monitor urine-specific gravity

55. Which of the following findings would indicate to the nurse that Ella's endocrine disturbance is improving with treatment?

    A. Serum sodium is decreasing

    B. Peripheral edema is decreasing

    C. Serum glucose is decreasing

    D. Urinary output is decreasing

Mrs. Orlando is a Latino female with known history of atherosclerotic heart disease, hypertension, and chronic congestive heart failure (CHF). She is being admitted now with recurrence of symptoms of CHF.

56. All of the following would be expected symptoms of CHF *except*

    A. Rapid, shallow, difficult respirations

    B. Polyuria

    C. Peripheral edema

    D. Pulmonary congestion and rales

57. The physician has ordered Mrs. Orlando to receive 80 mg of Lasix (furosemide) IV twice a day. The nurse notes that the patient's K^+ level is 3.0. The nurse should

    A. Administer the Lasix 80 mg IV as ordered

    B. Administer half the dose of Lasix (40 mg) IV

    C. Offer the patient potassium-rich foods and fluids after administering Lasix 80 mg IV

    D. Withhold the drug and notify the physician of the serum K^+ level

58. Mrs. Orlando demonstrates frequent bouts of dyspnea and fatigue as well as periodic confusion and disorientation. Which of the following nursing measures would have the *greatest* priority for Mrs. Orlando?

    A. Encourage her to turn, cough, and deep breathe every 2 hr

    B. Restrict oral fluids to 2000 cc/24 hr

    C. Administer O_2 therapy per nasal cannula and maintain side rails up

    D. Monitor arterial blood gases and urine output regularly

59. Mrs. Orlando is placed on restricted fluids. Which of the following electrolyte minerals should likewise be restricted for Mrs. Orlando?

    A. Calcium

    B. Potassium

    C. Sodium

    D. Chloride

60. The nurse notes that Mrs. Orlando's cardiac output is markedly decreased. Which of the following prescribed medications would *most* help to bring the patient's cardiac output to within normal range?

   A. Nitroglycerin

   B. Inderal

   C. Digoxin

   D. Procardia

61. Mrs. Orlando has been receiving digoxin 250 mg IV PUSH daily. Which of the following findings would indicate that the Digoxin has been effective in treating the patient's congestive heart failure?

   A. Apical heart rate is 120 beats/min

   B. BP is 138/86

   C. Urine output is 3000 cc/24 hr

   D. Rales auscultated in lower lung lobes

62. Which of the following would serve as the *best* indicator that Mrs. Orlando's CHF is resolving?

   A. Urinary output is averaging 400 cc/shift.

   B. Respiratory rate ranges from 16 to 24 breaths/min.

   C. Loss of 4 kg of body weight since initiation of CHF treatment.

   D. Central venous pressure (CVP) reading is ranging from 5.5 to 7.0.

Mrs. Orlando's CHF has responded poorly to treatment, and she is becoming increasingly disoriented and combative with nursing staff. Her BUN is 188 and her creatinine is 5.3. She is diagnosed with acute renal failure secondary to congestive heart failure.

63. The evening nurse discovers Mrs. Orlando attempting to climb out of bed. Mrs. Orlando tells the nurse that she "needs to go shopping" and that she "can catch the bus in the hallway." The most appropriate *initial* response would be

   A. Administer PRN sedation

   B. Notify the physician of the patient's behavior and request an order for soft restraints

   C. Notify the family of the patient's behavior and request that a family member stay at the patient's bedside through the night

   D. Keep the side rails in the upright position and attempt to reorient the patient

64. Mrs. Orlando's urinary output is to be measured hourly. In light of her acute renal failure, the nurse would expect which of the following findings in relation to urine output?

A. Oliguria; dark, concentrated urine, low specific gravity

B. Polyuria, pale yellow urine, high specific gravity

C. Oliguria; dark amber urine; high specific gravity

D. Polyuria; bloody-tinged urine; low specific gravity

Kay Long is a 68-year-old female admitted with diagnosis of fractured left hip.

65. X-ray of Kay's left femur reveals 40% demineralization with decreased density of bone. The nurse should recognize that these findings are indicative of which of the following bone disorders?

A. Osteoporosis

B. Osteoarthritis

C. Osteomalacia

D. Ostemyelitis

66. Demineralization of Kay's bone places her at risk for

A. Infection

B. Ankylosis

C. Hemorrhage

D. Fracture

67. Prior to open reduction and pinning of her fractured femur, Kay is placed in Buck's extension traction. The *chief* purpose of this preoperative treatment is to

A. Immobilize the extremity to prevent further demage

B. Reduce muscle spasms associated with her fracture

C. Reduce pin in the affected extremity

D. Improve alignment and position of fracture fragments prior to surgery

68. The physician has ordered that Kay receive atropine 0.2 mg preoperatively. The label reads gr 1/150 = ml. The nurse should administer

A. 0.2 ml

B. 0.5 ml

C. 1.0 ml

D. 1.5 ml

69. Following open reduction and pinning of the fracture, the nurse should place Kay in which of the following positions postoperatively?

A. Supine with legs adducted

B. Lateral with legs elevated

C. Supine with legs abducted

D. Side-lying with legs internally rotated

70. Sixteen hours postoperatively, Kay complains of pain in the lower extremity. The nurse should

A. Reposition the patient and elevate the head of the bed

B. Medicate the patient with the prescribed analgesia

C. Notify the physician of the patient's status

D. Elevate the affected leg on 2 pillows

Ira Lumen, 35 years old, goes to the STD (sexually transmitted disease) clinic with complaints of persistent dry cough, night sweats, "feeling feverish," and a "purplish" genital lesion. He is sexually active with multiple partners and is fearful that he has contracted AIDS.

71. Your understanding of those persons who are at risk for contracting AIDS include all of the following *except*

A. Homosexual men

B. IV drug abusers

C. Blood donors

D. Prostitutes

72. Priority assessment of the client should include

A. Environmental allergies

B. Dietary preferences

C. Previous physical injuries

D. Receipt of blood transfusion within the last 3 years

73. Ira is scheduled for HIV (human immunodeficiency virus) testing. This test represents

A. Definitive diagnosis of AIDS

B. Exposure to the virus with development of antibodies

C. Confirmation of IV drug abuse

D. Presence of AIDS-related complex

74. Ira's HIV test is positive. He is admitted and treated for *Pneumocystis carinii pneumonia.* During his hospitalization, he is depressed and fearful. As the nurse caring for Ira, your *best* therapeutic intervention would be

A. Avoid dealing with the depression because it takes a long time to resolve

B. Assist the client to understand that his illness is caused by a virus, not something he has done

C. Make the client understand that a cure is near at hand

D. Refer the client to the chaplain for ongoing spiritual support

75. You diagnose Ira as having anxiety, related to alterations in sexuality. Your care plan would include all of the following principles *except*

   A. Sexuality is more comprehensive than sexual intercourse alone.

   B. Alternative forms of sexual expression can be gratifying.

   C. No real change in sexual activity is necessary.

   D. Responsible behavior related to sexual activity is essential.

76. As you prepare Ira for discharge, he begins to ask questions about living in a household with other people. Client teaching would include

   A. Cleaning up of spills of body fluids with a weak chlorine bleach solution

   B. Avoiding sharing dinnerware with others

   C. Laundering clothing and bed linens separately

   D. Participating in unprotected sexual activity

Diane Z., a 45-year-old college student, is admitted to the hospital for diabetic acidosis.

77. The cause of Diane's symptoms is a

   A. Sudden increase in the concentration of cholesterol in the extracellular compartment

   B. Physiological phenomenon following the ingestion of too much highly acidic food

   C. Rise in the pH of the blood to a point above 7.5

   D. Decrease in the pH of the blood to a point below 7.32

78. Several laboratory tests are done. Diane's symptoms lead the nurse to expect the blood test to reveal

   A. Low sugar, decreased acidity, low CO_2 combining power

   B. Elevated sugar, normal acidity, high CO_2 combining power

   C. Elevated sugar, increased acidity, low CO_2 combining power

   D. Low sugar, increased acidity, high CO_2 combining power

79. The type of insulin that will be used during the emergency treatment of the acidosis and until Diane is eating regularly is

   A. Isophane insulin suspension (NPH insulin)

   B. Insulin injection (regular insulin)

   C. Insulin zinc suspension (lente insulin)

   D. Protamine zinc insulin suspension

80. A primary objective in caring for Diana is to restore potassium balance. Which of the following nursing measures is most important during this process?

    A. Accurately assess urinary output

    B. Encourage vigorous fluid intake

    C. Observe carefully for signs of diaphoresis

    D. Correct faulty eating and drinking habits

John Davis, aged 32, had been painting the inside of an enclosed cylinder, when an explosion occurred. He sustained partial and full thickness burns over the entire upper portion of his body, including both arms. He was admitted to the burn unit in critical condition.

81. Mr. Davis' burns are considered to be severe. Which one of the following aspects of nursing care should receive the highest priority?

    A. Maintaining adequate urinary output

    B. Maintaining the patient's blood pressure

    C. Establishing an adequate airway

    D. Administration of antibiotic therapy

82. Mr. Davis was not pulled from the enclosed space for approximately 45 minutes. Which of the following might indicate that Mr. Davis suffered from an inhalation injury?

    A. Absence of carboxyhemoglobin level

    B. Hoarseness and the presence of soot in Mr. Davis' mouth and nose

    C. Pain in Mr. Davis' neck

    D. Burns on his chest

83. While you are caring for Mr. Davis, he states that his pain is excruciating and he needs pain medication immediately. What is the appropriate route of narcotic administration?

    A. Intramuscularly

    B. Intravenously

    C. Orally

    D. Subcutaneously

84. The primary shift in the location of body fluids in a serious burn is from

    A. Interstitial to intravascular space

    B. Intracellular to interstitial space

    C. Interstitial to intracellular space

    D. Intravascular to interstitial space

85. Mr. Davis' intravenous fluid needs have been calculated to equal 10,000 cc the first 24 hours. How much fluid is needed for the first 8 hours according to the Parkland formula?

    A. 3333 cc

    B. 5000 cc

    C. 2500 cc

    D. 7500 cc

Mr. Thomas is brought into the emergency room in acute respiratory distress. He is awake but very confused and agitated. His cheeks appear very rosy, and his respiratory rate is 48 breaths/min. You note that Mr. Thomas is barrel chested, and is purse-lip breathing. He is unable to give a medical history because of his shortness of breath and infusion. His wife, who accompanied him to the hospital, does state that he has emphysema. The nurse caring for Mr. Thomas assesses the need for O_2 therapy.

86. Which of the following O_2 delivery systems would be contraindicated?

    A. O_2 per venturi mask set at 24% FIO_2

    B. A simple O_2 mask set at 4 liters of O_2

    C. A nasal cannula set at 6 liters of O_2

    D. A nasal cannula set at 2 liters of O_2

87. Which of the following results best indicate that the breathing exercises were effective?

    A. Mr. Thomas is breathing slower and easier

    B. Blood gases have returned to normal range

    C. Skin is warm and dry to touch

    D. Mr. Thomas is no longer anxious

88. An adequate nursing assessment of Mr. Thomas would include recognizing early signs of mild hypoxia, which include

    A. Drowsiness, mental obtundation, and cyanosis

    B. Restlessness, anxiety, and mild confusion

    C. Ringing in the ears, diaphoresis, and syncope

    D. Blurred vision, vertigo, and ataxia

89. Which of the following breathing exercises would be most beneficial for Mr. Thomas?

    A. Drawing a deep breath up through a straw

    B. Blowing bubbles forcefully through a straw into a glass of water

    C. Inhaling forcefully, holding inspired air, then releasing air quickly

    D. Inhaling deeply, then slowly blowing a feather across the table

90. Which of the following short-term goals should the nurse pursue first for Mr. Thomas?

    A. Decrease his anxiety and restlessness

    B. Maintain patent airway and respiratory management

    C. Prepare his family for stresses involved in his care

    D. Do a thorough respiratory assessment

WOMEN'S HEALTH EXAM B

Susan Anderson is a 27-year-old female, gravida I, para 0, *who is being seen in the OB clinic for her first prenatal visit with the nurse midwife.*

1. Which of the following assessments would *not* be routine in an initial prenatal visit?

   A. Blood pressure

   B. Weight

   C. Fundal height

   D. Pelvic exam

2. Susan states that her periods were very irregular, so an ultrasound to estimate gestation is planned. The nurse should prepare Susan for this by instructing her to

   A. Limit oral intake 4 hours prior to the test

   B. Empty her bladder fully, just prior to the scheduled test time

   C. Drink several large glasses of fluid prior to the test

   D. Maintain NPO from midnight prior to the test

3. Ultrasonography determines that Susan is 11 weeks pregnant. During this period, Susan will *most* likely experience

   A. Ankle edema

   B. Frequency

   C. Braxton Hicks' contractions

   D. Hemorrhoids

4. As pregnancy progresses, all of the following cardiovascular changes occur *except*
   A. Increased stroke volume
   B. Increased cardiac output
   C. Increased heart rate
   D. Increased peripheral vascular resistance

5. At a subsequent prenatal visit, Susan asks the nurse midwife, "When will I be able to feel the baby move?" The nurse is aware that fetal movement is most often first experienced
   A. Late in the first trimester
   B. Early in the second trimester
   C. In the middle of the second trimester
   D. Late in the second trimester

6. Susan complains of constipation. The nurse should recommend which of the following?
   A. Take 30 cc of mineral oil as needed
   B. Increase fiber and fluids in the diet
   C. Discontinue prenatal iron supplements
   D. Use Fleets enema qhs, as needed

7. Pregnancy continues to progress normally, and Susan is now 41 weeks. The nurse midwife suggests a nonstress test. The primary purpose of this test is to evaluate
   A. Fetal readiness for delivery
   B. Fetal response to uterine contractions
   C. Adequacy of placental function
   D. Spontaneity of fetal movement

8. At 42 weeks gestation, the decision is made to induce Susan's labor. Susan appears apprehensive and tells the nurse, "I've heard this is very painful. I don't know if I can handle induced labor." The *most* appropriate response would be,
   A. "Tell me more about your concerns."
   B. "I can understand that you're frightened by the induction."
   C. "Let me take a few minutes to explain this procedure to you."
   D. "It may be more painful, but your labor will not last as long."

9. While the IV oxytocin drip is infusing, Susan develops hypertonic uterine contractions. The fetal monitor shows late decelerations. The nurse's first response should be

   A. Turn the patient on her left side

   B. Administer O_2 per mask

   C. Stop the oxytocin infusion

   D. Notify the physician

Angela Barron, gravida I, para 0, is admitted to the Labor and Delivery Unit in early, active labor. She is dilated 3 cm and is experiencing contractions every 3 minutes.

10. Which of the following provides the *most* conclusive evidence that Angela's amniotic membranes have ruptured?

    A. The patient experiences a leakage of fluid from the vagina.

    B. Nitrazine Paper test of patient's urine changes color.

    C. A sonogram reveals minimal amniotic fluid.

    D. Microscopic examination of the fluid reveals a ferning pattern.

11. The nurse notes a run of late decelerations on the fetal monitor. Which of the following actions should be taken first?

    A. Administer O_2 per mask

    B. Increase IV fluid flow rate

    C. Reposition the patient to left, lateral position

    D. Notify physician of change in fetal status

12. Angela's labor accelerates, and vaginal exam shows cervical dilatation of 5 cm. She says to the nurse, "Please, give me something for the pain!" Which of the following should guide the nurse's decision about analgesia administration?

    A. Analgesia at this point in labor may interfere with effective, uterine contractions.

    B. Analgesia is contraindicated in light of the previous pattern of fetal heart rate deceleration.

    C. Angela's labor is too advanced to benefit from analgesia.

    D. Analgesia at this point in labor is appropriate.

13. Angela has delivered a live male infant. The nurse midwife is preparing for delivery of the placenta. Angela is now in which stage of labor?

    A. First stage

    B. Second stage

    C. Third stage

    D. Fourth stage

14. Angela is transferred to the mother-baby recovery room. At 1 hour postpartum, she is still unable to void. Which of the following nursing interventions should be considered *first*?

    A. Straight catheter for residual

    B. Encourage oral intake of fluids

    C. Palpate bladder for distention and position

    D. Check perineum for swelling or hematoma

15. Angela complains, "My IV hurts." The nurse examines the insertion site for evidence of infiltration. Which of the following observations would support her suspicions?

    A. Localized redness and swelling

    B. Warmth and edema

    C. Tenderness and decreased flow rate

    D. Pallor and coolness

Angela is transferred to the postpartum unit, and her baby is transferred to newborn nursery.

16. Which of the following assessments of Baby Boy Barron should the nursery nurse consider abnormal?

    A. Baby cries and kicks when exposed to cool air.

    B. Baby's respiratory rate is 48 respirations/min at rest.

    C. Baby's urine is pale in color and odorless.

    D. Baby's heart rate is 90 beats/min during sleep.

17. The nurse strokes Baby Boy Barron's cheek and notes that the infant turns his head in that direction. He is exhibiting which of the following newborn reflexes?

    A. Swallowing

    B. Rooting

    C. Placing

    D. Sucking

18. Angela has selected "rooming in" for herself and her baby. The *main* goal of this is to

    A. Provide the nurses with an opportunity to observe maternal-infant interaction

B. Initiate the maternal-infant attachment process

C. Assist the mother in developing a realistic understanding of the responsibilities of infant care

D. Allow the mother practice to develop good child-care skills

19. The nurse is teaching Angela umbilical cord care. Which of the following instructions is correct?

A. Apply warm, moist compresses to the cord stump at frequent intervals.

B. Cleanse the cord stump with Betadine and sterile water each morning.

C. Apply alcohol to the cord stump to promote drying.

D. Gently massage the cord stump to facilitate detachment.

20. Angela develops a postpartum infection, and IV antibiotics are initiated. Her baby's pediatrician orders breast-feeding to be discontinued temporarily. Which of the following actions would be *most* helpful in maintaining Angela's breast milk supply?

A. Wear a firm-support brassiere

B. Increase intake of calcium-rich food and fluids

C. Manually express breast milk at regularily scheduled intervals

D. Apply warm compresses frequently

21. One week after discharge, Angela's husband calls the postpartum unit and asks the nurse, "Is it normal for my wife to cry at the drop of a hat? I'm worried I've done something to upset her." The nurse's *best* initial response would be:

A. "Have you noticed any pattern to her periods of crying?"

B. "Try not to worry about it. I'm sure it's just the postpartum blues."

C. "Can you think of something you may have done to upset her?"

D. "Let's consider some of the ways you can decrease her depression."

Lori Benson, 28 years old, is 9 weeks pregnant and experiencing severe "morning sickness." She is hospitalized for supportive therapy.

22. In light of Lori's diagnosis of hyperemesis gravidarum, the nurse should anticipate which of the following acid-base imbalances?

A. Respiratory acidosis

B. Respiratory alkalosis

C. Metabolic acidosis

D. Metabolic alkalosis

23. Which of the following series of symptoms correlates with a diagnosis of dehydration?
    A. Slow, bounding pulse and poor skin turgor
    B. Soft, sunken eyeballs and decreased respiration
    C. Increasing blood pressure and elevated temperature
    D. Dry, hot skin and oliguria

24. Which of the following classifications of medication would be *most* indicated for Lori?
    A. Anticholinergic
    B. Antispasmodic
    C. Antiemetic
    D. Antibiotic

25. Lori's serum potassium is 3.0. Which of the following developments causes the nurse the *most* concern?
    A. Decreased level of consciousness
    B. Decreased cardiac output
    C. Decreased muscle tone
    D. Decreased arterial blood pressure

26. Lori is to receive 1000 cc of D_5W, IV, every 6 hours. The IV equipment drop factor is 10. Lori should receive
    A. 18 drops/min
    B. 21 drops/min
    C. 28 drops/min
    D. 32 drops/min

27. Lori's physician places her on hyperalimentation therapy. The *primary* purpose of this therapy is to
    A. Increase Lori's weight
    B. Prevent electrolyte imbalance
    C. Arrest metabolism of stored body fat and prevent ketosis
    D. Ensure adequate nutrition to the developing fetus

Karen Asher is a 28-year-old gravida I, para 0 at 37 weeks gestation who comes to the Emergency Department with a 2-hour history of vaginal bleeding.

28. Karen's admission vital signs are T 99, P 120, R 26, BP 90/50. In light of Karen's vaginal bleeding, the nurse should suspect

A. Hypovolemovic shock

B. Septic shock

C. Neurogenic shock

D. Cardiogenic shock

29. The physician suspects placenta previa. The symptom that would distinguish placenta previa from abruptio placentae is

A. Abdominal pain and cramping

B. Painless vaginal bleeding

C. Swelling and firmness of the abdomen

D. Pelvic heaviness and congestion

30. Which of the following orders should the nurse implement *first?*

A. O$_2$ per face mask at 6 L/min

B. Apply fetal monitor

C. Initiate IV fluids

D. Cross and type for 3 units whole blood

31. The fetal monitor indicates a rate of 184. The nurse recognizes that the fetal heart rate indicates

A. Fetal bradycardia

B. Fetal compensation

C. Fetal anoxia

D. Normal fetal heart function

32. Karen is transferred immediately to the delivery site in preparation for emergency cesarean section. She grabs the nurse's hand frantically asking, "What's happening to me?" The *most* appropriate initial response of the nurse should be:

A. "You've had some bleeding. The doctor wants to watch how your baby is doing."

B. "We're going to perform a C-section. I'm sure everything will work out okay."

C. "You seem to be in early labor. We will keep a close watch on you."

D. "We're moving you to Labor and Delivery. Your doctor feels a C-section is necessary for you and your baby."

33. In preparation for Karen's cesarean-section, the nurse should

A. Administer a cleansing enema

B. Insert a Foley catheter

C. Prep and shave abdomen

D. Check cervical dilatation by vaginal exam

34. During the preparation, Karen says to the nurse, "Everything is happening so fast. Is my baby going to die?" The *best* nursing response is
   A. "I'm sure you're very frightened by this. We're working as fast as we can."
   B. "Do you think your baby is going to die?"
   C. "Your baby's chances are best if we can deliver you now."
   D. "I know this must be hard for you. Would you like me to call the chaplain?"

35. During the anesthesia induction, the nurse notes that FHTs have fallen to 80. The nurse understands these FHTs are
   A. Responding to general anesthesia induction
   B. Indicating fetal hypoxia
   C. Returning to normal parameters from prior readings
   D. Indicating probable umbilical cord compression

36. A live male infant is delivered. The attending nurse's *immediate* intervention would be
   A. Suction the baby
   B. Assess Apgar score
   C. Oxygenate the baby
   D. Credé the baby's eyes

Rita Hayes is a 24-year-old married female experiencing her first pregnancy.

37. Rita and her spouse plan to attend Lamaze classes. The *primary* goal of Lamaze is to
   A. Facilitate a painless labor and delivery
   B. Teach breathing techniques that promote adequate fetal oxygenation
   C. Expose the male partner to the process of labor and delivery
   D. Enhance the laboring couple's ability to cope during labor

38. Rita is planning to breast-feed her baby. In preparation for breast-feeding, she should be encouraged to
   A. Rub her nipples briskly with a rough washcloth
   B. Wear a supportive brassiere
   C. Apply warm compresses to her breasts twice daily
   D. Increase dietary calcium

39. Rita's husband accompanies her during a seventh month prenatal visit. He asks the nurse practitioner, "Is it still okay to have sex?" The best response is

A. It's best to avoid intercourse in the third trimester.

B. Intercourse increases the risk of preterm labor.

C. Intercourse increases the risk of infection.

D. There is no reason to stop having intercourse as long as you both are comfortable.

Following an uneventful pregnancy, Rita delivers a full-term 8-lb baby girl. It is noted in the delivery room that the infant has bilateral cleft lip and palate.

40. Rita asks the postpartum nurse, "Can I still breast-feed my baby?" In light of the infant's anomaly, the nurse should recognize all of the following *except:*

A. The baby's ability to breast-feed may be inhibited.

B. The baby may experience difficulties with adequate oxygenation.

C. The baby's swallowing may be improved with prosthetic devices.

D. The baby will require gavage feedings until surgical correction is performed.

41. The nurse observes the interaction between Rita and her baby. Which of the following behaviors would indicate the *most* serious impairment of maternal–infant attachment?

A. Rita refers to the baby as "it."

B. Rita and her husband have not yet chosen a name for the baby.

C. Rita appears to be fearful when holding the baby.

D. Rita has refused all visitors except her husband.

Mary Cox is a 32-year-old female with a 7-year history of infertility. She is being followed in the clinic to determine the cause and to treat her infertility.

42. All of the following elements of Mary's history would contribute to infertility *except*

A. A 4-year history of oral contraceptive use

B. Endometriosis

C. Pelvic inflammatory disease

D. Obesity

43. The nurse discovers Mary crying. Mary tells the nurse, "I never thought I'd have so much trouble getting pregnant. My sister has three children, and she's 2 years younger than me." The most appropriate, initial response would be

A. "But at least you're going to get help with your problem now."

B. "Try not to compare yourself with your sister. I can see how much that upsets you."

C. "It must be difficult for you."

D. "Pregnancy may take longer for you, but think of how happy you'll be when you are pregnant."

44. Mary's husband is also going to undergo infertility testing. Which of the following diagnostic findings would be most associated with infertility?

A. Decreased sperm count

B. Sperm immobility

C. Decreased amount of ejaculate

D. Presence of bacteria in the seminal fluid

45. Mary is scheduled to undergo 1-day, diagnostic, laparoscopic surgery. The nurse should instruct Mary to

A. Avoid oral fluids 2 hours before the procedure

B. Limit strenuous, physical activity for 1 week after surgery

C. Anticipate mild cramping and abdominal discomfort following the procedure

D. Plan to remain in the recovery room until her vaginal bleeding stops

46. Mary conceives by means of artificial insemination. In her seventh week, she calls her physician's office complaining of sudden sharp pain in her lower left abdominal quadrant. The nurse suspects ectopic pregnancy. The nurse should instruct Mary to

A. Remain in bed with feet elevated for 24 hours

B. Limit physical activity and call back if vaginal bleeding occurs

C. Visit the physician that day for a pelvic exam

D. Go to the hospital immediately for an ultrasound

47. An ectopic pregnancy is comfirmed by ultrasound, and Mary undergoes surgery. Postoperatively, the most significant nursing diagnosis that the nurse must consider is

A. Alteration in comfort, pain

B. Fluid-volume deficit

C. Impaired individual coping, grief

D. Alteration in oxygenation

Barbara Borg is a 25-year-old, gravida I, para 0, female, 35 weeks pregnant. She is admitted to the antepartum unit with the diagnosis of pregnancy-induced hypertension. Her admission vital signs include T = 37.2, P = 88, R = 20, BP = 140/90.

48. Additional symptoms that would support a diagnosis of pregnancy-induced hypertension include
    A. Glucosuria and weight gain
    B. Tachycardia and diplopia
    C. Proteinuria and edema
    D. "Moon face" and polyuria

49. Which of the following interventions would be *most* beneficial to Barbara at this point?
    A. Provision of a quiet, darkened environment to decrease stimulation
    B. Restriction of sodium and fluids in the diet to decrease fluid retention
    C. Restriction of visitors to promote rest
    D. Administration of diuretics to decrease fluid overload

50. Barbara has been hospitalized for 3 days. Which of the following observations is *most* indicative of a worsening condition?
    A. Absence of deep tendon reflexes
    B. Clonus
    C. Nervousness and irritability
    D. Disorientation

51. Which of the following medications would *most* likely be administered to Barbara at this point?
    A. Aldomet
    B. Lasix
    C. Magnesium sulfate
    D. Calcium gluconate

52. In light of her worsening condition, the decision is made to deliver Barbara by cesarean section. In the first 24 hours postoperatively, the nurse should pay closest attention to which of the following?
    A. Drainage from the abdominal dressing
    B. Vital signs
    C. Neurological status
    D. Color and amount of lochia

Karen Elliot, 16 years old, is brought to the emergency room by her friend, complaining of abdominal pain and vaginal bleeding. She confides in the nurse that she thinks she's pregnant. Spontaneous abortion is suspected.

53. Pregnancy is confirmed, and Karen tells the nurse, "Please don't call my parents. I don't want them to know." The nurse should recognize that

A. Parents of a minor must be notified before treatment can be initiated.

B. Karen's parents must be notified, but their consent is not necessary for treatment.

C. For any minor, an attending physician or hospital administrator may sign consent for treatment.

D. Karen may receive treatment without parental knowledge or consent.

54. On pelvic exam, it is noted that Karen's cervix is dilated to 3 cm. This finding is *most* indicative of which type of spontaneous abortion?

A. Threatened

B. Imminent

C. Incomplete

D. Missed

55. Based on an understanding of spontaneous abortion, the nurse should anticipate that Karen will undergo

A. Saline induction

B. Vacuum extraction

C. Dilatation and curettage

D. Laparotomy

56. During discharge teaching, the nurse explains to Karen that she should notify her physician if she experiences which of the following?

A. Vaginal bleeding

B. Abdominal pain or cramping

C. Nausea and vomiting

D. Elevated temperature

Sally Brown, 28 years old, has been using an IUD for contraception for the past 4 years. She has decided to have it removed and is consulting the nurse to discuss birth control alternatives.

57. Which of the following elements of Sally's health history would contraindicate the use of oral contraceptives?

A. Dysmenorrhea

B. Diabetes mellitus

C. Hypertension

D. Pelvic inflammatory disease

58. Sally expresses interest in a diaphragm but fears it will not protect her adequately. The nurse should explain that

A. Diaphragms are effective but closely associated with toxic shock syndrome.

B. Diaphragms may be easily dislodged during intercourse.

C. Diaphragms need to remain in place for 2 hours following intercourse.

D. Diaphragms should be refitted after weight gain or pregnancy.

59. Sally explains that she is sexually active with multiple partners. She asks, "Will the diaphragm protect me from getting VD?" The nurse's *best* response would be which of the following?

   A. "Limiting your sexual contacts is the best protection."

   B. "Research shows that many sexually transmitted diseases are prevented by continual use of the diaphragm."

   C. "The use of a condom by the male partner is a good form of protection."

   D. "Diaphragms may actually increase the risk of venereal infection."

60. Sally decides to use a diaphragm for contraception. Which form of patient instruction would be *most* effective to teach Sally how to use it?

   A. Show her a videotape

   B. Provide her with a booklet with diagrams

   C. Involve her in an instructional class

   D. Encourage her to practice insertion, following a brief explanation

Emma is a 37-year-old mother of four admitted for an abdominal hysterectomy for uterine leiomyomas (fibroids) confirmed by ultrasound.

61. Which of the following series of symptoms would be *most* associated with uterine leiomyomas?

   A. Pelvic discomfort, purulent vaginal discharge, fever

   B. Pelvic heaviness, urgency, stress incontinence

   C. Menometrorrhagia, abdominal heaviness, anemia

   D. Amenorrhea, uterine cramping, weight loss

62. The nurse notes that Emma's preoperative blood work indicates a hemoglobin value of 8.2. The nurse should

   A. Encourage Emma to eat foods rich in iron

   B. Place Emma in protective isolation

   C. Position Emma with the head of the bed elevated 90 degrees

   D. Notify Emma's surgeon regarding the hemoglobin value

63. Preoperatively, Emma should be instructed on all of the following *except*
    A. Turning, coughing, and deep breathing exercises
    B. Splinting of the abdomen with a pillow during coughing
    C. Use of estrogen replacement medication following surgery
    D. Purpose and appearance of a Hemovac drain following surgery

64. Emma is to receive Robinul (glycopyrrolate) 0.1 mg preoperatively. The nurse should explain to Emma that this medication will
    A. Relax her abdominal muscles prior to surgery
    B. Cause her to feel drowsy or sleepy
    C. Cause her to experience dry mouth and thirst
    D. Help her to empty her bladder fully before surgery

Emma undergoes surgery for abdominal hysterectomy and is transferred to the postoperative recovery room.

65. Which of the following should the recovery room nurse check *first* in Emma's chart upon her arrival in the recovery room?
    A. Total blood loss during the procedure
    B. Sponge and instrument count following the procedure
    C. Total length of time for the procedure
    D. Anesthetics and drugs used during the procedure

66. Which of the following nursing actions in the immediate postoperative period has the *highest* priority for Emma's care?
    A. Check vital signs every 15 minutes
    B. Check I & O every 30 minutes
    C. Check level of consciousness
    D. Check for patent airway

67. Emma's Recovery Room admission BP was 100/62. Her present reading one-half hour later is 80/40. The *most* appropriate nursing action would be to
    A. Notify the surgeon and anesthesiologist of the reading
    B. Increase the drip rate of IV fluids
    C. Assess abdominal dressing for evidence of bleeding
    D. Apply O_2 per facial mask at 9L/min

68. The recovery room nurse is aware that Emma received Sublimaze (fentanyl citrate) prior to her operative procedure. Since Emma's respiratory

rate is 8 respirations/min, the nurse would likely administer which of the following medications?

   A. Innovar

   B. Ketamine

   C. Acetine

   D. Narcan

69. Emma is returned to her room on the postoperative unit following her surgery. She is to receive Ilopan (dexpanthenol) 250 mg every 8 hours. The primary purpose of this medication is to

   A. Increase urinary output by diuretic effect

   B. Decrease postoperative bleeding by a coagulation effect

   C. Provide for hormone replacement following surgery

   D. Decrease abdominal distention by increasing peristalsis

70. The Ilopan injection medication label reads 500 mg = 1 mL. The nurse should administer

   A. 0.3 mL

   B. 0.5 mL

   C. 0.8 mL

   D. 1.0 mL

71. Which of the following observations of Emma on her operative day should the nurse consider abnormal?

   A. Moderate amount sanguinous drainage noted in vaginal Hemovac

   B. Complaints of tenderness and discomfort in the lower abdomen

   C. Complaints of dizziness upon getting out of bed for the first time

   D. Urine output of 300 cc pinkish-tinged urine for the last 8 hours

72. Which of the following menus would be appropriate for Emma in order to increase her intake of iron following surgery?

   A. Ham and cheese sandwich, fresh fruit, salad, milk

   B. Lettuce salad with tomato, chicken noodle soup, apple

   C. Ham and eggs, dried cereal, milk

   D. Hamburger patty, canned corn, mashed potatoes

73. On her third postoperative day, Emma complains to the nurse of gas pains. Which of the following nursing instructions would be *most* beneficial to Emma?

   A. Encourage Emma to drink additional fluids

B. Administer a Fleet's enema to Emma as ordered.

C. Encourage Emma to ambulate as much as tolerated.

D. Instruct Emma to select bland, non-gas-forming foods for her menu.

Janet Addison, a 28-year-old mother of two, seeks medical treatment and health counseling for premenstrual syndrome (PMS).

74. In order to verify PMS, a thorough history is critical. Which of the following questions by the nurse would provide the *most* valuable information about Janet's experience with PMS?

    A. "Do you experience pelvic pain or cramping during your menstrual period?"

    B. "Have you noticed that your menstrual flow is heavier than usual?"

    C. "Are you aware of any mood changes that occur just prior to your period?"

    D. "Do you experience weight gain, headaches, or depression prior to your period?"

75. Which of the following comments by Janet during a health history would be *most* closely associated with PMS?

    A. "I had my first period at age 10."

    B. "The weight gain and bloating have worsened since my second child was born."

    C. "I often feel depressed and nervous during my periods."

    D. "I've noticed a real loss of libido in the past few months."

76. All of the following elements of client lifestyle are associated with PMS *except*

    A. Poor nutritional habits with excessive intake of caffeine and sugars

    B. Sedentary lifestyle with little regular exercise

    C. High stress occupations or professional roles

    D. Poor personal hygiene practices

77. Janet's physician prescribes vitamin B_6 therapy. The nurse explains to Janet that the purpose of this therapy is to

    A. Decrease lower abdominal cramping and discomfort

    B. Increase energy level and libido

    C. Increase blood progesterone and promote diuresis

    D. Reduce breast tenderness

78. The nurse should encourage Janet to alter her diet in which of the following ways?

A. Increase protein, increase fat, decrease sugar

B. Increase fat, decrease carbohydrate, decrease salt

C. Increase protein, increase carbohydrate, decrease salt

D. Increase carbohydrate, increase fat, decrease sugar

Betty White is a 56-year-old female admitted for diagnostic work-up of a lump in her left breast.

79. All of the following initial signs and symptoms are suggestive of breast malignancy *except*

    A. Breast dimpling

    B. Breast tenderness and pain

    C. Peau d'orange

    D. Nipple retraction

80. Of all of these elements of Mrs. White's health history, which is *most* associated with the development of breast malignancy?

    A. Over 40 years of age

    B. Menstruation began at age 10 and continued through age 50.

    C. Caucasian race

    D. Maternal history of breast carcinoma

81. Mrs. White's breast biopsy indicates the presence of malignant cells, and mastectomy is performed. Which of the following nursing diagnoses would probably have the *most* significance for Mrs. White in relation to her surgery?

    A. Alteration in fluid balance, potential deficit

    B. Activity intolerance

    C. Disturbance in self-concept

    D. Alterations in patterns of elimination

82. All of the following actions should be included in Mrs. White's postoperative care plan *except*

    A. No venipuncture on left arm

    B. No BP assessment on left arm

    C. Elevate left arm on pillows

    D. Exercise left arm and shoulder 1 day postoperatively

83. The nurse notices that Mrs. White closes her eyes during her mastectomy dressing changes and seems very unwilling to participate in her self-care. Mrs. White says, "I just can't face looking at it yet." The *most* appropriate response for the nurse would be

A. "It's perfectly natural to feel uneasy about this type of surgery at first."

B. "I'll stay with you and perhaps we can look at your wound together."

C. "This surgery has been very traumatic for you, hasn't it Mrs. White?"

D. "You seem concerned about your incision."

Ellen is a 21-year-old college student who complains to the clinic nurse of vaginal irritation and discharge. A diagnosis of vaginitis is suspected.

84. The clinical nurse asks Ellen if she has noted a creamy white, curd-like discharge adhering to the vaginal walls. The nurse is assessing for a classic symptom of

A. *Trichomonas*

B. *Gardnerella*

C. *Candida*

D. *Chlamydia*

85. Ellen tells the nurse that her vaginal discharge is greyish colored with an unpleasant odor. In preparation for a wet mount slide test to determine the vaginal organism, the nurse should

A. Irrigate Ellen's vaginal tract with sterile water prior to the vaginal exam

B. Cleanse Ellen's vagina with Betadine solution prior to the vaginal exam

C. Lubricate the speculum with water-soluble lubricant (K-Y Jelly) prior to insertion of the speculum

D. Place Ellen in lithotomy position and provide the physician with a sterile glove

86. Ellen expresses some pelvic discomfort during the vaginal examination. In order to reduce the client's discomfort, the nurse should

A. Encourage Ellen to bear down as if to have a bowel movement

B. Instruct Ellen to hold her breath to relax her abdominal muscles

C. Tell Ellen to take slow deep breaths through her mouth

D. Provide Ellen with a mild analgesic upon completion of the examination

87. The examining physician explains to Ellen that she has *Gardnerella* vaginitis, a sexually transmitted disease. Ellen begins to cry quietly and says to the nurse, "I feel so embarrassed! You must think I'm a terrible person!" Which of the following would be the *most* appropriate response of the nurse?

A. "Please don't feel embarrassed. This type of infection is quite common."

B. "Are you feeling guilty about having a venereal disease?"

C. "Try to calm yourself. I will keep your problem very confidential."

D. "This must be difficult for you. Would you like to talk about it privately?"

88. The physician tells Ellen that her sexual partner must be notified of the *Gardnerella* infection. The *chief* purpose of notifying the sexual partner is to

A. Encourage the sexual partner to seek medical attention if he shows signs of the infection

B. Provide counseling to the sexual partner on use of the condom to prevent infection

C. Inform the sexual partner of signs and symptoms of the infection to be watchful for

D. Prevent reinfection of Ellen by her sexual partner in future intercourse

89. Ellen is placed on Flagyl (metronidazole) therapy. The nurse should instruct the client to be watchful for which of the following signs that would indicate superinfection secondary to Flagyl therapy?

A. Abdominal cramping and diarrhea

B. Dry mouth and metallic taste

C. Vomiting and muscle weakness

D. White-coated "furry" tongue and fever

90. The nurse will know that Flagyl therapy has been effective for Ellen when

A. Ellen's vaginal itching and irritation have ceased

B. Ellen's vaginal swelling and erythema disappear

C. Ellen's sexual partner remains asymptomatic for a 6-week period

D. Ellen's vaginal tract culture is negative a week after therapy

CHILD HEALTH EXAM

Leo Joyce is a 14-month-old male who is admitted by his parents to the pediatric unit with suspected intussusception.

1. The nurse is aware that intussusception is characterized by which of the following pathophysiological changes?
   A. Telescoping of a portion of the bowel into another
   B. Inflammation and ulceration of the lining of a section of bowel
   C. Loss of peristaltic activity secondary to absence of ganglion cells
   D. Stenosis of the circular muscle of the pylorus

2. Which of the following comments by the parents in the nursing admission history would *most* suggest intussusception?
   A. "I've noticed his stools are a different color than usual."
   B. "He screams and draws up his legs when I touch his tummy."
   C. "He's had projectile vomiting for the last 2 days."
   D. "He's been running a temperature on and off for the last 5 days."

3. Which of these measures should be the *first* priority for Leo's nurse?
   A. Initiate IV fluid therapy to improve hydration
   B. Administer Tylenol for pain relief
   C. Insert a nasogastric tube for abdominal decompression
   D. Test stool sample for occult blood

4. Leo's physician treats the intussusception with barium enema. Which of the following observations by the nurse would provide the *most* conclusive evidence that the barium enema treatment was successful?

   A. Hyperactive bowel sounds noted

   B. Barium-colored stools noted in diaper

   C. Diminished abdominal pain

   D. Temperature normal

5. Barium enema is not successful, and Leo undergoes surgery for bowel resection. Immediately postop, the nurse's *first* priority intervention is

   A. Monitor vital signs

   B. Provide pain relief

   C. Monitor incision for evidence of bleeding

   D. Measure Gomco suction nasogastric tube drainage

6. The nurse caring for Leo notes that his IV insertion site appears swollen and pale and is cool to the touch. Based on these findings, the nurse should suspect which of the following?

   A. Infiltration

   B. Phlebitis

   C. Thrombus

   D. Air embolus

7. On the second postoperative day, Mrs. Joyce tells the nurse that Leo's abdomen "is becoming very full and round." The nurse should understand that this abdominal distention is likely a result of which of these?

   A. Probable development of acute peritonitis

   B. Expected shifts of body fluids to the abdominal cavity

   C. Accumulation of free air in the abdominal cavity following surgery

   D. Retention of residual from the enema

8. Leo weighs 22 pounds. Leo's physician orders vancomycin antibiotic 40 mg/kg of body weight per day to be given IV every 6 hours. The nurse should administer how many mg per dose?

   A. 60 mg

   B. 80 mg

   C. 100 mg

   D. 120 mg

Kevin Lewis, a 3 year old attending daily preschool, complains to his mother that he is feeling tired, achy, and warm. She notes an elevated temperature and a few reddish blisterlike lesions on his chest. Kevin's mother suspects chickenpox.

9. Which of the following schedules of symptoms would support a diagnosis of chickenpox (varicella)?

    A. Chills, headache, malaise

    B. Nausea, vomiting, diarrhea

    C. Koplik's spots, photophobia, fever

    D. Sore throat, chills and fever

10. Which of these statements is true concerning the communication of chickenpox (varicella)?

    A. It is one of the *most* contagious of diseases.

    B. It is a relatively contagious disease.

    C. It is one of the least contagious diseases.

    D. It is a noncontagious disease.

11. As a result of her exposure to Kevin's chickenpox, Mrs. Lewis may develop in the future symptoms of which disorder below?

    A. Roseola

    B. Scabies

    C. Shingles

    D. Hepatitis

12. Which of the following home-care measures should the clinic nurse instruct Mrs. Lewis to use for Kevin?

    A. Avoid bright indoor lights or sunlight for 2 weeks

    B. Isolate Kevin from siblings and playmates for 2 to 3 weeks

    C. Administer Benadryl as ordered for its antihistamine effect

    D. Administer Tylenol gr every 4 hours as needed for fever and aches

Melissa Edwin is a 2-year-old girl who is found by her mother to have ingested an undetermined amount of a household cleaner. Mrs. Edwin immediately dials the Poison Control Center of the neighborhood hospital.

13. Which of the following data should the Poison Control Center nurse consider the *most* essential?

    A. Type of ingestion

    B. Time of ingestion

    C. Amount of ingestion

    D. Number of previous ingestions

14. If inducing vomiting was indicated for Melissa's ingestion, the nurse would encourage Mrs. Edwin to administer which of the following?

    A. Syrup of ipecac

    B. Tannic acid

    C. Charcoal salts

    D. Milk

15. Upon the arrival of Melissa in the emergency room, which of the following actions should be employed initially?

    A. Prepare necessary equipment for gastric lavage

    B. Initiate IV therapy to promote diuresis

    C. Prepare activiated charcoal solution to antidote the ingested material

    D. Assess vital signs to establish a baseline

16. After Melissa has been stabilized, the nurse should provide counseling to Mrs. Edwin to prevent recurrence of an accidental ingestion. All the following statements concerning accidental ingestion are true *except:*

    A. Accidental ingestion occurs most frequently in children under age 5.

    B. Seventy-five percent of all accidental ingestion could be prevented by keeping materials out of reach.

    C. Children learn from their first ingestion and seldom repeat ingestions in the future.

    D. Investigation of nonedible materials by young children are believed to be an unconscious call for more attention and concern from the parent towards the child.

Mrs. Hartford has brought her 18-month-old daughter Rosie to a neurologist for consultation. She relates in a health history that Rosie has "very stiff muscles" and has shown very little spontaneous movement since birth. Although Mrs. Hartford excused this, thinking her daughter "was just lazy" since she was "such a fat baby at birth," she is now concerned because Rosie cannot yet sit upright without support and likewise is unable to stand or walk. A tentative diagnosis of cerebral palsy is made.

17. All of the following data from Mrs. Hartford's health history would support a diagnosis of cerebral palsy *except*

    A. Thirty-hour first stage labor with Rosie

    B. Cesarean-section delivery of Rosie

    C. Meconiun-stained amoniotic fluid with Rosie

    D. Toxemia of pregnancy with Rosie

18. Mrs. Hartford's comment that Rosie was "such a fat baby at birth" is significant towards a positive diagnosis of cerebral palsy because

    A. Large babies are associated with diabetes, which is closely related with the development of cerebral palsy.
    B. Large-for-gestational age babies are more prone to neurologic and respiratory disorders.
    C. A large baby may have precipitated a more difficult labor and delivery that could have contributed to the development of cerebral palsy.
    D. Large-for-gestational age infants are prone to hydrocephalus.

19. According to growth and development standards, at what age should Rosie have been able to sit upright without support?

    A. 4 months
    B. 5 months
    C. 8 months
    D. 10 months

20. Which of the following would be a realistic goal for a child with cerebral palsy?

    A. The child will ambulate independently by age 3.
    B. The child will avoid physical activity to reduce risk of self-induced injury.
    C. The child will dress himself without assistance by age 4.
    D. The child will engage in regular exercise to prevent contracture formation in extremities.

Mrs. Bivens brings her 6-month-old daughter Jill to a Well Baby Clinic for routine physical examination.

21. Jill was born 3 weeks premature, weighing 4 lb, 14 oz. Her present weight is 11 lb, 2 oz. The nurse should recognize that Jill's weight gain is

    A. Excessive, since birth weight is normally not doubled until 8 to 9 months of age.
    B. Excessive, since Jill was a premature infant with low birth weight.
    C. Within normal limits, since premature infants may show accelerated growth rates for the first months of life.
    D. Inadequate, since Jill should have tripled her birth weight by the sixth month.

22. Mrs. Bivens reports that Jill takes her bottle formula well but cries soon after feedings. She states, "I don't think she's getting enough to eat." The

physician plans to begin Jill on solid foods. Which of these food groups would likely be introduced *first?*

A. Vegetables

B. Fruit

C. Cereal

D. Meat

23. At age 6 months, Jill should have been immunized with all the following *except*

A. Oral polio

B. Diphtheria

C. Tetanus

D. Measles

24. The nurse administering an immunization to Jill would *most* likely use which of the following sites?

A. Dorsal gluteal

B. Vastus lateralis

C. Deltoid

D. Abdominal

Nine-year-old Buddy Jackson is admitted to the hospital for treatment of acute hyperglycemia and apparent ketoacidosis.

25. Which of the following laboratory tests is *least* associated with ketoacidosis?

A. Glucose 580

B. *p*H 7.31

C. Urine ketones large

D. Hemoglobin 6.4

26. The attending physician has ordered that Buddy is to receive 12 units insulin by IV route. Which of the following types of insulin would the nurse prepare to administer?

A. Lente

B. Regular

C. Humulin N

D. NPH

27. Because of the acute hyperglycemia, Buddy appears dehydrated with hot, dry, flushed skin and dry mucous membranes. Of the following interventions, which should the nurse consider the *first* priority?

    A. Initiate IV fluids as ordered

    B. Record intake and output

    C. Insert indwelling urinary catheter

    D. Measure urine specific gravity

28. Buddy recovers and begins attending diabetic classes with his family. The nurse should explain that all of the following increases the need for insulin *except*

    A. Infectious processes

    B. Increased activity and exercises

    C. Increased caloric intake

    D. Psychic or emotional stress

29. Buddy's parents should be taught that a symptom of hyperglycemia is

    A. Nervous, tremulous behavior

    B. Headache

    C. Frequent urination

    D. Slow pulse rate

Amy Foster is a 2½-year-old girl admitted to the hospital for treatment of cancer.

30. As her mother prepares to leave the hospital to return home, Amy begins to cry and scream loudly, trying to climb over the rails of her bed. The nurse should recognize that Amy's behavior is typical of which stage of separation anxiety?

    A. Protest

    B. Anger

    C. Despair

    D. Denial

31. Which of the following comments by the nurse would be most appropriate in response to Amy's behavior?

    A. "It's okay, dear, Mommy will be back to see you tomorrow."

    B. "Would you like me to put the television on for you?"

    C. "It's sad when Mommy leaves, isn't it? Crying may help you feel better."

    D. "Don't cry, Amy. I'll take very good care of you."

32. All of the following actions by the nurse would help Amy's adjustment to separation *except*

    A. Have a favorite toy or blanket brought in from Amy's house

    B. Provide Amy toys that help her express aggression such as modeling clay or punching balls

    C. Place pictures of family members and parents near Amy's bedside

    D. Engage Amy in competitive games such as cards or checkers

33. On Amy's fifth day of hospitalization, her mother is alarmed to find her daughter sucking her thumb while watching T.V. Mrs. Foster tells the nurse, "I'm worried about her! She hasn't sucked her thumb since she was a baby!" The nurse should recognize that Amy's thumb-sucking behavior is typical of which of the following defense mechanisms?

    A. Suppression

    B. Isolation

    C. Compensation

    D. Regression

34. In the middle of the night, Amy awakes from sleep crying out that she has a "very bad dream with ghosts and monsters." Which of the following nursing interventions would be most helpful to Amy?

    A. Amy should be allowed to stay awake and play with quiet toys until she falls back to sleep.

    B. Nurse should tell Amy that monsters and ghosts are not real and attempt to comfort her.

    C. Nurse should turn a small light on in the room and close Amy's door to reduce stimulation.

    D. Amy's physician should be notified and an order for sleep medication requested.

Allison Kelsey, aged 7, undergoes closed reduction of a complete fracture of her right radius. A fiberglass cast is applied in the cast room.

35. All of the following would be expected signs of a fractured extremity *except*

    A. False motion

    B. Crepitus

    C. Pain and tenderness

    D. Diminished radial pulse

36. Mrs. Kelsey explains that Allison injured her arm after falling from the top of a slide in their backyard. The nurse should chart Allison's fracture as which of the following?

    A. Spontaneous

    B. Pathologic

    C. Traumatic

    D. Pyrogenic

37. The nurse provides instruction on cast care to Allison and her mother. Which of the following statements by the nurse is correct?

    A. "Do not wiggle or move the fingers of your right hand for 2 to 3 weeks."

    B. "Observe your cast daily for any cracks or stains."

    C. "If your arm is sore, apply hot moist towels to the cast for several hours."

    D. "The doctor will remove the cast in 1 to 2 weeks."

38. Mrs. Kelsey should be instructed to notify Allison's physician if she notices which of the following?

    A. Pinkish coloration of fingernails

    B. Itching sensation of casted arm

    C. Slight swelling of fingertips

    D. Numbness and tingling of affected extremities

39. Which of the following nutrients should Mrs. Kelsey encourage to improve bone healing in Allison?

    A. Vitamin C

    B. Vitamin D

    C. Iron

    D. Magnesium

Mrs. Kathy Murphy calls her son Danny's Pediatric Nurse Practitioner with concern over her son's difficulty with respirations and "barking" cough. The PNP suspects laryngotracheobronchitis (LTB).

40. The characteristic "crowing" sound of respirations in LTB is

    A. Stridor

    B. Rhonchi

    C. Wheeze

    D. Rales

41. Which of the following comments by Mrs. Murphy to the Nurse Practitioner most strongly supports a diagnosis of LTB?

    A. "He's been very lethargic and drowsy these last few days."

    B. "His older sister has had asthma since she was 7 years old."

    C. "He seems to cough much more when he's lying down."

    D. "He had the flu a week ago."

42. The Nurse Practitioner recognizes that the primary goal of treatment of LTB is airway dilation. This goal is best achieved by instructing Mrs. Murphy to do which of the following?

    A. Place Danny in a hot, steamy shower stall

    B. Position Danny for sleep sitting up in a comfortable chair

    C. Place a cool moist humidifier in Danny's room

    D. Administer an over-the-counter cough suppressant

43. Mrs. Murphy should be instructed to watch for signs of worsening respiratory status, including which of the following?

    A. Low-grade fever

    B. Productive cough

    C. Restlessness

    D. Hoarse voice

44. Danny shows signs of acute respiratory embarrassment, and his mother brings him to the emergency room. Which of the following changes in vital signs would the nurse expect to note?

    A. Bradycardia, tachypnea

    B. Bradycardia, bradypnea

    C. Tachycardia, tachypnea

    D. Tachycardia, bradypnea

45. After completing a respiratory assessment, the nurse receiving Danny in the emergency room should plan to implement which of the following measures?

    A. Administer 100% O_2 therapy

    B. Initiate continuous cardiac monitoring

    C. Administer a preparation of epinephrine

    D. Assemble equipment for emergency tracheostomy

46. Danny's condition stabilizes, and he is admitted to the pediatric unit for further treatment. Which of the following nursing plans would *not* be appropriate for Danny?

A. Administering humidified O_2 by means of a croup tent to increase oxygenation

B. Encourage frequent play periods to decrease restlessness

C. Assess vitals frequently to monitor respiratory status

D. Encourage oral fluids to liquify secretions

Five-year-old Patrick visits the pediatric clinic for a prekindergarten physical examination.

47. Which of the following techniques would be most appropriate to use in testing Patrick's vision?

A. Ask Patrick to identify pictures from a storybook at near and far distances

B. Ask Patrick to read large print simple words from a close distance

C. Ask Patrick to focus on objects in the room such as light switch or table

D. Ask Patrick to identify shapes on a chart at a set distance

48. Which of the following behaviors would indicate a possible lag in Patrick's development?

A. Hops and skips well for several seconds

B. Prints some letters of name backwards

C. Laces shoes but cannot tie bow

D. Incorrectly identifies right arm from left

49. As part of a Wellness Program, the clinic nurse instructs Patrick's parents on health issues for their child. The nurse should explain that the leading cause of death for children Patrick's age is

A. Communicable diseases

B. Cancer

C. Accidents

D. Nutritional deficiencies

50. Patrick's mother complains that he seems to have a poor appetite and eats very little at meals. Which of the following suggestions by the clinic nurse would be *most* helpful in improving Patrick's nutritional intake?

A. Allow Patrick to eat whenever he wishes during the day

B. Serve Patrick's foods on special plates and bowls with cartoon decorations

C. Encourage Patrick to taste a few bites of a large variety of new foods

D. Supplement Patrick's intake at meals with several snacks throughout the day

51. Patrick receives a DPT booster injection. The physician has ordered Pat to receive *15* mg of acetaminophen (Tylenol) per kg of body weight at home if fever develops. Patrick weighs 36 lb. The nurse calculates the total dosage to be
    A. 180 mg
    B. 220 mg
    C. 240 mg
    D. 260 mg

52. If each tablet of Tylenol contained 1 grain, Patrick's parent would need to administer how many tablets for the correct dose?
    A. 2
    B. 3
    C. 4
    D. 5

Lucas Fitz is a 7-year-old boy admitted to the pediatric unit for treatment of multiple burns and lacerations. Child abuse has been confirmed.

53. As an abused child, Lucas is *most* likely to demonstrate which of the following types of behavior?
    A. Hostile and physically aggressive
    B. Withdrawn and suspicious
    C. Angry and excitable
    D. Emotional and overly dependent

54. Which of the following nursing actions would be *most* beneficial to Lucas during his hospitalization?
    A. Encourage Lucas to socialize with other children in the unit's playroom
    B. Allow no visitation by family members
    C. Assign one nurse per shift to care for Lucas
    D. Have a nurse or aide in attendance at Lucas' bedside at all times

55. A conference between the health care team and Lucas' parents is conducted. Which of the following comments by the parents should the nurse consider the most alarming?
    A. "He always wants to be by himself. He rarely talks to anyone."
    B. "Why should I care about him? He doesn't love us!"
    C. "He's so lazy. I have to scream at him to get him to clean his room!"
    D. "He's just impossible at times! What are we to do with him?"

Andy Mitchell, age 5, is newly diagnosed with acute lymphocytic leukemia.

56. The nurse should recognize that Andy would likely have which of the following sets of symptoms?
    A. Joint pain, fatigue
    B. Weight loss, diarrhea
    C. Swollen lymphic glands, anorexia
    D. Recurrent headache, fever

57. The nurse caring for Andy should plan which of the following strategies for his rest and activity?
    A. Maintain complete bed rest
    B. Plan care to allow for frequent rest periods
    C. Limit play periods to one-half hour per shift
    D. Limit visitation to a few hours only

58. Andy is placed on a chemotherapy protocol. Which of the following actions by the nurse would most help to reduce nausea and vomiting associated with chemotherapy treatments?
    A. Restrict all oral foods and fluids
    B. Administer ordered antiemetic prior to chemotherapy
    C. Encourage a high-protein, high-residue diet
    D. Allow Andy to pick any foods that he enjoys

59. Andy complains of severe joint pain. Which of the following medications should the nurse plan to administer?
    A. Vistaril
    B. Morphine
    C. Tylenol with codeine
    D. Valium

60. As part of the discharge teaching, Andy's parents should be instructed to do which of the following?
    A. The catheter insertion site must be washed daily and a gauze dressing applied.
    B. The catheter must be irrigated four times daily with sterile saline.
    C. They must make sure that clamps are readily available at all times.
    D. They should gently reinsert the catheter in the event it becomes dislodged.

Mrs. Santori, mother of 7-year-old Matthew, explains to the pediatrician, "You know, my son still wets his bed at night. He wakes up in the morning wet and then hides his sheets and pajamas. I want to help him, but I don't know what to do."

61. The pediatric office nurse should be aware that night time bladder control is normally accomplished by
    A. Ages 18 to 24 months
    B. Ages 24 to 28 months
    C. Ages 30 to 36 months
    D. Ages 36 to 40 months

62. The nurse should explain to Mrs. Santori, that all the following are accepted possible etiologies of enuresis (bed wetting) *except*
    A. Enuresis is caused by excessive periods of deep sleep in the child's sleep cycle.
    B. Enuresis may develop from overly vigorous toilet training practices when the child is not physiologically ready.
    C. Enuresis may be associated with urinary tract infection or congenital defect of the urinary tract.
    D. Enuresis may result from a subconscious drive for greater parental attention and affection towards the child.

63. Which of the following coping mechanisms is Matthew utilizing to decrease his anxiety over bedwetting?
    A. Denial
    B. Repression
    C. Suppression
    D. Sublimation

64. The office nurse interviews Matthew about his bedwetting problem. He says to her, "Oh please, don't tell anyone! My friends will think I'm a real sissy if they find out!" The nurse understands that Matthew's concern is probably based on which of the following?
    A. During this age period, peer group acceptance is of greatest importance to Matthew.
    B. Matthew is frightened that the nurse cannot be trusted and may reveal his problem to others.
    C. Matthew feels he is coping successfully with his problem and does not wish any help from the nurse.
    D. Matthew is self-conscious about discussing this personal problem with a member of the opposite sex.

65. All of the following are appropriate strategies to improve Matthew's night-time bladder control *except*

    A. Limit fluid intake after 6:00 PM each evening

    B. Awaken the child during his sleep cycle to void

    C. Encourage the child to share his feelings about his bedwetting

    D. Send him for a week at summer camp with his friends

Michael Washington is a 14-year-old with sickle cell anemia. Diagnosed at birth, this is his 23rd admission for sickle cell disease.

66. The nurse caring for Michael should have which of the following understandings about the etiology of sickle cell disease?

    A. It is related to fetal trauma during the birthing process.

    B. It is usually caused by an acute viral infection.

    C. It is a genetically linked disorder inherited from parents.

    D. It is associated with poor nutritional intake of iron.

67. Michael is in sickle cell crisis. All of the following signs and symptoms would suggest crisis *except*

    A. Acute abdominal pain

    B. Fatigue and shortness of breath

    C. Severe joint pain

    D. Anorexia and weight loss

68. In preparing a plan of care for Michael in crisis, the nurse recognizes that his *most* immediate need is for which of the following?

    A. Hydration

    B. Pain control

    C. Prevention of joint contracture

    D. Emotional support

69. In view of Michael's level of pain and potential for bleeding, the nurse would likely administer which of the following analgesics?

    A. A.S.A.

    B. Empirin #3

    C. Percodan

    D. Morphine

70. Michael's crisis has resolved, and his level of activity is increasing. He has been caught by nurses several times smoking in the stairwells. Which of

these would be the *most* appropriate response of the nurse caring for Michael?

A. Allow Michael to smoke, but restrict to designated smoking areas.

B. Discuss with Michael the risks of smoking in light of his diagnosis.

C. Notify Michael's parents to discuss appropriate disciplinary measures.

D. Remove the cigarettes from Michael's room.

Kenneth Levy is a 2-week-old male infant diagnosed with transposition of great vessels. He has been hospitalized since birth, undergoing a Rashkind procedure on his second day of life.

71. Kenneth's nurse should understand that the Rashkind procedure was performed to accomplish which of the following?

A. Creation of an atrial-septal defect to allow for arterial-venous mixing

B. Primary correction of the underlying defect

C. Reduction of blood flow from the pulmonary artery to the lungs

D. Reduction of stroke volume and cardiac output

72. Which of the following nursing diagnoses would be of *greatest* priority for Kenneth postprocedure?

A. Alteration in comfort

B. Potential for infection

C. Knowledge deficit

D. Alteration in cardiac output

73. Comfort measures are especially important in Kenneth's care for which of the following reasons?

A. Kenneth has undergone a significant psychic-emotional stress secondary to the trauma of surgery.

B. Normal maternal-infant bonding has been interrupted because of hospitalization

C. Discomfort and associated crying will increase O_2 consumption by body cells.

D. Excessive forceful crying may cause damage to the surgical site.

74. Nutritional management of Kenneth should focus on all of the following *except*

A. Small, frequent feedings

B. Use of a low-sodium formula

C. Limited stimulation during feedings

D. Supplementing with glucose water in between feedings

75. Kenneth is to be discharged soon on digoxin. Which of the following would alert Mrs. Levy to the development of digoxin toxicity?

    A. Consistent baseline heart rate of 120

    B. Projectile vomiting

    C. Persistent diarrhea

    D. Facial twitching

76. Mrs. Levy is learning infant CPR. Which of the following instructions by the nurse would be correct?

    A. Placement of fingers one-finger breadth below the nipple line

    B. Hyperinflation of the lungs with 2 quick breaths

    C. Hyperextension of the neck using chin thrust method

    D. Compression and ventilation ratio of 15:2

77. On the day prior to Kenneth's discharge, Mrs. Levy says to the nurse, "I don't think I can take him home. I'm just not ready for this!" Which of the following would be the best *initial* response of the nurse?

    A. "The Rashkind procedure was successful. We don't anticipate any difficulties at home."

    B. "I can certainly understand how terribly frightened you must be to have Kenneth at home."

    C. "Would you feel more comfortable if we delayed discharge for another week or so?"

    D. "You seem concerned about the discharge. Can you tell me more of what you are feeling?"

78. Which of the following nursing actions would *most* help Mrs. Levy to cope with Kenneth's impending discharge?

    A. Review and practice CPR technique

    B. Arrange for visiting nurse to come to the home

    C. Discuss the possibility of a 24-hour rooming-in of parents and child

    D. Phone the physician to arrange for delay of discharge

Steven Smith is a 7-year-old male with hydrocephalus, secondary to aqueductal stenosis. He has been admitted for evaluation and treatment of a suspected shunt malfunction.

79. Which of the following presenting symptoms *most* strongly suggests increased intracranial pressure in Steven?

    A. Increasing head circumference

    B. Behavioral changes

C. Decreased appetite

D. Heart rate = 76 beats/min

80. A CT scan confirms shunt malfunction, and Steven is scheduled for a shunt revision. Considering Steven's age and developmental level, which of the following aspects of his impending surgery will likely cause him the most concern?

A. Part of his head will need to be shaved to prepare the operative site.

B. He will need to receive a preoperative injection.

C. He won't be able to go back to school until he's recovered from his surgery.

D. He might suffer some residual brain damage as a result of the surgery.

81. In developing a plan of care for Steven, which of the following nursing diagnoses is most important to consider during the first 24 hours postoperatively?

A. Potential cognitive impairment, related to hydrocephalus and increased ICP

B. Alteration in nutrition: less than body requirements, related to NPO status postoperatively

C. Social isolation, related to hospitalization and separation from family and friends

D. Potential for infection, related to surgical incision and entry into the central nervous system

82. The nurse finds Mrs. Smith crying in the parent's lounge. She states, "The doctor told me Steven's shunt was probably malfunctioning for months. I must be a terrible mother if I can't even tell when my child's in trouble." The nurse's best initial response would be which of the following?

A. "Of course you aren't a terrible mother. Anyone could make a mistake like that."

B. "Let's figure out what you need to learn so that this won't ever happen again."

C. "As kids get older, the signs and symptoms of shunt malfunction can change. If you'd like, we can talk about these."

D. "You seem upset. Are you worried that you aren't going to be able to tell when he's in trouble in the future?"

83. The physician has ordered an analgesic for Steven, as needed for complaint of postoperative pain. Which of the following observations is not indicative of a 7-year-old child in pain?

A. Changes in facial expression

B. Ability to participate in play activities

C. Pulse = 100 bpm; BP = 120/78

D. Increase in number and length of sleep periods

84. Steven has been on anticonvulsant drug therapy for the last several years. What evidence would give the best indication that Steven is cognitively ready to accept responsibility for and to start learning self-medication?

    A. Steven brings his medication to his mother and reminds her that his "seizure medicine" is due.

    B. Steven knows the name of his medication and can identify it in a PDR color photograph.

    C. Steven can accurately explain what kind of medication he is taking and why.

    D. None. Seven year olds are too young to self-medicate.

During a routine physical examination, it is discovered that Cathy Gorman, age 12, has a 25-degree curvature of her spine. A diagnosis of scoliosis is made.

85. Upon physical examination, each of the following can be seen with scoliosis except:

    A. Lateral curvature of the spine

    B. Rotary deformity of the pelvis

    C. Accentuation of the cervical curvature

    D. Flank asymmetry when bent at the waist

86. Cathy is fitted for a Milwaukee brace. In order to provide patient teaching, the nurse must recognize that the primary goal of therapy is to

    A. Halt progression of the curvature

    B. Replace surgical correction

    C. Prevent the development of kyphosis

    D. Prevent muscle atrophy

87. Which of the following areas of patient teaching should the nurse have as a priority at this time?

    A. Explanation of external realignment therapy

    B. Demonstration of exercises

    C. Modification of lifestyles

    D. Promotion of positive self-image

While the pediatric nurse practitioner is teaching Cathy how to apply the brace, Cathy says, "This thing is horrible. Everyone is going to laugh at me."

88. Each of the following instructions provided by the nurse will help Cathy to be more accepting of the brace while promoting a positive self-image *except*

    A. Encourage her to wear brightly colored sweaters and blouses with high collars

    B. Recommend that she may occasionally remove the brace for special social occasions

    C. Emphasize positive aspects and eventual outcome of therapy

    D. Encourage involvement in activities that are compatible with her limitations

Michael Gorman, aged 4 months, is brought to the Pediatric Clinic for a routine well-care visit. The pediatric nurse practitioner performs an evaluation of his motor development.

89. The pediatric nurse practitioner would expect to see mastery of which of the following gross motor skills?

    A. While in prone position, he lifts his head and chest and bears weight on his forearm.

    B. He rolls easily from his back to his abdomen.

    C. He sits alone, leaning on his hands for support.

    D. He willfully rolls from his abdomen to his back.

90. The nurse should recognize which of the following as an example of fine motor skills development at age 4 months?

    A. He uses the pincher grasp to pick up small objects.

    B. Hands are predominately closed.

    C. He can transfer objects from one hand to another.

    D. He is unable to voluntarily grasp an object.

MENTAL HEALTH EXAM *D*

Samuel Torres is a 36-year-old factory worker admitted to the psychophysiologic unit for treatment of alcohol abuse. At the time of admission, Mr. Torres is acutely intoxicated.

1. Which of the following statements of Mr. Torres' wife would provide the nurse conducting an intake interview with the *most* valuable information about Mr. Torres' alcohol abuse?

    A. "He was laid off from his job 6 weeks ago, and that upset him a great deal. He always drinks when he's upset."

    B. "His drinking seems much worse now than in the past. He's so difficult to handle now."

    C. "I've tried hiding some of his bottles from him, but he gets so mad at me, I'm afraid he'll hurt me or the children."

    D. "He's had two blackouts in the last week—doesn't know where he's been or what he has done."

2. In this acute period of intoxication, the nursing diagnosis of great priority for Mr. Torres would be

    A. Ineffective individual coping

    B. Potential for injury

    C. Potential fluid volume

    D. Alteration in comfort

3. All of the following are psychological characteristics of alcohol-abusive patients *except*

335

   A. Personal insecurity

   B. Tendency to overuse denial as a defense mechanism

   C. Overdeveloped, punitive super-ego

   D. Inability to form close and lasting affection ties

4. Which of the following observed symptoms of Mr. Torres during withdrawal from alcohol should be of *greatest* concern to the nurse?

   A. Tachycardia

   B. Hypertension

   C. Nausea and vomiting

   D. Seizures

5. During withdrawal, Mr. Torres is becoming increasingly agitated and physically aggressive. Which of the following nursing interventions would be most appropriate?

   A. Place Mr. Torres in a quiet, darkened private room

   B. Place Mr. Torres in soft restraints

   C. Ambulate Mr. Torres around the unit

   D. Pad the bed side rails and place an airway at bedside

6. Which of the following types of medication would the nurse most likely administer to Mr. Torres during the withdrawal period?

   A. Narcotic analgesic

   B. Barbiturate

   C. Anti-cholinergic

   D. Anti-anxiety

7. One week later, Mr. Torres has completed withdrawal and is receiving treatment for alcohol abuse. Which of the following questions by the nurse would provide the most valuable information about his past alcohol abuse?

   A. "Mr. Torres, how much did you drink?"

   B. "Did you ever drink when you were alone?"

   C. "Have you ever forgotten what you were doing while you were drinking?"

   D. "Have you ever missed work because of your drinking?"

8. Which of the following comments by Mr. Torres best illustrates his acceptance of an alcohol abuse problem?

   A. "I can realize now that I may have a drinking problem."

   B. "I'm going to change. I feel like I can deal with life again."

C. "I think I've learned to control my drinking now."

D. "I need help to give up drinking for the rest of my life."

Debbie, a 16-year-old student, is admitted to the psychophysiologic unit in a semiconsciousness state with a history of a 58-pound weight loss in 3 months. Preliminary diagnosis is acute anorexia nervosa.

9. Which of the following admission lab values should the nurse caring for Debbie consider the *most* critical?

   A. Glucose, 80

   B. Potassium, 3.0

   C. Sodium, 144

   D. Hemoglobin, 10

10. Which vital sign would provide the *most* essential information in light of Debbie's current lab values?

    A. Temperature

    B. Pulse

    C. Respirations

    D. Blood pressure

11. Additional assessments of Debbie during this acute stage should include all of the following *except*

    A. Urine output

    B. Level of consciousness

    C. Skin turgor

    D. Urine Dextrostix

12. The nursing diagnosis of highest priority for Debbie in her acute anorexic episode would be

    A. Alteration in nutrition: less than body requirements

    B. Alteration in health maintenance

    C. Fluid-volume deficit

    D. Disturbance in self-concept

13. All of the following are common characteristics of anorexia nervosa *except*

    A. Preoccupation with food

    B. Fear of developing sexuality

    C. Independence from parental and peer pressures

    D. Distorted body image

14. The nurse recognizes that anorexic behavior often stems from the client's desire
    A. For self-abuse or self-mutilation
    B. To punish herself for past behavior through starvation
    C. To gain control over an aspect of her life
    D. To express hatred towards her parents

15. The nurse should recognize that Debbie has recovered from her psychic conflicts associated with anorexia when she
    A. Demonstrates an increase in weight
    B. Demonstrates serum electrolytes within normal parameters
    C. Reduces her exercise regimen to only once per day
    D. Makes a date with a companion for dinner

Mrs. Lucille Sturn is a 52-year-old widow admitted to the psychiatric hospital with a diagnosis of obsessive-compulsive reaction. Mrs. Sturn spends hours carrying out a routine of washing her hands, toilet facilities, and the sink. She is careful to wash all food and dishes before she eats.

16. Mrs. Sturn's obsessive-compulsive behavior is characterized by an overuse of which of the following?
    A. Sublimation
    B. Conversation
    C. Undoing
    D. Suppression

17. Mrs. Sturns says to the nurse, "I have so much cleaning to do. Germs, you know, they're everywhere." Which of the following explanations of Mrs. Sturn's compulsive washing is most accurate?
    A. It serves to keep the client distracted from her real fears.
    B. It serves to decrease anxiety by eliminating the obsession.
    C. It helps the client to control or modify her obsession.
    D. It represents a symbolic method through which the client can face her fear.

18. One realistic goal for Mrs. Sturn is that she will
    A. Express insight into obsessive thoughts
    B. Accept limits on ritualistic behaviors
    C. Initiate new forms of activity
    D. Stop ritualistic and repetitive behaviors

19. On the third day of Mrs. Sturn's hospitalization the nurse notes that Lucille is repeatedly late to group sessions and activities. Which of the following comments by the nurse to Lucille would be *most* appropriate?

    A. "Lucille, you must realize that these washing behaviors are unnecessary."

    B. "Lucille, I will have to limit you to one session of washing per day."

    C. "Lucille, you'll need to start earlier so you can complete your washing in time to go to group sessions."

    D. "Lucille, you will only get better if you go to your sessions. You'll have to control your washing routines."

20. Which of the following statements indicates a realistic short-term measure of improvement in Mrs. Sturn?

    A. "Wow, I never realized how ridiculous I was acting!"

    B. "I'll do whatever you think is best, nurse."

    C. "I wish I knew why I feel so anxious and scared all the time."

    D. "I should be able to get my cleaning done more quickly tomorrow."

Helen Black, aged 24, is admitted to the psychiatric unit by her mother who reports bizarre behavior of 2 days' duration. After returning from church services, the patient began to mumble repeatedly "I'm sorry," as she wept quietly.

21. While orienting the patient to the unit, the nurse observes her wide-eyed facial expression and hesitant demeanor. Helen stops abruptly and refuses to move saying "The devil, the devil—he's here and he'll get me!" The best response by the nurse would be

    A. "This is a hospital. You're here to get well and forget those kinds of thoughts."

    B. "I'll introduce you to the other patients. Once you get acquainted, you'll forget about the devil."

    C. "Helen, I think you're frightened. We will keep you safe here."

    D. "The devil isn't here, Helen. Just look around. Do you see him?"

22. Over the next several days, Helen becomes increasingly nonverbal and refuses to eat. She often glances about as if terrified and secludes herself in her room. The *most* helpful approach by the nurse would be

    A. Maintain consistent contact and provide continued verbal input even if she does not respond

    B. Allow her to be alone for greater periods of time, since she seems more comfortable away from others

    C. Insist she mix with other patients and set limits on how much time she can spend in her room

    D. Prevent any further regression by requiring her to assume greater responsibility for her care

23. Helen is diagnosed as suffering from schizophrenia, catatonic type. While giving her AM care, the nurse notes her tendency to sustain unusual body postures and abnormal muscle tone. The nursing diagnosis of *lowest* priority for this patient at present is

    A. Potential alteration in skin integrity

    B. Potential alteration in mobility

    C. Alteration in communication

    D. Alteration in socialization

24. The motor behaviors described above are sometimes referred to as posturing or waxy flexibility. Other common symptoms seen in patients with this type of schizophrenia include

    A. An apparent indifference to surroundings and lack of response to stimuli

    B. Silly, nonsensible speech and frequent giggling

    C. Tendency to believe others are "out to get them"

    D. Delusions of grandeur and history of chronically poor interpersonal skills

25. The medications *most* commonly prescribed to treat this condition are

    A. Stimulants such as caffeine or amphetamine

    B. Major tranquilizers like Haldol

    C. Minor tranquilizers like Valium

    D. Sedatives or soporifics such as chloral hydrate

26. Patients such as Helen often require extensive and supportive nursing care. All of the following complications are potential risks of the illness *except*

    A. Aspiration pneumonia

    B. Malnutrition and weight loss

    C. Decubitus ulcers

    D. Flaccid paralysis

27. Improvement in Helen's clinical picture would most likely be demonstrated *first* by which behavior?

    A. Gradual increase in amount of verbal production

B. Ability to discuss her fears and concerns with the nurse

C. Increased awareness of environment

D. Return of spontaneous motor movements

28. Helen's condition begins to improve slowly. What nursing intervention would be appropriate in attempting to form a working relationship with her now?

   A. Spend time discussing her recent family problems with her

   B. Engage in conversations about religion and her beliefs

   C. Ask her to help choose what she will wear on each day

   D. Begin family therapy sessions

29. Helen finally begins to verbalize with the nurse. She expresses great fear that God will punish her, since "He hates all sinners, and I am the worst of all." Such delusional beliefs are best handled by:

   A. Reasoning with the patient so she may see she neither is a sinner nor will God harm her

   B. Interrupting immediately and telling the patient she must not speak of this again

   C. Responding to the guilty feelings that played a role in the delusions formation

   D. Asking a member of the clergy to visit the patient

30. This admission is Ms. Black's first psychiatric hospitalization. Which of the following factors would be *most* associated with a poor prognosis?

   A. A rapid onset of symptoms

   B. High IQ and steady employment in the past

   C. History of good relationships

   D. Strong familial history of schizophrenia

Margaret Wilson, aged 26, enters the emergency room for treatment of an acute overdose of Elavil (amitriptyline).

31. Margaret is very lethargic but rousable on admission. Gastric lavage is performed, and vital signs are stable when she is transferred to ICU for close observation. Of *greatest* concern during the next 48 hours would be

   A. WBC of 6000

   B. EKG changes

   C. K+ value of 3.6

   D. Slightly elevated TPR

32. Margaret tells the ICU nurse, "I'm sorry I didn't die. Life is useless. Why did you have to save me?" The *best* response of the nurse would be
    A. "You know you don't mean that."
    B. "It's our job Margaret. Nothing is ever that bad."
    C. "I know you're feeling hopeless. Tell me what's happening."
    D. "Let's concentrate on getting well. In a few days you'll feel differently."

33. Further history indicates Margaret has been seeing a psychiatrist for depressive symptoms and has been diagnosed as having borderline personality disorder. The nurse would be *most* surprised to learn that this patient
    A. Believes she has been chosen by God to be his special messenger on earth
    B. Has a history of episodic substance abuse
    C. Has made other suicide attempts
    D. Has a pattern of unstable, intense relationships with others

34. Upon transfer to the psychiatric unit, Margaret is informed by the admitting nurse that it will be necessary to check her belongings for any unsafe or banned items. She begins to scream angrily, "What's the matter with you? I'm upset. Get away from me!" The nurse should *first*
    A. Administer emergency tranquilizers as ordered
    B. Place Margaret in seclusion and restraints
    C. Eliminate the belongings search so as to avoid upsetting her
    D. Set verbal limits on her behavior

35. Margaret requests a weekend pass 2 days after transfer to the psychiatric unit. Ms. Grant, her primary nurse, informs her following the treatment team meeting that the pass has not been approved. Margaret responds angrily, "They all hate me, they're so mean! I know you'd have let me go. You're the only decent nurse here!" The nurse's *best* response is
    A. "I would have approved it, but you're right—I'm only one voice."
    B. "I don't think the others realize how hard you've been trying."
    C. "Margaret, you'll never get a pass behaving this way."
    D. "This was the team's decision. Let's talk about why we feel it's not appropriate now."

36. Margaret's behavior in this situation illustrates the use of which defense mechanism?
    A. Splitting
    B. Reaction formation

C. Conversion

D. Repression

37. Margaret's physician resumes her regular dosage of Elavil. Which effect of this medication might the staff and patient expect to see *first?*

   A. Elevated mood

   B. Improved reality testing

   C. Improved sleep pattern

   D. Fewer hallucinations and delusions

John Reynolds, a 24-year-old male, is ordered by the court to undergo psychiatric evaluation after arrest for robbery and assault. During admission to the unit he comments to the nurse, "Don't worry, sweetie, I'll only be here a short time. This was all my lawyer's idea, but it sure beats jail."

38. These statements would *best* illustrate the defense mechanism of

   A. Rationalization

   B. Regression

   C. Sublimation

   D. Splitting

39. John's tentative diagnosis is sociopathic personality disorder. What factor in the patient's history would be *least* consistent with this diagnosis?

   A. Early childhood deprivation and neglect

   B. Previous incarceration for stealing and vandalism

   C. Prior diagnosis of childhood conduct disorder

   D. Symptom onset following an identifiable loss

40. The nurse would likely observe John's interacting with other patient's by

   A. Attempting to monopolize conversations and being intrusive

   B. Being superficially pleasant and appearing interested in them

   C. Avoiding most contact and refusing to join in group activities

   D. Demonstrating poor social skills and little awareness of the milieu

41. In developing an effective nurse-patient relationship with John, the nurse should

   A. Anticipate that with support and nurturance he may well recognize the degree of his illness

   B. Expect attempts to test limits and recognize their importance for him

   C. Capitalize upon his highly developed intelligence and level of insight

    D. Allow him a high degree of autonomy and self direction to increase motivation

42. In planning realistic long-term goals, the nurse should recall that patients with John's diagnosis
    A. Often require life-long medication therapy
    B. Rarely function autonomously in the community
    C. Usually seek treatment because of their emotional distress
    D. Are referred for psychiatric intervention repeatedly by others

43. A unit search is conducted after another patient reports to the staff he's been offered drugs by John. Small amounts of cocaine and marijuana are found. When approaching him with this information, the nurse would be *most* surprised if John:
    A. Threatens to sign out of the hospital
    B. Shrugs his shoulders and makes light of the whole affair
    C. Becomes tearful and subsequently expresses real remorse
    D. Becomes angry and demands to know "Who told you?".

44. John returns from a pass 4 hours late. He hands the nurse a bouquet of flowers and says, "I'm sorry I was late, but I knew you'd understand. Can't we just keep this our little secret?" The nurse should
    A. Focus her interaction with John on how relationships with others can be beneficial to him
    B. Keep the flowers but explain to him that any further tardiness will be reported
    C. Return the flowers and talk with John about the consequences of violating rules
    D. Not report the tardiness since John is signaling the nurse he's trying to develop a relationship

John Meyers, aged 36, is admitted into the emergency room following an ingestion of rat poison. The primary ingredient of the product was warfarin. After being stabilized, he is transferred to psychiatry.

45. Given the ingested substance, which of the following symptoms might the nurse be most alert for?
    A. Nausea and vomiting
    B. Complaint of sore throat
    C. Bleeding gums and bruising easily
    D. Fever and headaches

46. John is presently unable or unwilling to provide any history or information about the circumstances of his ingestion. In evaluating appropriate unit placement and/or privileges for him, the nurse should be *most* concerned about:
    A. Allowing as much independence as possible
    B. Providing a calm, comfortable environment
    C. Maintaining safety and security
    D. The presence of other peers of similar age

47. What nursing intervention would be *most* appropriate at this time?
    A. Placing the patient in restraints and seclusion
    B. Limiting his contacts with other patients
    C. Observing him closely and instituting suicide precautions
    D. Involving him in recreational groups

48. John's family provides information about his behavior prior to the ingestion. Which symptom would be *most* suggestive of an acute organic mental illness?
    A. Sudden difficulties with memory and orientation
    B. Auditory hallucinations
    C. Elaborate delusions
    D. Withdrawal from others over a long period of time

49. John tells the nurse he ate rat poison so he could kill himself "before I fall into enemy hands." In evaluating his suicidal risk, the nurse should recall
    A. As a male, he is less likely to successfully kill himself than if he were female.
    B. Direct questioning about suicide should be avoided, since he may learn of new ways to try to kill himself.
    C. Delusional, psychotic people are at risk because of poor reality testing and impaired judgment.
    D. Having failed in his attempt, he is unlikely to consider suicide again.

50. Which piece of information from John would tend to suggest he made a suicidal gesture and not a true attempt?
    A. He is surprised he did not succeed.
    B. He ingested the poison and immediately called for help.
    C. He ingested enough poison to constitute far more than a lethal dose.
    D. He timed his ingestion to coincide with a period when he would not be discovered.

John's family describe him as a loner who seemed "out of time" with the rest of the world. Past records indicate he has been hospitalized 13 times for treatment of psychiatric illness since age 19. He has never followed up with outpatient care. His current diagnosis is schizophrenia, chronic undifferentiated type.

51. John is placed on Prolixin Decanoate (IM) for symptomatic treatment of illness. This medication is often chosen particularly for patients
    A. Who have difficulty taking daily medication
    B. Who are demonstrating symptoms of tardive dyskinesia
    C. Who have become overly dependent on tranquilizers for relief of anxiety
    D. Who have liver disease and cannot metabolize other major tranquilizers

52. Which of the following effects of antipsychotic medications would John's nurse be likely to consider a contraindication to further use?
    A. Drowsiness and decrease in resting blood pressure
    B. Tremors of the upper extremities and rigid facial expression
    C. Dry mouth and blurring of vision
    D. Facial grimacing and involuntary movements of fingers and toes

53. John's acute symptoms of psychosis have now remitted. All of the following are reasonable goals of nursing therapy *except*
    A. Helping the client verbalize insight into his deep-seated conflicts
    B. Improving his social skills so he may more comfortably function in the milieu
    C. Educating the patient about his medications and need for continued follow-up
    D. Helping the client gain some sense of worth and accomplishment in activity groups

54. John is to be discharged to a specialized deinstitutionalization program in the community. After learning he has been accepted for placement, the nurse notices he begins to regress and becomes very dependent upon the staff. What should the nurse do first?
    A. Postpone discharge, since he is clearly not ready.
    B. Describe the observed behavior and discuss it with John.
    C. Suggest increasing the dosage of medication to his physician.
    D. Ignore the behavior unless John comments on it himself.

55. Clients such as John often experience marked anxiety when changes or separations occur in their lives. This is because

    A. They have punitive superegos.

    B. They have few ego strengths.

    C. Hospitalization has deprived them of their civil rights.

    D. Psychotropic drugs diminish motivation.

Charles Humbert, aged 23, is admitted by the emergency room with acute dehydration. He has been experiencing frequent episodes of loose, bloody stools for 2 weeks. He has a 5-year history of ulcerative colitis.

56. Which of the following classes of medication would generally be contraindicated in Charles' treatment?

    A. Steroids

    B. Opiates

    C. Sulfa drugs

    D. Anticoagulants

57. Charles' fluid and electrolyte balance is restored, but he continues to have bloody diarrhea. The nurse notes, despite instruction to the contrary, that he flushes the toilet after each BM. The *least* likely explanation for this behavior is

    A. He is embarrassed by the odor.

    B. He is denying or minimizing his illness.

    C. He is malingering.

    D. He is seeking a means of exercising control.

58. Due to his debilitated state and need for complete GI rest, Charles is at severe nutritional risk. His doctor orders total parenteral nutrition (TPN) to be administered via a central line. The advantage of *this* type of administration as compared with the use of a peripheral line is

    A. It permits administration of more concentrated solutions.

    B. It carries less risk of infection and bleeding.

    C. It does not require use of sterile technique in dressing changes.

    D. The rate of infusion no longer requires monitoring.

59. After seeing his physician who suggests the need for total colectomy and ileostomy, the nurse finds Charles dressed and packing his suitcase. He angrily states, "Take this IV out—I'm not staying here any more! He can't be serious. I'd never agree to such a thing!" The nurse should *first*

A. Tell Charles he cannot leave and call hospital security

B. Point out to him that the surgery may be quite beneficial

C. Recognize that Charles feels overwhelmed and ask what happened

D. Remove the TPN line and obtain an AMA form

60. Charles begins to sob, ''Why are you doing this to me?'' I'm not a bad person!'' The nurse should respond

A. ''Do you think you're a bad person?''

B. ''It doesn't seem fair. No one expects or wants something like this.''

C. ''Charles, we're not doing it to you. Your illness has made this necessary.''

D. ''It would help if you'd realize we only want what's best for you.''

61. Charles sits down on his bed and weeps softly. He turns to the nurse and asks, ''Someone told me about vitamin therapy treatments. They use all-natural substances and have cured people like me. Isn't it at least worth a try?'' The nurse would *best* respond

A. ''Unorthodox treatments rarely ''cure'' people. You'd be wasting valuable time.''

B. ''If it were me, I'd look into it. You can always have surgery later if it doesn't work.''

C. ''I can understand wanting to consider all the options. I think you need time to ask questions and think through the decision.''

D. ''You really have no choice. Your doctor has exhausted all the possibilities with measures he's found useful in similar cases.''

62. Subsequently, Charles elects to have the recommended surgery. Twenty-four hours into his postoperative course he suddenly becomes markedly febrile and has an elevated white count (WBCs = 16,000). His physician orders removal of the central line and discontinues TPN. The nurse knows this is because

A. The presence of a central line may limit Charles' ability to deep breathe effectively.

B. Antibiotics can safely be administered by peripheral IVs.

C. Nutrient-rich solutions offer a ready medium for bacterial growth.

D. Charles' remaining GI tract is now functional, and antibiotics are better absorbed via the PO route.

63. Later in the day, Charles reports to the night nurse he has seen bugs crawling up the wall opposite his bed. His mood also seems labile; at times he cries fretfully, and at other times he seems easily irritated. The nurse might well interpret these symptoms as evidence of

A. Impending functional psychosis

B. Latent schizophrenia

C. Acute organic brain syndrome

D. Adjustment disorder

64. Ms. Jones, the ostomy nurse, has observed Mr. Humbert's withdrawn, silent manner during their postoperative contacts. Seemingly, his physical condition is steadily improving, but he continues to keep his eyes averted from the stoma and incision site. He also answers her questions regarding previous teaching with a shrug of his shoulders. The best *initial* approach to these difficulties would be:

A. Supply Mr. Humbert with written materials regarding ostomy care since he seems unable to retain verbal information

B. Insist that Mr. Humbert look at his wound and stoma during the next visit

C. Give Mr. Humbert feedback about his observed behavior and ask him for his perceptions

D. Inform Mr. Humbert he will begin caring for his ostomy independently tomorrow and that the nursing staff will not assist him

Margaret Blue, aged 21, enters the hospital complaining of episodes of shortness of breath, feelings of panic, and syncope. She is admitted to the general medical floor. She fears she may be suffering from a heart condition although these symptoms began approximately 1 month ago.

65. Given her history and an essentially normal physical exam, what cardiac problem might Margaret be at greatest risk for?

A. Congestive failure

B. Mitral value prolapse

C. Ventricular septal defect

D. Coronary artery disease

66. As part of the diagnostic work-up, cardiac and psychiatric consultants are ordered for Margaret. She asks the nurse, "Just because I get anxious when this happens doesn't mean I'm crazy, does it?" The nurse's *best* response is

A. "Ask the doctor. I don't know why they've called the psychiatrist."

B. "Now don't get upset. That will only make things worse."

C. "You mentioned feeling anxious and it's important to look at all of your symptoms."

D. "Anxiety can be helped with medication. Maybe that's why the psychiatrist has been called."

67. Margaret is subsequently diagnosed as suffering from a conversion disorder. All of the following data from the nursing history would support this diagnosis *except*
    A. Margaret's mother has been in daily contact with her since symptoms began.
    B. Margaret recently curtailed her visits to her dying grandmother as they were too "upsetting."
    C. Margaret's symptoms have become so severe she can no longer function at work.
    D. Margaret admits she can "bring on" an attack.

68. In formulating an approach to Margaret's in-hospital nursing care, the nurse will
    A. Ignore further physical complaints since they are a function of psychologic disturbance
    B. Recognize that her complaints are based on a conscious need to avoid conflict
    C. Emphasize the need for Margaret to acknowledge that her symptoms are not physiologically based
    D. Express the belief physical symptoms will subside while encouraging gradual resumption of normal activities

69. Which of the following short-term goals would *not* be a reasonable expectation for Margaret?
    A. She will verbalize the conflict experienced which led to the development of conversion symptoms.
    B. She will gradually resume her normal daily activities.
    C. She will utilize others' assistance in reality testing about her symptoms.
    D. She will engage in conversations about topics other than physical complaints.

70. Upon discharge, Margaret is asked to return for outpatient follow-up with the nurse psychotherapist. Therapeutic goals would dictate what frequency of appointments?
    A. Daily contacts to ease the transition from hospital to home
    B. Weekly assistance to provide support and minimize feelings of abandonment
    C. Monthly appointments for medication monitoring
    D. Appointments whenever physical symptoms increase

The psychiatric nurse clinician is called to the emergency room to see Hugh Thomas, aged 31, an attorney. He has no prior history of psychiatric illness and the triage form lists his complaint as "trouble sleeping."

71. As the nurse enters the room, she observes Hugh shouting at his wife very angrily. He suddenly turns around and says, "OK lady, what's your problem? I don't have one—my wife here does!" The *best* response for the nurse at this point is

    A. "Why don't I talk with her then? You can wait outside if you'd like."

    B. "Mr. Thomas, get a hold of yourself. That's no way to behave."

    C. "I was told you've been having some sleep difficulties. Why don't you tell me about that."

    D. "You don't have to talk to me if you don't want to. I'm just here to help."

72. Mr. Thomas begins to speak rapidly before the nurse can respond to his initial outburst. He paces and seems unaware that he is jumping from topic to topic. This behavior is called

    A. Echololia

    B. Flight of ideas

    C. Word salad

    D. Thought broadcasting

73. Mrs. Thomas tearfully states, "This just isn't like him. I can't believe the change." Which of the following questions would the nurse be *least* likely to ask *next?*

    A. "When did you notice the change?"

    B. "What is your husband usually like?"

    C. "What's different about his behavior?"

    D. "Have the two of you been getting along recently?"

74. Hugh is normally described as very sociable, confident, hard working, and successful. Given his history and the observations thus far, which diagnosis would the nurse tend to *eliminate?*

    A. Acute organic brain syndrome

    B. Schizophrenia

    C. Manic depressive illness

    D. Drug intoxication or withdrawal

75. Hugh's wife notes he had seemed "low" the past several weeks following the death of a close friend. Which of the following sleep disturbances are *not* typically seen with depressed patients?

    A. Sleeping more than usual

    B. Early morning awakening

    C. Difficulty staying asleep

    D. Unable to fall asleep

76. Following a complete assessment, the nurse recommends psychiatric admission for Mr. Thomas. His tentative diagnosis is mania. Which of the following behavioral descriptions in the evaluation notes would *best* support this diagnosis?

    A. Difficulty with concentration, poor judgment, and intrusiveness

    B. Mutism, expansive mood, and irritability

    C. Loss of pleasure in usual hobbies and poor grooming

    D. Fatigue, dysphoria, and ideas of reference

77. Early during Hugh's hospital stay he complains loudly to the staff and patient group, "This place is *so* boring! There's nothing to do here!" Which of the following activities would be most appropriate for him?

    A. Playing chess with another intelligent person

    B. One-to-one conversation with a depressed elderly man

    C. Reading the newspaper to fellow patients

    D. Involvement in an exercise group led by the staff

78. Lithium carbonate is prescribed for Hugh. His most recent lithium level of 2.3 mEq/L means the nurse should anticipate

    A. An increase in the prescribed dosage

    B. A decrease in the prescribed dosage

    C. Holding further lithium until the level is verified

    D. No change in the prescribed medication regimen

79. Just prior to discharge, Hugh attends the unit "medication group." He remarks, "I hate that lithium. I feel so slow. It's a drag having no energy." What feedback from a group or staff member would likely be *most* helpful?

    A. "That's what it's supposed to do. Your doctor ordered it, and you'd better take it."

    B. "I believe you. But, I've noticed you seem to finish activities you start since you've been on the lithium."

    C. "Maybe you don't need it anymore. Why don't you ask your doctor if you can cut down?"

    D. "You're just beginning to realize how depressed you were underneath all that hyperactivity."

80. The nurse should be *most* concerned if Hugh were to complain about the following symptom of lithium use

    A. "How come my hands sort of shake nurse?"

    B. "I can't seem to walk right. I stagger like a drunk."

    C. "Gosh, I'm always so thirsty."

    D. "Is it normal to feel sort of nauseated on this medication?"

Mr. and Mrs. Johnson and their 7-year-old son Billy are seen by the nurse psychotherapist. Billy has been absent from school a great deal and is diagnosed by the pediatrician as school-phobic.

81. In treating school phobia the nurse will recall
    A. The goal is to return the suffering child to the classroom as soon as possible.
    B. The child's intrapsychic problems are related to traumas suffered in the classroom.
    C. Unlike other phobic disorders, sufferers don't experience typical signs and symptoms of anxiety.
    D. As a systemic problem, the only focus of attention and intervention will be family dynamics.

82. When asking each member of the family about the problem, Mr. Johnson replies, "Get this kid back in school where he belongs. My wife just babies him!" The nurse's next response should be
    A. "You sound very angry Mr. Johnson. Can you tell me more about that?"
    B. "You want to see Billy back in school? What keeps that from happening?"
    C. "That seems pretty simplistic. What part do you play in the difficulty?"
    D. "Mrs. Johnson, is that true? Do you baby Billy?"

83. Mrs. Johnson angrily retorts, "You're such a bully! Why do you pick on him so?" The interaction thus far best illustrates which family dynamic?
    A. Emotional cut off
    B. Transference
    C. Triangling
    D. Double bind

84. In formulating a treatment approach with the Johnsons, all of the following interventions would likely be considered *except*
    A. A trial of psychoactive medication such as imipramine (Tofranil)
    B. Rewarding Billy for each day he attends school
    C. Switching Billy to a different teacher and classroom
    D. Having Mrs. Johnson accompany Billy to school and remain in the classroom

85. After working with the family for several weeks, Mr. Johnson raises the issue of discontinuing sessions. Which of the following outcomes could the nurse utilize as the *basic* criterion for determing the success of therapy?

    A. Billy no longer complains of symptoms each morning and attends school regularly.

    B. Mrs. Johnson allows Billy to be more independent.

    C. Mr. Johnson describes why Billy's school phobia developed.

    D. The Johnsons verbalize an understanding of their marital conflicts.

Mrs. Ruth Bosworth reports to the community mental health center requesting counseling. She feels she needs help in coping with her mother, Mrs. Cosgrove, who has Alzheimer's disease.

86. Mrs. Bosworth has asked her mother to move into her home rather than maintaining a separate apartment. Which of the following explanations would help the nurse understand this decision *most* readily?

    A. "I could tell by the look on her face she was afraid to be alone."

    B. "I used to find burned food on the stove she'd completely forgotten."

    C. "It's only right. I'm her daughter and it's my duty to care for her."

    D. "A change of scenery will do her good. I'm sure she's forgetful because she's alone."

87. Mrs. Bosworth states, "I should have known something was wrong a long time ago. She seemed nervous and restless. Could that have been related to her Alzheimer's?" The nurse would likely respond

    A. "No, Alzheimer's is a physical problem in brain functioning. Being nervous is different."

    B. "I don't think so. Were there upsetting things happening to her then?"

    C. "It's possible. People sometimes sense they're not functioning quite as well and get anxious about it."

    D. "Your mother probably already knew of her difficulties but couldn't admit it."

88. Information from Mrs. Cosgrove's physician suggests a mild to moderate level of cognitive impairment. If she were to be hospitalized, what behavior might the daughter be likely to report after visiting her mother?

    A. "She seems much better. I guess the change of scenery really worked miracles."

    B. "She's more content there. Maybe she's been depressed at home."

    C. "She seems worse to me. She was confused about where she was the whole time."

    D. "I couldn't see any difference. She was still a little forgetful just like at home."

89. Mrs. Cosgrove does move into the daughter's home. To facilitate the transition and maximize her ability to function, it would be helpful to do all of the following *except*

    A. Bring along as many of her personal possessions as possible and place them in her room

    B. Encourage her to maintain her usual daily routine in the new setting

    C. Plan new and varied activities for her to keep her highly stimulated

    D. Plan the move in advance and make the shift from one home to the other gradually

90. The nurse therapist is considering the possibility of forming a support group for the family members of Alzheimer's patients. The benefits provided would include all of the following *except*

    A. A "night off" when caretakers would be freed of usual responsibilities and able to socialize

    B. Assistance with problem solving and a means of sharing information about resources

    C. Decreasing feelings of isolation and providing support in coping with a difficult situation

    D. Opportunities to explore past and current conflicts with the affected family member

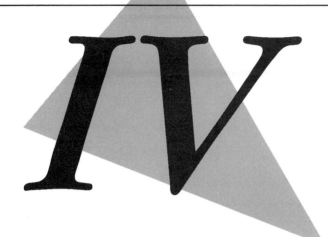

ITEM
RATIONALES
FOR
COMPREHENSIVE
REASONING
EXERCISES

ADULT HEALTH TEST ITEM RATIONALES

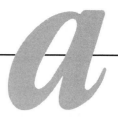

1. The intended response is **B.** An increased intracranial pressure presses on the brain stem, where the vital signs are regulated. The changes that occur with increased intracranial pressure include a decrease in pulse and respirations with an increase in systolic blood pressure and temperature.

2. The intervention that will help reduce intracranial pressure is elevating the head of the bed 30 degrees, since the action promotes venous drainage and decreases the total volume within the intracranial vault (response **D**).

3. The most effective way to prevent a joint from developing ankylosis (contracture) is to keep the joint moving. Thus, passive range of motion (PROM) exercises are indicated for the CVA patient (response **C**).

4. The intended response is **D.** The credé method is application of gentle pressure by massaging the bladder, which stimulates the bladder muscle to expel retained urine, thus helping to prevent urinary retention.

5. The intended response is **D.** Responses **A, B,** and **C** are unrealistic for the post-CVA patient, requiring that he have a greater level of independence than is probable following this brain injury. Ambulation with assistance and tripod cane is realistic, since external supports are provided to bolster independence.

6. The intended response is **D.** The progressive muscle weakness affecting the diaphragm resulting in respiratory arrest signifies its priority importance.

7. The correct order for suctioning of the patient with endotracheal tube in place is response **D.** Suctioning an endotracheal tube requires sterile tech-

nique. The mouth is then to be considered cleaner than the nose. Thus, going from sterile to very clean to clean is considered the proper order for the suctioning process.

8. The most valid indicator that Chet no longer requires mechanical ventilation is response **B.** A normal arterial blood pH with a decreasing O_2 flow indicates that the patient's respiratory status is satisfactory for removal of mechanical ventilation. Attempts of the patient to assist the ventilator (response **A**) or extubate himself (response **D**) are not accurate enough evidence to support discontinuation of ventilation. A respiratory rate of 32 breaths/min is much too rapid to indicate adequate pulmonary function.

9. The intended response is **D.** Although all the listed nursing diagnoses are important for the patient with ALS, the nurse's priority concern is always effectiveness of airway and ventilation, and since this disease involves degeneration of nerve impulses, respirations are ultimately affected.

10. The most serious concern in Wayne's progressive disease is pneumonia, which often results in death. Thus, the intended response is focused on preventing respiratory complications by turning, coughing, and deep breathing (response **A**).

11. The correct response is **C,** since an isotonic solution such as 0.9 or normal saline must *always* be used in irrigation of a nasogastric tube in order to prevent undue removal of sodium and acids from the stomach, which could result in fluid and electrolyte and acid-base imbalances in the patient.

12. The process of nasogastric tube insertion is not a pleasant one, and the nurse should anticipate that the patient will experience gagging sensations as the tube courses through the esophageal tract. However, symptoms of coughing and gasping indicate possible misplacement of the tube in trachea or lung, and thus, the tube should be removed. The correct response is **D,** and following the tube removal, the patient should be allowed to rest briefly so that he may fully oxygenate before the procedure is restarted.

13. The presence of dark brown "coffee ground" coloration (response **D**) in gastric drainage indicates the need for a Hemoccult test, used to determine the presence of blood in gastric drainage.

14. Potassium is poorly stored in the human body and must be supplied with a daily oral intake of potassium-rich foods. Since the patient is NPO, the nurse should take special note of her potassium serum values, response **B.**

15. The intended response is **C,** since the continuous passing of watery stools precipitates a fluid and electrolyte imbalance with fluid deficit. Assessing for skin turgor and mucous membrane moisture will alert the nurse to evi-

dence of dehydration associated with continuous fluid loss with stools. The other interventions listed are also fitting, but response **C** is the priority.

16. The intended response is **C,** because adequate hydration and regular exercise are very important for regular bowel elimination. Response **A** is incorrect, because daily bowel movements are not necessary nor realistic for all clients. Response **B** is incorrect since daily laxative use is inappropriate for regulation of elimination, often leading to laxative dependence and loss of normal bowel function and tone. Avoiding foods high in bulk, response **D,** is exactly opposite of what the client should do to attain bowel regularity, since bulk foods facilitate bowel evacuation.

17. The intended response is **A,** since chlamydial infections are sexually transmitted. The symptoms in response **B** are incorrect, with pain and fever being more associated with the disease. Although dysuria is common, hematuria (response **C**) is not. Response **D** describes symptoms of a different sexually transmitted disease, herpes simplex II.

18. The major goal for the scrotal support postoperatively is **A,** to reduce swelling, which will reduce congestion associated with the surgery and thus reduce discomfort.

19. The patient reflects his understanding of the sexually transmitted nature of the disease and the best measure to prevent reinfection in response **D,** the wearing of a condom during sexual intercourse. In response **A,** he only seeks attention for reinfection and does not prevent it. Response **B** is incorrect, since reinfection can occur even if the patient has taken the full course of antibiotic therapy. Response **C** shows an understanding of sexual transmission of the disease, but does not effectively prevent reinfection because partners could harbor the disease without his knowledge.

20. The intended response is **D.** The patient should be instructed to apply *cold* compresses to the affected area to reduce swelling and discomfort.

21. The intended response is **A.** Commonly, a grand mal seizure is preceded by an unusual sensory illusion called an "aura." If the patient has repeated seizure episodes, he may come to anticipate the onset of a seizure by the experience of aura that precedes the actual seizure activity.

22. All the nursing interventions listed are correct steps in providing seizure precautions *except* for response **A,** the intended response. A padded tongue blade, once a staple in seizure management, is no longer used with patients experiencing seizure because it may actually act as an airway obstruction during seizure. An oral airway would provide both protection to the tongue from biting behavior as well as an airway during seizure activity. The airway

should only be inserted if the patient has not already entered into seizure activity.

23. Snoring and labored respirations, response **D,** would cause the nurse caring for the postictal patient the greatest concern since these would indicate possible airway obstruction from the tongue or accumulation of oral fluids in the mouth. The nurse noting labored respirations after seizure should immediately assess the patient's airway patency for possible obstruction.

24. The most valuable implementation in the postictal phase is response **D,** turning the patient onto his left side to open the airway. This position will provide for greatest patency of the trachea and bronchus and is thus the most critical action for the nurse following the patient's seizure. The actions listed in responses **A, B,** and **C** are all appropriate, but should follow the positioning of the patient onto his left side.

25. The patient is most likely to experience apnea during the tonic phase of seizure, response **C.** During this phase, the patient's muscles are in a state of rigid contraction, and the patient may not be able to breathe effectively with respiratory muscles in spasm.

26. The intended response is **B.** Alcohol should be avoided by the patient taking Dilantin, because alcohol reduces the effectiveness of the anticonvulsant action of the drug, thus making the patient much more susceptible to recurrence of seizure activity.

27. The intended response is **C,** since turning the patient and staying with him in attendance during the seizure is both the most effective and simplest management for the family member to learn and implement. Although response **D** is appropriate management postictal and knowing emergency phone numbers in response **A** would likewise be beneficial, response **C** is still the most helpful, most valuable response.

28. The intended response is **C,** since chest pain usually occurs after physical or emotional stress in stable angina. The patient's description of chest pain occurring even in a resting state strongly suggests *unstable* angina, a much more serious form of this cardiac condition.

29. The intended response is **C.** Onset of menopause and irregular nutrition have little to do with the onset of anginal pain. A positive family history of cardiac disease is certainly important, but most important is the patient's history of cigarette smoking, a *primary* risk factor for the development of coronary artery disease.

30. The intended response is **D,** since digoxin is the least likely of the listed medications to decrease onset and severity of anginal pain associated with coronary artery disease.

31. Patient instruction on the actions and uses of nitrate medication is critical to ensure compliance with therapy. The patient should know to place the nitroglycerine tablet under her tongue when chest pain occurs, response **A**. Response **B** is incorrect, since the medication can be repeated every 5 min as necessary up to 3 tablets. Response **C** is incorrect since this medication is a vasodilator, which would cause skin to become warm and flushed. Response **D** is incorrect, because headache and dizziness are common side-effects of the vasodilating action of this drug, and the medication should not be discontinued by the patient in response to these common side-effects.

32. The intended response is **C**, the diet lowest in saturated fat, sodium, and cholesterol. Since animal meats are rich in saturated fat and cholesterol, response **A** and **B** are incorrect. Response **B** is likewise high in sodium, as is response **D**, containing dairy products that are sodium-rich.

33. The intended response is **B** underlying the basic principle that an open airway is essential for life. Postoperative swelling or bleeding at the surgical site could easily present an airway obstruction for the patient; thus, this observation is *most* critical and of greatest priority.

34. A basic principle of medical and surgical asepsis is thorough handwashing before contact with patient or equipment. **A** is the intended response, so that the nurse providing care to the tracheostomy patient reduces the risk of transmission of microbes from other areas of the hospital onto either patient or equipment utilized with that patient. Following handwashing, the nurse should perform the remaining steps in this order: open necessary kits and dressings, pour sterile solutions, apply sterile gloves.

35. The patient receiving tracheostomy care would be most appropriately placed in the semi-Fowler's position, response **C**. This position affords easiest access to the stoma site and also allows for better ventilation of the patient during the procedure.

36. Suctioning is a process that removes accumulating secretions from the respiratory tract. In doing so, however, it also draws out necessary O_2, predisposing the patient being suctioned to O_2 loss and CO_2 narcosis. In light of this, the nurse preparing to suction the patient should hyperoxygenate the patient first, either by O_2 per cuff or by Ambu bag lung inflation. Thus, the correct response is **C**.

37. Families caring for the patient with tracheostomy at home must learn the basics of CPR, response **D**, should airway obstruction occur in the home. Although all the remaining responses are important in tracheostomy care, the teaching of CPR to the family members should be viewed as highest priority.

38. The intended response is **A**, since pulse rate will escalate in respiratory distress as a compensatory effort by the heart to circulate more essential O_2 to body cells. It should be noted that response **B**, restlessness, is often the *earliest* sign of respiratory distress, and family members should be alert for that symptom when caring for the tracheostomy patient in the home.

39. The intended response is **C**, since the cardiac arrthymias associated with cocaine toxicity are most life-threatening. Cocaine is a powerful amphetamine that causes increased cardiac stimulation, resulting in tachy rate and potentially life-threatening arrhythmia. Responses **A, B, D** are likewise associated with cocaine toxicity, but **C** is of greatest significance to the nurse caring for the patient.

40. The nurse should *not* want to elevate the head of the bed in this situation, since this would increase cardiac muscle. In this *except* question, then, the intended response is **C**. The patient should be monitored continuously in response **A** because he is already demonstrating tachy rate. Oxygen administration in response **B** is indicated to improve oxygenation status in light of the patient's vital signs. Initiation of IV therapy routes in response **D** is critical to provide access for needed fluids and medication administration.

41. The intended response is **A**, since the maintenance of a patent airway for the patient is most critical. Again, the principle of airway and its necessity for life is underlined in this question. All other nursing interventions listed are likewise appropriate, but response **A** is the priority.

42. The patient experiencing cocaine toxicity and withdrawal is undergoing a state of neuromuscular hyperexcitability. The patient should be gently reoriented to his surroundings and allowed visitors who may provide comfort to him. Restraints are inappropriate, since they will likely simply increase the patient's agitation and combative behavior. The treatment of choice is response **D**, placing the patient in a large, open, quiet area with someone in constant attendance. This question could have been answered solely on the basis of having someone remain with the patient at all times, mentioned only in response **D**.

43. The intended response is **C**. Response **A** is incorrect, since the rapid heart rate could signal dehydration. Response **B** is likewise incorrect because both systolic and diastolic values indicate a decreased circulating blood volume, which could evidence fluid deficit or dehydration. Response **D** is incorrect because a central venous pressure of 1 indicates low right atrium filling pressure, indicating fluid volume deficit. Only response **C**, urine output of 75 cc/hour, indicates that an adequate fluid volume has been established, which would allow for body cooling and subsequent reduction of core body temperature.

44. The intended response is **A,** since a positive skin test for TB does not mandate a lung tissue biopsy. Persons with previous exposure to TB may react positively to a TB skin test without actually having the disease. For this reason, any reactions to skin tests not considered negative *should* be followed up, but through either a chest x-ray or a sputum culture for acid-fast bacillus (AFB), *not* through a lung biopsy.

45. The intended response is **B,** since a positive sputum test for AFB is the most reliable indicator of active tuberculosis. Response **C,** chest x-ray may be used, but will not provide differential diagnosis. Responses **A** and **D** are inappropriate.

46. Because tuberculosis is transmitted by droplet nuclei in coughed sputum and respiratory secretions, the patient with active TB would likely be placed in respiratory isolation, requiring that the caregivers and visitors wear masks when in contact with the infected patient. Even more important to isolating the TB bacterium is to enforce response **B,** instructing the patient to cover his mouth during coughing and wash his hands often to prevent contamination of self or others.

47. Since TB is a contagious disease, the patient's family could, in fact, have acquired the infection from the patient. For that reason, response **D,** involving testing of family members, is an important nursing intervention for control of disease transmission and early detection of other potentially infected persons. Response **B** is incorrect because it delays testing until symptoms develop in family members, which increases the possibility that they will, in the meantime, infect others. Chest x-ray is not necessary every 6 months, thus making response **C** incorrect. Response **A** is incorrect because the disease is clearly contagious, being bacterial in origin.

48. The intended response is **D,** because long-term maintenance therapy against TB is important to prevent reoccurrence of active TB with its associated symptoms. Proper reinforcement of the need to remain on medications for an extended length of time is critical, because the patient is very likely to discontinue medication therapy once his symptoms subside, and yet he is still very likely to suffer a relapse with the disease.

49. All of the listed symptoms are associated with TB except **C,** the intended response. Hematemesis, blood in emesis, is not associated with this respiratory disease, thus making it the intended response.

50. Although all of the actions identified by the patient will assist him in coping with his TB, the *most essential* action is to remain on medication prescribed for long-term TB management, response **D.**

51. The intended response is **A**. In this item the reader is simply asked to associate the disease name diabetes insipidus to the deficiency state of ADH production. Response **B**, diabetes mellitus, is a deficiency or absence of insulin production. Cushing's syndrome is an abnormality of the adrenal glands. Graves' disease is an abnormality of the thyroid.

52. Because the patient does not manufacture adequate amounts of antidiuretic hormone, the body cannot retain fluids, and excessive loss of fluid by urination is a cardinal sign. Since the patient loses excess fluid, she experiences excessive thirst; thus, response **B**, polydypsia, is the correct response. Responses **A** and **D** are incorrect, since they would typify the patient with fluid volume excess. Response **C** is incorrect, since patients with diabetes insipidus experience polyuria.

53. The intended response is **A,** since body stores of K^+ are poor, and through excessive urination, most of the body's K^+ would be lost, resulting in a hypokalemic state.

54. Fluid loss is so extreme in diabetes insipidus that the patient requires substantial fluid replacement to maintain fluid balance in the body. Thus, the intended response is **B,** since in this *except* question, limiting fluids would be contraindicated and potentially harmful to the patient.

55. In this evaluation question, the nurse should recognize that the patient's status is improving when her urinary output decreases, thus restoring fluid balance in the body and the process of excessive urination caused by ADH deficiency is controlled. The intended response, then, is **D**.

56. The intended response is **B,** since patients experiencing congestive heart failure (CHF) do not adequately perfuse the kidneys, causing a decrease in renal output. All other symptoms listed are classing for CHF.

57. The purpose of Lasix therapy in CHF is to increase urinary elimination of excess fluids in the body. However, Lasix is a diuretic that is not potassium-sparing and in this situation, it is most likely that Lasix has caused a low serum K^+ level, 3.0—with 3.5 to 5.0 being normal serum levels. For this reason, the nurse should withhold the drug temporarily and notify the physician of the patient's hypokalemic state. The correct response is **D**.

58. Although all interventions identified are appropriate for the patient with CHF, the one of priority for the patient suffering from respiratory embarrassment secondary to CHF is response **C**. The periods of dyspnea and periodic confusion are indications of inadequate oxygenation, calling for O_2 replacement therapy.

59. Sodium, response **C,** should be restricted in addition to fluids, because sodium will tend to cause fluid retention, which would further complicate an already overworked, failing heart, thus worsening the congestion in the heart.

60. The medication that would most affect cardiac output is digoxin, response **C.** Digoxin increases the contractility of the cardiac muscle, thus increasing the strength and force of contraction, which will increase the output of blood from the left ventricle into systemic circulation.

61. If digoxin has been effective, cardiac output with secondary perfusion to the kidneys will be increased. Increased arterial perfusion to the kidneys will result in increased urinary output, response **C,** which will help to remove excess fluids and thus reduce congestion within the heart. Response **A** is incorrect because digoxin *slows* heart rate. Digoxin should likewise *decrease* blood pressure as fluids are excreted in urine, making response **B** incorrect. The auscultation of rales in the lungs would indicate continued congestion within the heart with back-up of fluids to the lungs, evidence that digoxin has *not* yet been effective for the patient's CHF.

62. The *best* indicator that the CHF is resolving is that there is less pressure within the right atrium, with a corresponding central venous pressure reading within normal parameters, response **D.** (Normal venous pressure is 4 to 10 mm Hg.)

63. The intended response is **D,** since the patient's behavior clearly indicates safety risks that would be handled best *initially* by upright rails and call light within reach. It is very probable that the confusion is related to the elevating levels of waste products in the patient's blood circulating to the brain and impairing mental function.

64. The patient in renal failure would show symptoms of response **C,** oliguria with dark amber color and high specific gravity.

65. The x-ray findings of demineralization typify the bone condition of osteoporosis, response **A.** Because of the decalcification of the bone, the bone has less density and mass, causing it to lose tensile strength and to be more easily fractured.

66. Fracture, response **D,** is a common complication of osteoporosis, since bone mass and strength are decreased secondary to loss of calcium.

67. The chief purpose of Buck's traction prior to hip fixation surgery is to improve alignment of the body fragments, which reduces the amount of bone and tissue manipulation in surgery, response **D.** Although the remaining responses are also true, the chief purpose is response **D.**

68. The patient should receive response **B**, 0.5 mL of atropine preoperatively.

> Amount desired—0.2 mg
>
> Amount available—gr 1/150 = 1/150 × 60 mg = 0.4 mg
>
> Unit of medication—1 mL
>
> $SOLUTION$ $\dfrac{0.2\ \text{mg:}}{0.4\ \text{mg}} \times 1\ \text{mL} = 0.5\ \text{mg} \times 1\ \text{mL} = 0.5\ \text{mL}$

See Chapter 22 for further assistance with this calculation problem.

69. To prevent dislocation of the hip, the patient should not be allowed to position the lower extremities in adduction. Thus, response **C**, supine with legs in abduction, is the correct response.

70. Since the patient is in her first day postoperative, left-extremity pain is expected, and should be medicated with postoperative analgesia as ordered. The intended response, then, is response **B**.

71. Since blood donors do not come into contact with the blood of others, the correct response is **C**.

72. The correct response is **D**. Prior to 1985 blood testing for HIV was not available to blood banks. Cases of transfusion-related AIDS exposure have been documented. Anyone who received blood or blood products prior to the current testing practices of blood banks may be at risk of having been exposed to the AIDS virus.

73. The correct response is **B**. HIV testing reveals that the person has been exposed to the AIDS virus and has developed antibodies to the virus. A positive result offers very little information regarding whether or not the client will go on to become symptomatic for AIDS.

74. The correct response is **B**. A virus is the identified cause of AIDS. Frequently clients diagnosed with AIDS or who test positive for HIV feel guilty about this disease. Societal views vary and can be prejudicial because AIDS has affected sexually active and IV drug users. Those who have participated in "high risk" behaviors associated with transmission of the virus may feel guilt associated with those practices or be victims of prejudice. This response factually explains what the cause of their illness is.

75. The intended response is **C**. The most effective available weapon against AIDS is education. Recognizing that behavioral changes are required to prevent transmission of the virus is the first step in behavior modification. Persons who are HIV-positive must be willing to change sexual practices in order to prevent transmission of the virus.

76. The intended response is **A.** The AIDS virus is known to be very fragile outside of the body. A diluted chlorine bleach and water solution has been found to be effective in killing the virus. Both of these items are common household items readily available.

77. Diabetes acidosis leads to urinary water loss, and additional loss of Na^+ and K^+. Hypovolemia and electrolyte imbalances occur. Glucose levels are very high in these clients, and free fatty acids are broken down resulting in acidosis. A pH of 7.32 reflects an acidic state in circulating blood. Thus **D** is the intended response.

78. The intended response is **C.** Glucose, unable to be metabolized without insulin, accumulates in the serum, causing hyperglycemia. Stored fats are metabolized rapidly for energy, resulting in release of free fatty acids into serum, causing acidosis.

79. Regular insulin is indicated because it is the most rapid acting of those listed. It is used to bring glucose levels down as quickly as possible, thereby correcting the underlying problem that is producing the acidosis.

80. The correct response is **A.** Attempts to restore potassium balance can result in hyperkalemia if adequate urinary output is not maintained.

81. The intended response is **C.** The nurse must be able to prioritize care. The concept of tissue perfusion relies on oxygenation. The nurse must be able to identify airway, breathing, and circulation. Without establishing airway and breathing, circulatory assistance will never be achieved.

82. The correct response is **B.** It is important to stress the respiratory effect that an inhalation injury has on the patient. It is apparent that the respiratory system affects the oxygenation-perfusion status of the patient when the ability of the lungs to function properly is altered. The nurse needs to identify the respiratory effects of an inhalation injury by noting signs and symptoms.

83. The correct response is **B.** The concept of circulation needs to be identified with a patient who has suffered a burn injury. One aspect that must be noted is the effect that the burn has within the vasculature. This effect has implications for drug administration, which can potentially lead to detrimental effects. Therefore, the nurse must be aware of these changes.

84. The correct response is **D.** The nurse needs to be aware of the fluid shifts that occur in a burn injury. The concept of circulation is utilized, since this shift leads to circulatory changes and has effects on the patient's stability. This definitely has implications on how to monitor, treat, and evaluate patient care.

85. The correct response is **B.** The concept of circulation is used to identify fluid loss, which occurs with burns, and the effect it has on the circulatory status. Therefore, a guideline used to identify fluid requirements is the Parkland formula. The Parkland formula identifies the increased fluid requirements needed in the first 24 hours. This is noted especially the first 8 hours, when half the fluid requirements are needed. This exemplifies the concept of burns creating a fluid shift from the intravascular to interstitial, with an eventual sealing of the leak with time. It also identifies the large fluid replacement that is needed with severe burns.

86. The intended response should be **C.** A high percentage of O_2 is contraindicated in patients with chronic lung disease because it can eliminate the hypoxic drive necessary to stimulate respiration. Too much O_2 can have an adverse effect on the patient's breathing. O_2 should be delivered to him by a venturi mask, a simple mask, or a nasal cannula at a low percentage of O_2.

87. All four goals are important. However, **B** is an immediate, life-sustaining measure. Therefore, it is the intended response.

88. When bronchoconstriction occurs, there is not enough oxygen-carrying capacity in the blood to adequately perfuse the body. This leads to improper oxygenation of the brain. The most common early symptoms manifested are restlessness, anxiety, and mild confusion, caused by lack of O_2 delivery to the brain. The correct response is **B.**

89. The intended response is **D.** Persons with emphysema have difficulty with the expiratory phase of breathing. Slow, controlled exhalation will strengthen the recoil mechanism of the alveoli.

90. The intended response is **B.** A normal pO_2 indicates that adequate oxygenation is taking place at the cellular level.

WOMEN's HEALTH EXAM ITEM RATIONALES

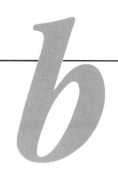

1. Response **C**, fundal height, would not be routine in an initial prenatal examination, since the uterus has probably not grown to sufficient height to be palpated by the examiner. Fundal height becomes a routine assessment in the second and third trimesters.

2. Ultrasonography requires that the bladder be filled with urine in order to better visualize the uterus during the procedure. For this reason, the patient is instructed to drink several large glasses of fluids, response **C**.

3. A classic feature of the latter part of the first trimester of pregnancy is urinary frequency, owing to the pressure of the growing uterus on the bladder. Thus, the intended response is **B**.

4. The cardiovascular change that is not expected in advancing pregnancy is **D**, increased peripheral vascular resistance.

5. Most females first experience fetal movement between the 15th and 20th week of pregnancy, the middle of the second trimester, response **C**.

6. The pregnant female experiencing constipation should increase fiber and fluids in the diet, response **B**. She should not use any stool softeners or laxatives unless specifically prescribed by the physician. Although the iron in prenatal vitamin-mineral supplements can be very constipating, the patient should *not* discontinue use of these necessary supplements.

7. The primary purpose of the nonstress test in pregnancy is to evaluate adequacy of placental function, response **C**.

8. In this situation, Susan is postterm and delivery by induction of labor is indicated. This is not an appropriate time to try to search out the patient's feelings. Rather, clear and direct information should be supplied to the patient to reduce her concerns and at the same time expedite the process of induction. The goal is best achieved in response **C**, the intended response.

9. Hypertonic contractions of the uterus coupled with late decelerations of fetal heart rate by the fetal monitor strongly suggest fetal distress. The nurse should immediately stop the infusion of oxytocin, response **C**.

10. The intended response is **D**. The ferning pattern of amniotic fluid is the definitive evidence of rupture of amniotic membranes.

11. Late decelerations indicate inadequate fetal oxygenation. In supine position, the weight of the uterus compresses the inferior vena cava, which decreases the blood supply to the right side of the heart. A position change to left lateral increases circulation of blood to the heart, which then improves uteroplacental circulation, thus improving fetal oxygenation. The intended response is therefore **C**.

12. At this point in labor, Angela would benefit from the administration of analgesia, since it would serve to reduce the pain of contractions, allow rest periods between contractions, and assist her to maintain control of the labor process, without interrupting the labor pattern. Therefore, the intended response is **D**.

13. The intended response is **C**. The stages of labor are as follows:

    Stage One—Dilatation of the cervix to 10 cm

    Stage Two—Delivery of the infant

    Stage Three—Delivery of the placenta

    Stage Four—The first 1 to 4 hours postpartum

14. Difficulty with voiding is a common problem postvaginal delivery. The nurse caring for Angela should *first* assess the bladder's distention and position to determine whether or not she is ready to void and if indeed a problem exists. Therefore, the intended response is **C**.

15. The intended response is **D**. The classic signs of infiltration of IV fluids include localized pallor, coolness, edema, and tenderness. Redness, warmth, swelling, and tenderness suggest phlebitis of the IV site.

16. The intended response is **D**. Normal newborn heart rate ranges from 120 to 160 beats/min, and thus a rate of 90 beats/min is too low. The newborn

will cry and kick when exposed to cool air in order to stimulate heat production in his body. The normal newborn respiratory rate ranges from 30 to 50 breaths/min at rest. Finally, newborns do not concentrate urine well, and thus the urine tends to be very pale in color without characteristic odor.

17. The intended response is **B.** The newborn uses the rooting reflex (*i.e.,* turning his head to the direction of mouth or cheek stimulation) in order to locate food.

18. The intended response is **C.** Although "rooming in" does facilitate **A, B,** and **D,** the primary reason is **C** because it is the best way to introduce the mother to 24-hour responsibility for her infant. There are other, better opportunities during the postpartum period to fulfill the other goals.

19. The intended response is **C.** The cord stump will detach spontaneously if it is allowed to dry. Application of alcohol to the cord stump promotes drying.

20. The intended response is **C.** The patient must express breast milk to continue stimulation of the letdown reflex. Manual expression of breast milk at regular intervals approximates the infant's own feeding schedule and will facilitate maintenance of the mother's breast milk supply during the period of time she is not able to breast-feed.

21. The intended response is **A.** Assessment of patterns of crying periods would provide necessary information in identifying the possibility of postpartum depression, secondary to hormonal influences.

22. The intended response is **D.** With recurrent bouts of emesis, the patient will lose acids from the stomach that may lead to a shift in the acid-base balance resulting in a metabolic alkalosis.

23. The patient with hyperemesis gravidarum is prone to acute dehydration because of fluid loss in recurrent emesis. The patient will exhibit dry, hot skin owing to the decrease in sweat production and subsequent cooling of the body. Likewise, the patient will demonstrate oliguria, as the kidneys attempt to retain needed fluids and thus reduce urine production. Thus, the correct response is **D.**

24. The medication of choice for the patient with hyperemesis gravidarum is **C,** an antiemetic medication to reduce or halt the frequency and intensity of vomiting.

25. A serum potassium level of 3.0 signals hypokalemia, with levels of 3.5 to 5.0 being normal. The nurse should be most concerned about decreased

stimulation to the cardiac muscle resulting in decreased contractility and subsequent cardiac output, response **B**.

26. The correct response is **C**. The calculations are as follows:

$$\frac{\text{Total amount of IV fluids 1000 cc}}{\text{Total time of infusion 6 hr} \times 60 \text{ min/hr} = 360 \text{ min}} \times \begin{matrix}\text{Drop}\\ \text{factor}\\ (10)\end{matrix}$$

$$\frac{1000}{360} \times 10 = 2.77 \times 10 = 27.7 = 28 \; \frac{\text{drops}}{\text{min}}$$

27. Although all the responses listed are potential benefits of hyperalimentation therapy, the primary purpose of this therapy for the patient is **C**, to arrest the process of fat destruction and ward off the potential for the development of subsequent metabolic acidosis or ketosis.

28. The intended response is **A**. Since the patient is experiencing vaginal bleeding, the most likely cause of the changes in vital signs is fluid loss or hypovolemia. The elevated pulse rate signifies the body's efforts to compensate the loss of circulating volume.

29. The intended response is **B**, since the hallmark feature of placenta previa is painless vaginal bleeding. The patient experiencing abruptio placenta would have moderate to severe pain and may not demonstrate any vaginal bleeding.

30. Although all these actions are necessary for the management of this patient, the action of greatest priority to be implemented *first* is **C**. IV fluids are required to support the patient's circulatory status and counteract the life-threatening effects of hypovolemic shock.

31. The elevation of fetal heart rate indicates fetal efforts toward compensation for the decreased circulating O_2 resulting from maternal hemorrhage and hypovolemic shock.

32. In this situation, the patient is experiencing a crisis episode, requiring direct and concise factual information from the nurse. Response **D** provides simple but honest information to the patient, which best supports her coping abilities.

33. The intended response is **B**, since the bladder must be decompressed by catheterization in order to better access the uterus for delivery of the baby. Response **D** is entirely incorrect, since any cervical stimulation could precipitate hemorrhage.

34. Response **A** catastrophizes the situation for the patient, making it even *more* frightening for her than it already is. Response **B** underlines the no-

tion of fetal death, increasing the patient's state of alarm and anxiety. Response **D** is inappropriate, since being in the situation does not allow for a conversation with spiritual workers. The intended response is **C**, since it provides the most direct and accurate information.

35. The intended response is **B.** Fetal hypoxia is occurring because fetal compensatory effort has failed.

36. The intended response is **A.** Suctioning the baby provides a patent airway, *always* the first priority for the nurse.

37. The intended response is **D.** Lamaze classes are intended to help laboring couples to anticipate and manage the predictable events of labor.

38. The intended response is **B.** The prenatal female requires the additional support of a well-fitted brassiere because the breasts are enlarged due to hormonal influences in preparation for lactation.

39. There is no research to indicate that sexual intercourse is harmful to either the pregnant female or fetus, and for that reason, the intended response is **D.**

40. The intended response is **D,** since many devices are available to insure adequate nutritional intake by the baby.

41. The intended response is **A.** The reference to the baby as "it," signifies Rita's failure to see the infant as a human being and her sense of detachment and isolation from the child.

42. The intended response is **A.** There remains no conclusive evidence that use of oral contraceptives later contributes to female infertility. The remaining responses are all associated with infertility.

43. The intended response is **C,** since this response best shows the nurse's concern for the patient's feelings and a value for what the patient is experiencing. Response **A** provides false reassurance. Response **B** is unrealistic, since the patient will likely continue to compare herself with others who are successful in conceiving. Since pregnancy is not guaranteed with infertility treatment, response **D** is likewise inappropriate.

44. The lab finding most associated with male infertility is response **B,** spermatic immobility, meaning that sperm cannot travel up to the female ova effectively enough to achieve fertilization.

45. The intended response is **C.** Some amount of pelvic and abdominal discomfort should be expected following laparoscopy. Response **A** is incorrect,

since the patient should be NPO from midnight on prior to the procedure. Activity most often is not limited after one or two days postoperatively (response **B**). The patient may be discharged from the outpatient recovery with some vaginal bleeding, and should be provided with a peri pad prior to discharge.

46. The possibility of ectopic pregnancy calls for immediate and direct action by the nurse and the medical team. The patient should be instructed to report to a hospital immediately, response **D**. Ultrasonography will provide information about the status and implantation of the fetus in order to attain differential diagnosis.

47. The intended response is **C**, since the loss of her pregnancy, no matter during what point of the pregnancy, will precipitate a grief reaction for Mary.

48. The intended response is **C**. Proteinuria and edema are closely associated with the fluid balance disturbances that occur in pregnancy-induced hypertension (PIH).

49. The appropriate nursing management of the patient with PIH is to reduce sensory stimuli in an effort to reduce stimulation to the patient, response **A**. The primary concern for this patient is the development of *seizures,* and thus environmental stimuli should be minimized.

50. Clonus, the presence of alternating muscular contraction and relaxation, is an ominous sign in the patient with PIH, and would clearly be a sign of a worsening condition in this patient. Thus, the intended response is **B**.

51. The intended response is **C**. Magnesium sulfate would be administered to Barbara at this point to prevent or control seizure activity related to the PIH. Responses **A** and **B** would only serve to alter fluid status. Response **D**, calcium gluconate, is the *antidote* for a possible overdose of the medication of choice, magnesium sulfate.

52. Although all listed responses are parts of the nursing assessments to be conducted on Barbara following her cesarean section, the assessment of greatest priority is **C**, neurological status, since the possibility of neurological problems still exists.

53. The intended response is **D**. Although there has been considerable discussion of the rights of minors in relation to pregnancy counseling and care, presently a minor who is pregnant may receive treatment related to the pregnancy or the termination of pregnancy without parental-guardian knowledge or consent.

54. Karen is experiencing an imminent (also referred to as inevitable) spontaneous abortion (response **B**), because cervical dilatation is present.

55. The nurse would expect Karen to undergo **C** dilatation and curettage (DC),
to remove any remaining fetal-placental matter. Responses **A** and **B** refer to
types of *induced* abortion. Response **D**, laparotomy, is not necessary in this
situation.

56. It is expected that Karen will experience some vaginal bleeding and pelvic
pain following the D and C surgery. Nausea and vomiting are common after-
effects of anesthesia used in surgery. Karen should notify her physician if
she experiences fever, since this symptom may indicate postoperative infection. Thus, the intended response is **D**.

57. The intended response is **C**, since the vascular changes associated with hypertension can be aggravated significantly by the routine use of oral contraceptives. The remaining responses are not contraindications for oral contraceptives; in fact, menstrual irregularities and dysmenorrhea are often
treated with hormone manipulation by oral contraceptive medications.

58. The only correct statement about the diaphragm as a contraceptive device
is **D**. Diaphragms are not associated with toxic shock (although tampon
usage has been correlated), are not easily dislodged during sexual intercourse, and should remain in place for several hours following intercourse.

59. The best response is **C**. Current thought suggests that the use of a condom
during sexual activity provides the most protection against the transmission
of sexually transmitted diseases.

60. In order to ensure the greatest efficacy of the diaphragm and the greatest
comfort and compliance of the women utilizing this method of contraception, the nurse would want the patient to engage in an active form of learning that involves her practice with the device. Thus, the intended response
is **D**.

61. The intended response is **C**, since these are classic symptoms and signs of
uterine fibroids. Response **A** suggests pelvic inflammatory disease (PID).
Response **B** suggests uterine prolapse. Response **D** is incorrect since the
three symptoms identified are unrelated to this diagnosis.

62. Since Emma is a preoperative patient, response **D** is the correct action for
the nurse. A hemoglobin of 8.2 is insufficient for the patient to undergo a
surgery that will involve blood loss. Response **A** is incorrect, since the iron
absorption will not be rapid enough to correct the low hemoglobin before
surgery. Response **B** is unrelated to hemoglobin—rather, isolation would

be considered for abnormal WBC values. Response **C** will offer no alleviation of the problem of low hemoglobin and is thus incorrect.

63. The intended response is **C.** Estrogen therapy is not indicated, since abdominal hysterectomy removes only the uterus, and thus the ovaries, which are responsible for estrogen production, remain intact.

64. Robinul, much like atropine, is used to dry secretions of the oral passages prior to surgery to reduce the risk of accidental aspiration. Thus, the intended response is **C.**

65. The intended response is **D,** since the patient may still be experiencing the effects of any anesthetics and medications used during the surgical procedure. The recovery room nurse should be alert for evidence of continued central nervous system depression, such as decreased respiratory and pulse rates. Responses **A, B,** and **C** are not as high in priority as response **D,** and are therefore incorrect.

66. Patent airway, response **D,** is always a very high priority for the nurse, since obstructed airway is a life-threatening occurrence. Since the patient has just undergone surgery, patent airway is of critical importance, ensuring that the patient is able to ventilate freely as she recovers from the effects of the surgical anesthesia.

67. The intended response is **A,** since the precipitous fall in blood pressure could indicate bleeding-hemorrhage in this immediate postoperative patient. Response **C** is not an adequate action for the nurse, since the bleeding may be occurring internally without outward evidence by drainage on the dressing. Responses **B** and **D** would only be appropriate actions *after* the surgeon had been notified of the patient's blood pressure and status.

68. Sublimaze is used in surgery to potentiate the effects of anesthesia. Since this medication has a CNS depressant effect, and the patient's depressed respiratory rate indicates excessive CNS depression, the nurse should administer Narcan, response **D,** to counteract the effects of the Sublimaze on the patient's respirations. The other responses are incorrect, since they all cause respiratory depression.

69. The intended response is **D,** since Ilopan acts to decrease abdominal distention by promoting peristalsis. Patients undergoing general anesthesia and abdominal surgery benefit from this medication, since both processes tend to hinder or even halt peristaltic waves in the bowel, predisposing the postoperative patient to serious elimination complications such as paralytic ileus or bowel obstruction.

70. The intended response is **B.** Since there are 500 mg in 1 mL of solution, there would be the desired 250 mg in half the amount of solution, or 0.5 mL.

71. The intended response is **D,** since such a low urine output could indicate fluid and electrolyte imbalance. Ideally, the patient should have at least 40 cc of urine output per hour to ensure adequate renal perfusion and function. This patient's output is less than that, and nursing actions to correct the imbalance should be considered once the source of the decreased output is identified. Responses **A, B,** and **C** are normal and expected findings for the 1-day postoperative hysterectomy patient.

72. The intended response is **C,** since this response provides the greatest amount of iron. Food sources rich in iron include meat, fish, poultry, eggs, green leafy vegetables, bread and cereal products.

73. The most effective way to encourage the passage of retained abdominal gas is through ambulation, response **C.** The remaining responses are not as efficient in solving this problem as ambulation, and are thus incorrect.

74. The intended response is **D,** since these are all classic symptoms of the forms of PMS. Response **A** is describing symptoms related to dysmenorrhea, which is not associated with PMS. Heavier menstrual flow is also not associated with PMS, since this is a symptom occurring during the period, not before the period. Response **C** is focusing on a symptom of PMS, but is not as specific as response **D,** and is therefore incorrect.

75. Response **B** is correct, since symptoms of PMS are often exacerbated following childbearing. Response **A** is unrelated to the syndrome. Response **C** addresses symptoms during the menstrual period, and premenstrual syndrome involves symptoms *prior* to the menstrual period. Response **D** is incorrect since many PMS patients report an *increase* in libido.

76. Response **D** is the intended response because it has no relationship with the syndrome. Research indicates that all the remaining responses have been correlated to PMS symptomotalogy.

77. Vitamin B_6 is often used in management of the PMS patient in order to increase blood progesterone levels and promote diuresis. It may also play a role in stabilizing mood of the premenstrual female. Therefore, the intended response is **C.**

78. Response **C** is the intended response, since early research shows that lowering the percentages of fat, refined sugar, caffeine, and alcohol in the diet may reduce some of the common symptoms of PMS. Responses **A, B,** and **D**

are thus incorrect, since they have not reduced the correct nutrients and foodstuffs.

79. The intended response is **B,** since pain and tenderness in the affected breast are not common initial symptoms of breast malignancy. Responses **A, C,** and **D** are all closely associated with breast cancer.

80. A maternal history of breast carcinoma is a significant risk factor for familial development of the disease. Thus, the intended response is **D.** Although females over age 40 are at higher risk than younger women, response **A** is incorrect because maternal history of the disease is still most significant. Likewise, early menarche and long menstrual life (response **B**) and caucasion race (response **C**) are likewise associated with the development of breast malignancy but are not as significant as a positive maternal history of the disease.

81. Since the patient has undergone surgery that is often considered at least somewhat disfiguring, the nurse should be sure to address disturbance in self-concept, response **C,** in the nursing care plan.

82. The operative arm should not be exercised so soon after mastectomy surgery, since this could cause trauma to the site and may increase extremity edema and pain. In this *except* question, then, the intended response is **D.**

83. In this situation, the patient is expressing her feeling of discomfort with her physical appearance, and issues of self-concept are certainly arising with each surgical dressing change. Response **A** notes the patient's feelings, but does nothing to help her work through them. Response **B** is overly direct and forces the patient to view the wound when she has already expressed her unreadiness to do so, magnifying her feelings of apprehension and anxiety. Response **C** *catastrophizes* the situation by suggesting to the patient that the surgery was "very traumatic." The intended response, then, is response **D,** an open-ended statement that centers on the nurse's observations of the patient's response to the wound and facilitates further expression of the patient's feelings.

84. The intended response is **C,** since characteristic symptoms of a candida infection are creamy, curdlike discharge adhering to vaginal walls, vaginal itching, and vaginal irritation.

85. In preparation for a wet mount slide of vaginal culture specimen, the nurse should position the patient in lithotomy position, response **D.** The vaginal tract should not be irrigated with any solution prior to examination (responses **A** and **B**) since this process might alter the culture findings. The speculum should not be lubricated in order not to interfere with culture findings.

86. The most effective way to decrease discomfort during a pelvic exam would be to instruct the patient to take slow deep breaths, which will help to relax muscles and decrease discomfort. Thus, response **C** is most appropriate.

87. The patient's reaction to a diagnosis of sexually transmitted disease is natural and expected. The nurse should recognize the patient's feeling of discomfort and provide her with an opportunity to express her feelings privately. Therefore, the most effective response is **D**, which conveys the nurse's appreciation of the patient's feelings and affords her an opportunity to express herself in private to avoid undue embarrassment.

88. Although notification of sexual partners would include all of the interventions listed, the chief purpose for notifying the sexual partners of the patient with sexually transmitted disease is to prevent unknowing reinfection in future sexual intercourse. Response **D**, then, is the intended response.

89. Flagyl is the appropriate antibiotic therapy for this diagnosis. However, a common side-effect of this medication is superinfection, an example of which is an overgrowth of *Candida albicans* on the tongue, causing it to have a "furry" appearance with accompanying low-grade fever. Although the other symptoms are also side-effects of Flagyl therapy, only response **D** involves symptoms of superinfection.

90. The intended response is **D**. Negative vaginal cultures would indicate that the disease has been effectively managed with medication therapy. The other responses are not reliable indicators of successful treatment.

CHILD HEALTH EXAM ITEM RATIONALES

1. The intended response is **A**. Intussusception involves a "telescoping" of one segment of the bowel into another, resulting in an obstruction of flow of intestinal content. Response **B** describes colitis; response **C** describes Hirschsprung's disease; and response **D** describes pyloric stenosis.

2. The intended response is **B**. Intussusception classically develops with severe abdominal pain, causing the child to scream and draw up his legs towards the chest during a pain spasm. Although bloody "current jelly" stools are associated with intussusception, response **A** is not as descriptive as response **B**. Vomiting is a later sign of the disease and is not as common as response **B**. Fever is not usually related to this disorder.

3. The nurse's first priority with Leo is to insert a nasogastric (Salem Sump, Levine) tube in order to decompress the abdomen, thus reducing abdominal pressure and pain. Thus, the correct response is **C**.

4. A common approach to management of intussusception is administration of barium enema in order to detelescope the segment of bowel involved. The most definitive evidence that this procedure is successful is the passage of barium-colored stools by the child, indicating that an obstruction of intestinal content flow no longer exists (response **B**).

5. During the immediate postoperative phase, the first priority of the nurse is always the timely and consistent measurement of vital signs (response **A**).

6. Coolness, swelling, and paleness of an IV insertion site suggest infiltration of the IV fluids into surrounding tissues, response **A**.

7. The intended response is **B**. The distention of the abdomen is related to the "third space" shifting of fluid into the abdominal cavity, an expected result of the disorder and surgery.

8. The nurse should administer **C**, 100 mg per dose.

   Leo's weight in pounds = 22, and 22 divided by 2.2 = 10 kg

   or 2.2 lb per kilogram.

   10 kg × 40 mg = 400 mg total dosage for 24 hr.

   400 divided by 4 for Q 6 hours dose = 100 mg/dose.

9. The intended response is **A**. The symptoms listed in response **B** are typical of influenza, and these gastrointestinal complaints are not typical of chickenpox. Symptoms in response **C** characterize measles. Response **D** describes respiratory symptoms typical of upper respiratory infections.

10. The intended response is **A**. Chickenpox (varicella) is one of the most contagious diseases of childhood, its causative virus being transmitted easily from host to host.

11. The adult caring for the child with chickenpox is at risk for the development of shingles, response **C**.

12. The intended response is **C**. Since the lesions of chickenpox cause itching, the child has a tendency to scratch the lesions, exacerbating his condition and leading to potential scarring. The administration of Benadryl is desirable for its anti-itching effect. Response **A** typifies management of the child with measles. Isolation of a child for a period of 2 to 3 weeks, response **B**, is unnecessary and undesirable. Tylenol may be given for symptomatic relief, but the dosage in response **D** is 10 grains (600 mg), an adult dosage.

13. The correct response is **A**. The type of ingestion is most important because it will determine the mode of treatment appropriate for the ingestion. For example, the patient who has ingested a caustic substance such as drain cleaner would *not* be encouraged to induce vomiting, since emesis of the caustic substance would cause further damage to the body's structure.

14. Syrup of ipecac, response **A,** is most often used when the induction of vomiting is indicated as a treatment measure in accidental ingestion.

15. The intended response is **D**. It is important for the admitting nurse to assess the patient's status following ingestion and establish a baseline from which to determine treatment and supportive measures.

16. Unfortunately, children do not seem to learn from their ingestions, often having repeat ingestions in the future. Thus, in this *except* question, the intended response is **C.**

17. The intended response is **B.** Since cerebral palsy is most related to fetal stress, especially during labor and delivery, a cesearean section delivery of the infant, which would minimize pressure to the fetal skull, would be least likely to be related to the development of this syndrome in the infant.

18. A large infant may have precipitated a more difficult labor and delivery, which increases the risk for fetal stress and the subsequent development of cerebral palsy. Thus, the intended response is **C.**

19. The intended response is **C.** The nurse must be aware that growth and development standards are broad enough to allow for individual differences in the development of children. Although a child may sit *with* spinal support at age 6 months, most are not able to sit *without* support until age 8 months. Based upon this standard, the nurse is then aware that Rosie is significantly lagging in her development.

20. The intended response is **D,** since exercise is critical to maintain muscle strength and joint mobility in the child with cerebral palsy. Response **A** is unrealistic, since the child may never accomplish ambulation. Response **B** is contraindicated, since limiting activity will foster greater muscle atrophy and loss of joint mobility. Response **C** is a substantial goal for a normal 4 year old, and is unrealistic for the child with cerebral palsy.

21. The intended response is **C,** since premature infants often gain weight more rapidly than full-term babies in the same period of time.

22. The correct response is **C,** since this food is most easily digested by the infant and is thus most desirable with which to start oral feedings of solid foods.

23. Jill should have been immunized with DPT (diphtheria, pertussis, tetanus) and OPV (oral polio vaccine) at 2-month intervals since birth. At age 6 months, though, she would not receive MMR (Measles, Mumps, Rubella). This vaccination is given between 12 months and 15 months of age. The intended response, then, is **D.**

24. The most commonly used site for injection in the infant is **B,** the vastus lateralis site of the thigh. Although the deltoid (response **C**) may be used, it is less desirable than the thigh since absorption is not as effective. The other two responses are inappropriate for use in childhood vaccination.

25. The intended response is **D.** Although the elevated blood glucose, decreased *p*H value, and presence of ketone bodies in the urine all suggest a

ketoacidotic state, the decreased hemoglobin value in response **D** is unrelated.

26. Since the insulin is to be given by intravenous (IV) route, the only type of insulin the nurse may use is regular insulin, response **B**. Additionally, a rapid action of the insulin is desired, and thus regular insulin is the only correct choice for the nurse.

27. It is expected that patients with acute hyperglycemia will develop signs and symptoms of dehydration because of the excessive fluid loss in polyuria. All responses are associated with fluid balance in the body; however, the intervention most critical (of highest priority) in this situation is response **A**, since initiation of IV fluid therapy will serve to help correct or reverse the underlying hypovolemic state.

28. The intended response is **B**, since exercise and activity can use increased utilization of carbohydrates for energy, *reducing* the need for insulin.

29. Response **C**, frequent urination, is a classic symptom of hyperglycemia. The remaining responses are associated with hypoglycemia, or low blood glucose.

30. The intended response is **A**. Protest is the first stage of separation anxiety in the hospitalized toddler, characterized by loud and frantic protesting of the parent's departure from the child's environment.

31. The intended response is **C**, since this response recognizes the child's concern over her mother's departure and encourages her to express her emotions through crying, a natural reaction for a toddler. **A** is incorrect, since the child at this age has no concept of time and cannot understand "tomorrow." **B** attempts to distract the child, which will likely increase her frustration because it ignores the central component of her fear. Finally, **D** is incorrect since it negates Amy's feelings of concern and suppresses her outlet of crying.

32. The intended response is **D**. Amy is too young to engage in competitive play and will likely experience even greater frustration with such activities. All other responses would be appropriate ways to reduce her concern and facilitate her adjustment to the hospital environment and separation from parents.

33. The intended response is **D**. Regression, the return to a behavior from an earlier developmental period, is a common coping mechanism of hospitalized children. Amy's thumb-sucking behavior is a common and expected event in a hospitalized toddler and should not be considered cause for alarm.

34. The intended response is **B.** Toddlers are prone to nightmares, and the nurse best manages the event by reinforcing that such things as ghosts and monsters are not real while remaining with the child to provide comfort and a greater sense of security. Sleep is too important to the toddler to allow her to remain awake to play (response A). Closing Amy's room door may increase her sense of aloneness and isolation, magnifying her fears (response C). Sedation is not indicated (response D).

35. The intended response is **D.** A diminished radial pulse would indicate decreased arterial perfusion of the extremity, an abnormal and serious finding. The remaining responses are all characteristic of fracture.

36. Because Allison's fracture is secondary to traumatic injury, the correct response is **C.** Spontaneous or pathologic fractures occur in the absence of trauma and are most often associated with bone disease such as osteoporosis or osteosarcoma. Response **D** is completely unrelated.

37. The intended response is **B.** Continued assessment of the casted extremity and the cast itself is an important aspect to this patient's care. The child should be encouraged to wiggle and move the fingers of the casted arm; thus response **A** is incorrect. Hot towels should not be applied to the cast and will likewise probably provide no pain relief (response **C**). Response **D** is incorrect, since the fracture will not heal within 1 or 2 weeks, but rather in several weeks.

38. Numbness and tingling of the affected extremity suggest pressure on the nerves of that arm, an abnormal and potentially serious finding. The remaining responses are all typical findings in the patient with a cast. Thus, the intended response is **D.**

39. The intended response is **B.** Vitamin D is essential for the absorption of calcium into the bone, a critical element for bone healing.

40. A characteristic sign of LTB is a loud, crowing sound with respiration termed stridor (response **A**), caused by a narrowing of the air passageways.

41. The intended response is **D,** since often a child will develop LTB as a sequela to a *Haemophilus influenzae* (flu). Responses **A** and **C** are not specific to suggest LTB, since these might be associated with many respiratory ailments. Response **B** is unrelated to LTB.

42. Cool, moist humidification of room air is the ideal method of dilation of airway passages. Hot, steamy areas have not proven as successful in the management of LTB, and may place the child at risk for burns. Thus, the intended response is **C.**

43. Response **C**, restlessness, indicates a worsening respiratory condition, indicating a decrease in O_2 supply to the tissues of the brain.

44. The intended response is **C**. The child in acute respiratory embarrassment will demonstrate an increased heart rate and an increased respiratory rate as a result of the body's effort to compensate for the diminished oxygenation.

45. The intended response is **C**. Epinephrine is commonly administered to improve the respiratory status of the child with acute LTB. Response **A** is incorrect, since only low concentrations of O_2 (less than 30%) would be administered. Cardiac monitoring is not indicated unless the child shows underlying cardiac abnormalities. Tracheostomy is no longer a common method of management of the respiratory distress of the child with LTB.

46. The nurse caring for Danny as he recovers from LTB would NOT want to encourage frequent play periods (response **B**), since this stimulation and activity will cause an increased use of O_2 by body cells. The goal of management for Danny at this time is O_2 *conservation*.

47. The intended response is **D**. The Snellen Eye Chart is used to test visual acuity for all ages; however, since Patrick may not yet be able to identify letters or words, he should be asked to identify shapes printed on the eye chart hung at a 20-foot distance from the child.

48. The intended response is **C**. Usually by age 5 years, the child can lace his shoes and correctly tie a bow in the laces. The remaining responses are all normal behaviors in the 5-year-old child.

49. The intended response is **C**. Accidents are the leading cause of death in children aged 2 through 5, and the parents should be encouraged to remove any potential sources of injury to their child, such as poisons or dangerous machinery that might be present in the home.

50. The intended response is **B**. Foods served on special dinnerware will likely seem much more attractive to the 5 year old. Appetite and intake vary widely in the age group, and the parents should expect that their child will go through periods when he simply does not wish to eat certain amounts or types of foods. However, parents should not allow the child to eat frequent snacks or have meals whenever he chooses. Likewise, the child should not be encouraged to try a large variety of new foods with small bites of each, since he will probably rebel and choose not to eat at all instead.

51. The intended response is **C**. Since 1 kg = 2.2 lb, Patrick's kilogram weight is approximately 16 kg $\times$ 15 mg = 240 mg total dosage.

52. The intended response is **C.** Since 1 grain = 60 mg, 4 tablets would provide the total correct dosage of 240 mg.

53. The intended response is **B.** It is common that children of abusive parents demonstrate withdrawn behavior, often demonstrating little emotional response to any stimulus. They are likewise often suspicious and uncomfortable, having difficulty in developing trusting relationships.

54. The intended response is **C.** Having one nurse per shift care for Lucas will facilitate the development of a trust relationship between nurse and patient, a critical need in the care of the abused child.

55. The intended response is **B.** The parent who believes that his child does not love him or like him is very prone to abusive behavior or the continuance of an abusive pattern.

56. The intended response is **A.** Patients with ALL develop joint pain secondary to an overcrowding of the joint by the huge numbers of immature white blood cells produced in this disease. Fatigue is associated with the anemia so common to the leukemic patient.

57. The intended response is **B.** Although the patient with ALL may experience fatigue, complete bed rest is too restrictive for the young child. Rather, periods of activity interspaced with rest periods is the ideal management. Restriction of play or visitation may precipitate or exacerbate feelings of isolation and depression in the child with ALL.

58. The intended response is **B.** The administration of anti-emetic medication prior to the initiation of chemotherapy would most help to reduce the distressing symptoms of gastrointestinal irritation. Allowing Andy to choose any food (response **D**), will not ensure adequate nutritional intake of necessary foods and fluids. NPO status (response **A**) would only be indicated if the nausea and vomiting become severe. A high-residue diet will increase bowel elimination, an undesired effect in the patient prone to diarrhea secondary to chemotherapy.

59. The intended response is **B.** Since Andy's pain is perceived as severe, potent analgesia should be administered.

60. The correct answer is **C.** Because the Hickmann is a central line, the risk for significant blood loss secondary to dislodging of the catheter cap is high. Clamps should be readily available to place on the open catheter to prevent blood loss.

61. The intended response is **D.** Even though daytime bladder control is often achieved in the second to third year of life, nighttime control is delayed normally until 3½ years or later.

62. Enuresis or bedwetting is not thought to be a subconscious behavior to attract greater parental attention. Thus, the intended response to this *except* question is **D.**

63. The intended response is **C.** Matthew is aware at the conscious level that he is wetting his bed but wishes to "hide" that reality from his awareness in an effort to reduce his anxiety over this behavior, a form of suppression as a defense mechanism.

64. During the school-age years, peer groups of the same sex take on special significance to the child. Matthew is probably very concerned that he would lose his peer group friends if they should find out about his bedwetting behavior. Thus, the intended response is **A.**

65. The only unacceptable strategy for dealing with Matthew's bedwetting in this *except* question would be response **D,** an unhelpful and potentially emotionally upsetting strategy that would probably serve only to expose his problem to others of his peer group.

66. The intended response is **C.** Sickle cell disease is a genetically linked disease inherited from parents who either have the disease or carry the trait for the disease. For this reason, couples with a history of sickle cell diseases are encouraged to seek genetic counseling prior to conception of future offspring.

67. Anorexia and weight loss, response **D,** are not typically associated with sickle cell crisis. The vaso-occlusive changes that occur as a result of the bunching of sickled red blood cells cause the remaining three symptoms: abdominal pain, joint pain, and shortness of breath.

68. The intended response is **A.** Because Michael is experiencing vaso-occlusion from the sickled cells, hydration, typically by means of IV therapy, is the priority measure in sickle cell crisis. The remaining responses, though important, are of secondary importance to hydration.

69. Michael should be medicated with response **D,** morphine sulfate. Reduction of the severe pain by morphine will likewise reduce O_2 consumption by the body, a desired effect in sickle cell crisis. The remaining responses are all incorrect, since these three medications all contain aspirin, which is contraindicated for the patient with potential for bleeding.

70. The intended response is **B.** Smoking poses a serious risk to the patient with sickle cell disease, since the oxygen-carrying capacity of RBCs is already quite compromised.

71. The intended response is **A**. The Rashkind procedure is used as a temporary measure to allow for mixing of arterial venous blood flow until such time as final surgical correction can be completed later in infancy.

72. Alteration in cardiac output, response **D**, is the intended response. Alteration in cardiac output is of prime importance to the nurse caring for the child with this cardiac malformation, even after the Rashkind procedure has been performed. Constant monitoring of the ability of the heart to adequately pump blood and perfuse the tissues of the body is a critical element of postprocedure care.

73. The intended response is **C**. Both pain and crying will cause the body to utilize greater amounts of O_2, an undesirable effect in the child with impaired cardiac output and O_2 transport.

74. In this *except* question, the intended response is **D**. Supplementing the routine formula feedings with additional glucose feedings will require that the infant use excess energy for feeding, thus increasing O_2 consumption by the body, an undesired effect.

75. A classic sign of digoxin toxicity is response **C**, persistent diarrhea.

76. The intended response is **A**. Current guidelines for infant CPR call for placement of fingers for chest compression at one finger-breadth below the nipple line. All remaining responses are incorrect for infant CPR.

77. Mrs. Levy is expressing an underlying fear of having her son at home in her care without the support of professionals, an expected and understandable concern in light of the child's diagnosis and related problems. In order to gather more information from Mrs. Levy so as to know the best way of helping her to cope with Kenneth's impending discharge, the nurse should focus on Mrs. Levy's feelings and encourage her to express herself more fully. Thus, the intended response is **D**.

78. The intended response is **C**. Arranging for the Levy family to stay with their son for a 24-hour period while still in the relative safety of the hospital environment will help the parents to recognize any genuine problems they may have with the infant's care and will likewise help to ease them into the role of care providers in anticipation of discharge.

79. Presenting symptoms of increased ICP are usually much more subtle in an older child than they are in an infant, frequently manifesting behavioral changes or a decrease in school performance. An older child's fontanels are closed, and although his cranial sutures are not completely fused, an increase in ICP will not cause an increase in head circumference. Decreased appetite may accompany increased ICP, but it may also accompany the flu.

Bradycardia is a *late* sign of increased ICP, but a heart rate of 76 in a 7 year old is within the normal limits of 75 to 100 bpm. Therefore, the correct answer is **B**.

80. The correct response is **C**. A 7-year-old child is most likely in Erikson's stage of "industry versus inferiority," where friends, school, and activities are most important. Response **A** speaks to body image concerns. Although these are very important, they tend to be more important to a child who is a little older. A bald spot on the head of a 7 year old probably won't make him want to stay home from school, as it probably would for a 12 year old. Response **B** is more common in toddlers and preschoolers. A 7 year old doesn't like shots, but can understand why he needs it and that the discomfort will be short-lived. Response **D** is high-level, abstract thinking, more characteristic of adolescents.

81. The correct response is **D**. The emphasis in this question is on the immediate postoperative period, where physical needs take precedence over more long-term, psychosocial issues. NPO for a short time after surgery is accepted practice following a shunt revision and is well tolerated under ordinary circumstances. However, potential infection is a serious concern, since infection in the central nervous system can have devastating short- and long-term consequences.

82. This mother needs two things from the nurse: (1) reassurance that she didn't hurt her child and that she is capable of taking good care of him and (2) help learning how to meet his needs. **C** is the correct response, because it does this without giving empty platitudes, introducing new worries, or assuming the nurse knows the mother's educational needs before the mother does.

83. Children express and deal with pain in a variety of ways. Although their normal behavior is usually affected, they can "play through their pain." Therefore, their ability to participate in play activities does not mean they aren't in pain. The correct response is **C** because, although children may demonstrate their pain through a change in their vital signs, the vital signs listed in this scenario are within normal limits for a 7 year old.

84. There is not a set age at which children are cognitively ready to accept major responsibility for their own care. In self-medication, it is important that a child be able to identify his medicine, have some idea of time so that he knows it is due, and recognize the importance of taking it appropriately. **A** is the correct response because it is the only answer that contains all these components.

85. **C** is the correct response. Accentuation of the cervical curvature is characteristic of lordosis. Each of the other responses is characteristic of scoliosis.

86. The purpose of therapy is to halt the progression of the curvature. Therefore, **A** is the correct response. Although the Milwaukee brace may prove to be successful at externally realigning the curvature in cases of mild scoliosis, it does not necessarily replace or prevent the need for internal realignment in the future. Muscle atrophy may actually be a complication of externa, realignment therapy; therefore, the brace must be left off for short periods of time. Wearers are instructed to do exercises to prevent atrophy. Kyphosis involves the curvature of the thoracic spine.

87. **D** is the correct response. Each of the responses involved key areas of teaching for the child with a Milwaukee brace. Cathy has verbalized concerns about peer acceptance. The nurse should recognize her need for support and encouragement. Teaching at this time should focus on helping Cathy to learn how to deal with the reactions of others.

88. **B** is the correct response. Each of the responses is appropriate recommendations except **B,** because the brace must be worn for 23 hours each day.

89. **A** is the correct response. A 4-month-old infant will lift his head and chest when in a prone position and bear weight on his forearms. Although he may accidentally roll unto his back, he will not be able to voluntarily do so until 5 months of age. At 6 months, infants accomplish the task of rolls from back to abdomen. It is not until 7 months that an infant can sit alone, using his hands for support.

90. A 4-month-old infant will hold an object in his hand, but he will be unable to willfully reach for and grasp it until 5 months. **D** is the correct response. At 1 month of age, the infant's hands are predominately closed. Infants will not master the transferring of objects from one hand to another until 7 months. Pincher grasp is not established until 10 months.

MENTAL HEALTH EXAM ITEM RATIONALES

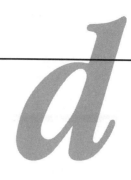

1. The intended response is **D**. Although all four responses might suggest to the nurse that the patient suffers from problem drinking, response **D** provides the most valuable information because it centers on the effect of alcohol abuse on the daily living of the patient. The loss of consciousness associated with "black out" spells certainly underlines the severity of the abusive behavior.

2. The intended response is **B**, since the acutely intoxicated patient is at high risk for self-induced injury, secondary to the loss of judgment, orientation, and behavior control associated with decreased cerebral function as well as the incoordination and poor depth perception associated with decreased cerebellar function.

3. The intended response is **C**. In Freudian theory, the superego functions to set limits on human behavior by ascribing "right" and "wrong" values to that behavior. The alcohol-abusive patient typically lacks such self-control because the superego is underdeveloped and thus unable to guide behavior.

4. The intended response is **D**. The patient undergoing withdrawal from alcohol is prone to developing delirium tremens, which may lead to seizure (convulsant) activity.

5. The intended response is **D**. Mr. Torre's agitation may well be signaling the onset of delirium tremens, which calls the nurse to implement seizure precautions such as upright side rails and bedside airway. A darkened room may cause the patient greater distress, since shadows could heighten hallucinatory experiences common to DTs. The patient is too unstable to be

ambulated, and he should not be placed in soft restraints, which might cause him greater self-injury should seizures occur.

6. The nurse would administer an anti-anxiety medication (response **D**) such as Librium or Valium, not only to calm the patient but also to ward off seizure activity during the detoxification period.

7. The intended response is **D,** since this response by the patient provides the nurse with the greatest amount of information about the influence of alcohol on the patient's life-style, indicating alcohol addiction.

8. The only response that indicates acceptance of an alcohol abuse problem is **D.** In this response, the patient recognizes that he must stop drinking any form of alcohol and maintain sobriety in order to overcome his alcohol addiction.

9. The lab value that should be considered most critical is **B.** A K$^+$ level of 3.0 indicates hypokalemia, a life-threatening electrolyte imbalance that could result in cardiac arrythmia and cardiac arrest.

10. Of the four vital signs, response **B,** pulse, is most essential in light of the patient's hypokalemic state. (Review chapter on fluids and electrolytes for further discussion of this topic if needed.)

11. The intended response is **D.** In this fasting state, Debbie may "spill" ketone bodies in her urine from the excess metabolism of body fat, but she would not "spill" glucose. The urine Dextrostix test, then, is not appropriate to the patient's situation.

12. The nursing diagnosis of highest priority is response **C,** fluid volume deficit, since fluid and associated electrolyte imbalance are most life-threatening to Debbie in her acute anorexic episode.

13. In this *except* question, the intended response is **C.** Anorexic patients tend to perceive excessive parental or peer pressure. All other responses correctly characterize the anorexic patient.

14. Anorexic behavior is believed to be centered in the patient's desire and perceived need for control, response **C.** The behavior is not thought to be intentional self-abuse or self-mutilation, nor is it a mode for punishment of self or others.

15. Debbie will evidence recovery from the psychic issues of anorexia when she is able to engage in eating patterns that are socially acceptable. Response **D,** making a date with a companion for dinner, suggests that the anorexic patient is able to engage in eating patterns in a more acceptable and correct fashion.

16. The intended response is **C,** since the obsessive-compulsive patient attempts to "undo" the underlying feelings that caused the obsession and may act out the associated compulsive behaviors.

17. The intended response is **C.** Although the patient explains her compulsive washing rituals by claiming that she is concerned about germs, the reality is that the patient is attempting to control her underlying obsession by conducting her compulsive rituals. Although the compulsive behavior may reduce her anxiety, the obsession will not be eliminated.

18. The intended response is **B.** The acceptable goal for the obsessive-compulsive patient is that she will accept some limitation on the compulsive behavior. It is unrealistic that the patient will surrender her compulsive rituals altogether.

19. The intended response is **C.** As stated in the above rationale, a realistic goal is for the patient to accept limitation on the ritual. The patient must learn to adjust such rituals in order to accept other responsibilities, such as attendance at therapy sessions.

20. The intended response is **C,** since the patient is evidencing an initial insight into the true source of her obsessive-compulsive behavior, anxiety.

21. The intended response is **C.** Other responses dismiss the patient's experience and fears or are subtly demeaning. The response assures her of safety and conveys staff sensitivity to her behavior and communication.

22. The intended response is **A.** While accepting the patient's current need for distance from others because of her fear, this approach assures Helen of the nurse's concern for her and her availability. It neither supports further regression nor expects adherence to standards she cannot presently meet.

23. The intended response is **D.** The other diagnosis would take priority since it addresses Maslow's lowest hierarchies—physical and safety needs. Without assurance that these needs are met, Helen can direct no energy or attention to socialization.

24. The intended response is **A.** Other responses are more consistent with other subtypes of schizophrenia—disorganized type (hebephrenia), paranoid type, or undifferentiated type.

25. The intended response is **B.** Haldol, a major tranquilizer or neuroleptic, would most likely be prescribed for Helen's immobilizing anxiety. Other drugs mentioned are of very limited or of no proven value in treatment of this acute psychotic process.

26. The intended response is **D.** The other options are all hazards associated with the prolonged immobility and apparent insensitivity to bodily sensa-

tions-functions seen in catatonic patients. Helen's current refusal to eat and move will predispose her to developing complications **A** to **C**. Without further intervention, she may well develop muscle contractures also.

27. The intended response is **C.** Improvement in the catatonic picture is often a slow, gradual process and has been likened to the thawing of an iceberg. Nurses have reported a subjective sense that such patients become more aware or seem to "be here" prior to actual observable motor movements or more apparent levels of increased functioning.

28. The intended response is **C.** A focus on concrete, day-to-day events is less threatening at this level of the patient's recovery. Eventually, with much effort on the part of the nurse and patient, other options may be approached.

29. The intended response is **C.** Delusions by definition are *fixed* false beliefs. No amount of reasoning by the nurse or clergy person will be likely to succeed in shaking Helen's belief. By recognizing her fears, the nurse does not indicate she shares Helen's belief, but can understand her feelings. To dismiss her verbal expressions invites a return to her previous silence.

30. The intended response is **D.** Options **B** and **C** would be assets or resources that might support Helen in her recovery. Rapid onset of symptoms is also often associated with a shorter recovery period and better subsequent adjustments. Strong family history of schizophrenia is often associated with repeated episodes of psychosis and a deteriorating course.

31. The intended response is **B.** One of the primary risks of overdose with tricyclic antidepressants such as Elavil are cardiac arrythmias. Thus EKG changes warrant close attention. Other values are within normal limits or of minimal concern.

32. The intended response is **C.** This option addresses the feelings being communicated by Margaret (covertly) and encourages further communication.

33. The intended response is **A.** This option would be more consistent with a disorder such as schizophrenia where delusions are more commonly seen. Delusions of a bizarre nature are generally not seen in borderline personality disorder. The other behaviors mentioned are common symptoms for borderline patients.

34. The intended response is **D.** Unless clearly a threat to safety, inappropriate behavior or patient's loss of control should be met *initially* with the least aggressive measure. If the patient cannot respond appropriately or regain control, then more active measures may be required. Option **C** conveys to Margaret that her feelings are unmanageable or terribly powerful and will only delay an inevitable confrontation.

35. The intended response is **D.** The scenario described illustrates the defense mechanism of splitting and Margaret's attempt to manage her feelings and anxiety through its use. It is vital the nurse avoid this trap of being "the good guy." Further, though Margaret's behavior is irritating, she deserves an opportunity to discuss the situation and her feelings with concerned others rather than being dismissed or depreciated.

36. The intended response is **A.** This defense mechanism is often seen in the borderline personality disorder.

37. The intended response is **C.** Although Elavil is an antidepressant and ultimately may improve mood, an early indication of effectiveness is evidence of improvement in the so-called vegetative signs such as sleep or appetite disturbance.

38. The intended response is **A.** John provides a "logical" explanation for his inappropriate behavior.

39. The intended response is **D.** All of the other factors are positively correlated with the subsequent diagnosis of sociopathy.

40. The intended response is **B.** Contrary to most lay expectations, sociopaths are often superficially pleasant and quite popular with other patients. They demonstrate keen awareness of the environment at the obvious and subtle levels. They may assume "leadership" roles within the patient group and appear sensitive and supportive to peers.

41. The intended response is **B.** Sociopaths are rarely insightful or genuinely interested in change since they do not share the same values as most of society. Adherence to rules is often only accomplished because of the consistent reinforcement of consequences associated with violation. Limits should be set firmly and consistently without punitive or personal investment.

42. The intended response is **D.** Sociopaths often come to psychiatric facilities by way of the legal system or other institutions. Prognosis is very poor for such individuals, since they experience little personal distress or anxiety.

43. The intended response is **C.** Remorse is rarely expressed by such individuals or evident only in terms of the consequences they themselves will suffer as a result of the inappropriate behavior.

44. The intended response is **C.** Consistent adherence to unit rules and regulations and a focus upon the consequences of their violation are most useful here. The nurse must keep in mind the only benefit seen by the sociopath in relation to others is the potential benefit he or she can obtain through them. The primary and consistent focus of such persons is *me*.

45. The intended response is **C.** Warfarin is an anticoagulant and as such, in excess, may produce symptoms of uncontrolled bleeding. Other symptoms are of a less serious nature and more explainable as a result of efforts to treat the ingestion.

46. The intended response is **C.** Until the nurse has information to the contrary, this ingestion must be regarded as a serious attempt at suicide or evidence of grossly impaired judgment. In either case, the patient's safety needs must be given priority over other considerations.

47. The intended response is **C.** The least restrictive approach possible, given concerns about safety, makes this the best response.

48. The intended response is **A.** An acute organic illness may first become evident in abrupt changes in overall orientation or other cognitive functions. Other symptoms listed are more suggestive of functional difficulties.

49. The intended response is **C.** Other responses all represent commonly held myths about suicide. Although we tend to think first of depressed patients as suicidal risks, psychotic individuals too are to be taken seriously.

50. The intended response is **B.** This behavior is more suggestive of ambivalence—a wish to die but the wish to live also. The other behaviors are all *serious* attempts with indications of ability to follow through on a well-constructed plan and act upon firm intentions to die.

51. The intended response is **A.** Because this drug is absorbed slowly, it can be administered by injection at longer intervals (every 2, 3, or 4 weeks). Thus, for patients with compliance problems of many types this may be the drug of choice.

52. The intended response is **D.** These symptoms may be indicative of tardive dyskinesia, a serious and possibly irreversible consequence of neuroleptic use. The other symptoms are also commonly seen with neuroleptics but may decrease with time or be treated with other medications or means.

53. The intended response is **A.** It is unlikely this goal could be achieved in an individual with such severe, chronic pathology. The other goals *are* potentially achievable and could improve the client's ability to function and could improve his quality of life.

54. The intended response is **B.** John deserves feedback about his behavior and an opportunity to share his perceptions, thoughts, and feelings. This approach validates his improved functional ability and autonomy.

55. The intended response is **B.** The ability to adapt successfully requires that one have resources to draw upon to sustain the self. Ego strengths develop

when the external world can gratify the individual and this sense of goodness be internalized to be drawn upon as needed. For a variety of reasons, the chronically impaired individual is unable to accomplish this task.

56. The intended response is **D.** All the other drugs listed are often prescribed to address specific symptoms of the illness—inflammation, hypermotility of the gastrointestinal tract, and risk of infection. Further, the likelihood of blood loss and anemia caused by the illness itself makes the risks of anticoagulant use very high for this patient.

57. The intended response is **C.** This illness is one that particularly assaults one's sense of body image, autonomy, and self-esteem. Thus, other responses offer explanations consistent with this understanding. Further, psychophysiological illnesses are disorders in which actual physiological alteration of the tissue or organs is seen. No symptoms need to be exaggerated here, nor is there a suggestion of an apparent reason or goal for which Charles would consciously seek to feign physical illness.

58. The intended response is **A.** Highly concentrated solutions utilized to provide high levels of nutrition are quite irritating to small, peripheral veins. The solution is more rapidly diluted and dispersed into circulation when delivered into the larger area of the right atrium. Each of the other responses is clearly false.

59. The intended response is **C.** This response recognizes the level of the patient's anxiety, seeks to maintain the flow of communication, and *begins* with the least intrusive or restrictive intervention. Further, at this point, a here and now orientation may be most helpful and manageable for the patient rather than a "logical" discussion of hypothetical benefits.

60. The intended response is **B.** It most clearly reflects the patient's communicated feeling and avoids exacerbating his sense of isolation and distance from others.

61. The intended response is **C.** Again, the ability to reflect the client's message reassures him he has been heard and is respected. It increases the chances the communication process can continue in an effective, reciprocal manner and respects his autonomy and capabilities.

62. The intended response is **C.** A hazard of TPN and central line use is the potential for infection and generalized sepsis. Other responses are clearly false or present as less likely sources of risk.

63. The intended response is **C.** There are multiple possible etiologies to support this assessment—fever, infectious processes, recent use of anesthetics or other drugs, postoperative fluid and electrolyte changes. The symptoms reported are also more consistent with an organic alteration.

64. The intended response is **C**. All other options make assumptions or inferences about the observations thus far. They are also based on the belief Mr. Humbert's behavior is willful or oppositional in some way and will tend to communicate this to him rather than conveying respect and interest.

65. The intended response is **B**. Given Margaret's age, the lack of physical findings, and a negative prior history, the other disorders are less likely.

66. The intended response is **C**. It both recognizes and restates what the patient has communicated—she gets anxious—and validates that she and her symptoms are taken seriously. Other responses tend to either catastrophize or dismiss the patient and her concern.

67. The intended response is **D**. The physical symptoms represent an *unconscious* conflict and thus are not under Margaret's voluntary control. Additionally, each of the other options suggests psychologic factors that may have influenced the onset or continuance of symptoms.

68. The intended response is **D**. A direct assault upon Margaret's unconscious defensive operations is unlikely to be helpful. Further, any complaint should be taken seriously and explored—patients with conversion disorder also experience physical problems. Answer **D** recognizes that the illness is an expression of conflict and supports the independent, functional abilities of the client while offering continued support and hope.

69. The intended response is **A**. The key words in the question are *short-term* goals. All other options do not demand insight and introspection, processes which require considerable time and effort. Thus, these goals could be achieved more rapidly.

70. The intended response is **B**. Many patients with this disorder have conflicting feelings around issues of dependence and independence. Options **A** and **C** tend to speak to the extremes of this spectrum. Option **D** runs the risk of providing reinforcement for the original "physical" presentation or "secondary gain."

71. The intended response is **C**. Businesslike and matter-of-factly it addresses the identified complaint and avoids judgments. Further, it implies the nurse's ability to control the situation, not withering in the face of the patient's anger or dismissing him as too difficult to deal with.

72. The intended response is **B**. The other symptoms are also usually associated with psychotic processes but are quite different from the rapid and confusing reporting of many thoughts or ideas seen in this symptom.

73. The intended response is **D**. It is least likely to yield concrete data helpful in making a diagnosis and most likely to elicit a defensive response.

74. The intended response is **B.** It would be rare to see such a late onset of schizophrenia in an individual without prior history. Further, a history of marriage and good social relations is also less consistent with this diagnosis. The alteration in sleep pattern is also more consistent with the other diagnoses.

75. The intended response is **D.** Although some depressed patients complain of insomnia, careful questioning often reveals they can get to sleep but often awaken during the night or early in the morning having considerable difficulty getting back to sleep. The overall total sleep time is often decreased in depressed patients, although some young depressives report hypersomnia.

76. The intended response is **A.** Manic patients are rarely mute and rarely complain of fatigue or an inability to enjoy pleasurable activities. All other behaviors are more typically seen in mania.

77. The intended response is **D.** This option offers a structured means of channeling the patient's high energy level without excessively demanding either concentration or self-control. Both of these latter abilities are often impaired during acute phases of the illness.

78. The intended response is **C.** The reported level is far in excess of therapeutic range and approaching dangerously toxic levels. The patient should be observed closely, lithium held until a second level is determined, and, subsequently, dosages altered if needed.

79. The intended response is **B.** The feedback provides concrete behavioral information as to a change since taking lithium. It allows the patient to consider the information and make his own decision without engaging in a power struggle, placating, or assaulting defenses.

80. The intended response is **B.** Although each of the patient's reported symptoms should be evaluated and addressed as a possible drug side-effect or other symptomatology, option **B** may be indicative of severe lithium toxicity. Gait disturbances and ataxic movements are signs of the neurotoxic effects of excessive amounts of the drug.

81. The intended response is **A.** With prolonged absence, the likelihood of greater anxiety and continuation of the problem increases. Interventions will not stop there, however. The other responses are also untrue.

82. The intended response is **B.** Other responses are likely to elicit anxiety and defensiveness. Option **B** restates Mr. Johnson's communication to let him know that he has been heard but offers further opportunity for exploration, suggesting the problem may be more complex.

83. The intended response is **C.** Billy is the third party who has become the focus of his parents' conflict. Through him they express feelings or issues that most likely relate to their relationship.

84. The intended response is **C.** Billy's symptoms are least likely to be improved by this approach, since his anxiety is more likely related to conflicts at home. Each of the other interventions has been shown to be effective singly or in combination.

85. The intended response is **A.** This criterion is measurable and speaks most specifically to the behavior for which the family sought assistance. Although the other options may be desirable, they do not necessarily mean the problem is resolved.

86. The intended response is **B.** This provides concrete evidence of a safety hazard for the mother. She needs supervision, and this may be provided in the daughter's home or through other similar means.

87. The intended response is **C.** There is no way of knowing what caused the mother's anxiety. However, it is not unusual to see mild to moderate levels of anxiety in patients with Alzheimer's before cognitive impairment is obvious.

88. The intended response is **C.** For those with cognitive impairments, the structure of and cues provided by a *familiar* environment are very helpful. Any change to a new and unfamiliar setting may well result in increased anxiety, confusion, and disorientation.

89. The intended response is **C.** The limitations of a cognitive impairment make changes more difficult to assimilate. Thus, preserving as much of the familiar as possible and making the change slowly should help minimize the trauma and anxiety.

90. The intended response is **D.** This option is more likely to be the focus of a therapeutic group that encourages insight and intrapsychic exploration.

Appendix A
National Council of State Boards of Nursing, Inc.
Boards of Nursing

Alabama

Executive Officer
Alabama Board of Nursing
Suite 203, 500 Eastern Blvd.
Montgomery, Alabama 36117   Tel: (205) 261-4060

Alaska

Executive Secretary
Alaska Board of Nursing
Dept. of Commerce and
Economic Development
Div. of Occupational Licensing
3601 C. Street, Suite 722
Anchorage, Alaska 99503   Tel: (907) 561-2878

For Licensing Information

Licensing Examiner
Board of Nursing
Pouch "D"
Juneau, Alaska 99811

American Samoa

Executive Secretary
American Samoa Health Service

Regulatory Board
Pago Pago, American Samoa 96799   Tel: (684) 633-1222 ext. 206

Arizona

Acting Executive Director
Arizona State Board of Nursing
5050 N. 19th Avenue, Suite 103
Phoenix, Arizona 85015   Tel: (602) 255-5092

Arkansas

Executive Director
Arkansas State Board of Nursing
University Towers Building, Suite
   800
Little Rock, Arkansas 72204   Tel: (501) 371-2751

California

Executive Officer
California Board of Registered Nursing
1030—13th Street, Suite 200
Sacramento, California 95814   Tel: (501) 371-2751

Executive Office
California Board of Vocational
   Nurse and Psychiatric
   Technician Examiners
1020 N. State, Room 406
Sacramento, California 95814   Tel: (916) 342-2715

Colorado

Program Administrator
Colorado Board of Nursing
State Services Bldg., Room 132
1525 Sherman Street
Denver, Colorado 80203   Tel: (303) 866-2871

Connecticut

Executive Officer
Connecticut Board of Examiners for
   Nursing

150 Washington Street
Hartford, Connecticut 06106   Tel: (203) 566-1041

For Licensing Information

Section Chief, Applications
Examinations and Licensure
Div. of Medical Quality Assurance
Connecticut Dept. of Health Services
150 Washington Street
Hartford, Connecticut 06106

Delaware

Executive Director
Delaware Board of Nursing
Margaret O'Neill Building
P.O. Box 1401
Dover, Delaware 19901   Tel: (302) 736-4752

District of Columbia

Contact Person
District of Columbia Board of Nursing
614 H. Street, N.W.
Washington, D.C. 20001   Tel: (202) 727-7468

Florida

Executive Director
Florida Board of Nursing
111 Coastline Drive, East
Jacksonville, Florida 32202   Tel: (904) 359-6331

Georgia

Executive Director
Georgia Board of Nursing
166 Pryor Street, S.W.
Atlanta, Georgia 30303   Tel: (404) 656-3943

Executive Director
Georgia State Board of Licensed
  Practical Nurses
166 Pryor Street, S.W.
Atlanta, Georgia 30303   Tel: (404) 656-3921

Guam

Nurse Examiner Administrator
Guam Board of Nurse Examiners
P.O. Box 2816
Agana, Guam 96910   Tel: (671) 734-4813

Hawaii

Executive Secretary
Hawaii Board of Nursing
P.O. Box 3469
Honolulu, Hawaii 96801   Tel: (808) 548-3086

Idaho

Executive Director
Idaho Board of Nursing
500 South 10th Street
Suite 102
Boise, Idaho 83720   Tel: (208) 334-3110

Illinois

Nursing Education Coordinator
Illinois Department of Registration
   and Education
320 West Washington Street 3rd
   Floor
Springfield, Illinois 62786   Tel: (217) 782-4386

Indiana

Board Administrator
Indiana State Board of Nursing
Health Professions Bureau
One American Square
Suite 1020, Box 82067
Indianapolis, Indiana 46282-0004   Tel: (317) 232-2960

Iowa

Executive Director
Iowa Board of Nursing
Executive Hills East
1223 East Court
Des Moines, Iowa 50319   Tel: (515) 281-3256

Kansas

Executive Administrator
Kansas Board of Nursing
Landon State Office Building
900 S.W. Jackson, Suite 551 S
Topeka, Kansas 66612-1256   Tel: (913) 296-4929

Kentucky

Executive Director
Kentucky Board of Nursing
4010 Dupont Circle, Suite 430
Louisville, Kentucky 40207   Tel: (502) 897-5143

Louisiana

Executive Director
Louisiana State Board of Nursing
907 Pere Marquette Building
150 Baronne Street
New Orleans, Louisiana 70112   Tel: (504) 568-5464

Executive Director
Louisiana State Board of Practical
    Nurse Examiners
Tidewaters Place
1440 Canal Street, Suite 2010
New Orleans, Louisiana 70112   Tel: (504) 568-6480

Maine

Executive Director
Maine State Board of Nursing
295 Water Street
Augusta, Maine 04330   Tel: (207) 289-5324

Maryland

Executive Director
Maryland Board of Examiners of
    Nurses
201 West Preston Street
Baltimore, Maryland 21201   Tel: (301) 225-5880

Massachusetts

Executive Secretary
Massachusetts Board of Registration
  in Nursing
Leverett Saltonstall Building
100 Cambridge Street, Room 1519
Boston, Massachusetts 02202   Tel: (617) 727-7393

Michigan

Nursing Consultant
Michigan Board of Nursing
Dept. of Licensing & Regulation
Ottawa Towers North
611 West Ottawa
P.O. Box 30018
Lansing, Michigan 48909   Tel: (517) 373-1600

Administrative Assistant
Michigan Board of Nursing
Dept. of Licensing & Regulation
Ottawa Towers North
611 West Ottawa
P.O. Box 30018
Lansing, Michigan 48909   Tel: (517) 373-1600

For Examination Information

Office of Testing Services   Tel: (517) 373-3877

Minnesota

Executive Director
Minnesota Board of Nursing
2700 University Avenue West, #108
St. Paul, Minnesota 55114   Tel: (612) 642-0572

Mississippi

Executive Director
Mississippi Board of Nursing
135 Bounds Street, Suite 101
Jackson, Mississippi 39206   Tel: (601) 354-7349

Missouri

Executive Director
Missouri State Board of Nursing

P.O. Box 656
3523 North Ten Mile Drive
Jefferson City, Missouri 65102   Tel: (314) 751-2334 ext. 141

Montana

Executive Secretary
Montana State Board of Nursing
Department of Commerce
Division of Business and Profes-
    sional Licensing
1424 9th Avenue
Helena, Montana 59620-0407   Tel: (406) 444-4279

Nebraska

Associate Director
Bureau of Examining Boards
Nebraska Department of Health
P.O. Box 95007   Tel: (402) 471-2001 or
Lincoln, Nebraska 68509   (402) 471-4358

Nevada

Executive Director
Nevada State Board of Nursing
1281 Terminal Way, Suite 116
Reno, Nevada 89502   Tel: (702) 786-2778

New Hampshire

Acting Executive Director
New Hampshire Board of Nursing
    Education & Nurse Registration
Department of Health and Human
    Services
78 Regional Drive
Building B, Room #7
Concord, New Hampshire 03301   Tel: (603) 271-2323

New Jersey

Executive Director
New Jersey Board of Nursing
1100 Raymond Blvd., Room 319
Newark, New Jersey 07102   Tel: (201) 648-2570

New Mexico

Executive Director
New Mexico Board of Nursing
4125 Carlisle N.E.
Albuquerque, New Mexico 87107   Tel: (505) 841-6524 ext. 28

New York

Supervisor/Nursing Education
New York State Board for Nursing
State Education Department
Cultural Education Center   Tel: (518) 474-3843 or
Room 3013   474-3844 or
Albany, New York 12230   474-3845

For Licensing Information

Supervisor
Division of Professional Licensing
     Services
State Education Department
Cultural Education Center
Albany, New York 12230   Tel: (518) 474-3817

North Carolina

Executive Director
North Carolina Board of Nursing
P.O. Box 2129
Raleigh, North Carolina 27602   Tel: (919) 828-0740

North Dakota

Executive Director
North Dakota Board of Nursing
Kirkwood Office Tower
Suite 504
7th Street South & Arbor Avenue
Bismarck, North Dakota 58501   Tel: (701) 224-2974

Northern Mariana Islands

Chairperson
Commonwealth Board of Nurse Ex-
     aminers
Public Health Center

Tel: (0-11-670) area code
     234-8950 or
     234-8951 or
     234-8952 or
     234-8953 or

P.O. Box 1458
Saipan, CM 96950

234-8954
Tel: 234-2018 or 2019

Public Health Center

Ohio

Executive Secretary
Ohio Board of Nursing Education
    and Nurse Registration
65 South Front Street
Suite 509
Columbus, Ohio 43266-0316

Tel: (614) 466-3947

Oklahoma

Executive Director
Oklahoma Board of Nurse Registra-
    tion & Nursing Education
2915 North Classen Boulevard
Suite 524
Oklahoma City, Oklahoma 73106

Tel: (405) 525-2076

Oregon

Executive Director
Oregon State Board of Nursing
1400 S.W. 5th Avenue, Room 904
Portland, Oregon 97201

Tel: (503) 229-5653

Pennsylvania

Executive Secretary
Pennsylvania Board of Nursing
Department of State
P.O. Box 2649
Harrisburg, Pennsylvania 17105

Tel: (717) 787-8503

Rhode Island

Executive Secretary
Rhode Island Board of Nursing Reg-
    istration & Nursing Education
Cannon Health Building
75 Davis Street, Room 104
Providence, Rhode Island 02908-
    2488

Tel: (401) 277-2827

South Carolina

Executive Director
State Board of Nursing for South
  Carolina
1777 St. Julian Place, Suite 102
Columbia, South Carolina 29204-
  2488   Tel: (803) 737-3800

Administration & Info: Tel: (803) 737-6594

Educational & Exam Svcs.:   Tel: (803) 737-6596

Legal & Disciplinary Svcs.:   Tel: (803) 737-6598

Accounting & Computer Svcs.: Tel: (803) 737-6598

South Dakota

Executive Secretary
South Dakota Board of Nursing
304 South Phillips Avenue, Suite 205
Sioux Falls, South Dakota 57102   Tel: (605) 334-1243

Tennessee

Executive Director
Tennessee State Board of Nursing
283 Plus Park Boulevard
Nashville, Tennessee 37217   Tel: (615) 367-6232

Texas

Executive Secretary
Board of Nurse Examiners for the
  State of Texas
1300 East Anderson Lane
Building C, Suite 225
Austin, Texas 78752   Tel: (512) 835-4880

Executive Director
Texas Board of Vocational Nurse
  Examiners
1300 East Anderson Lane
Building C, Suite 285
Austin, Texas 78752   Tel: (512) 835-2071

Utah

Executive Secretary and Nurse Con-
  sultant
Utah State Board of Nursing
Division of Occupational and Profes-
  sional Licensing
Heber M. Wells Building, 4th Floor
160 East 300 South
P.O. Box 45802
Salt Lake City, Utah 84145   Tel: (801) 530-6628

Vermont

Executive Director
Vermont State Board of Nursing
Redstone Building
26 Terrace Street
Montpelier, Vermont 05602   Tel: (802) 828-2396

Virgin Islands

Chairperson
Virgin Islands Board of Nurse Licen-
  sure
Division of Professional Licensing
P.O. Box 7309
Charlotte Amalie
St. Thomas, Virgin Islands 00801   Tel: (809) 774-9000 Ext. 132

Virginia

Executive Director
Virginia State Board of Nursing
1601 Rolling Hills Drive
Richmond, Virginia 23229-5005   Tel: (804) 662-9909

Washington

Executive Secretary
Washington State Board of Nursing
Department of Licensing
P.O. Box 9649
Olympia, Washington 98504   Tel: (206) 586-1923

For Licensing Information   Tel: (206) 753-3728

West Virginia

Executive Secretary
West Virginia Board of Examiners for
  Registered Nurses
922 Quarrier Street
Suite 309, Embleton Building
Charleston, West Virginia 25301   Tel: (304) 348-3596

Executive Secretary
West Virginia State Board of Examin-
  ers for Practical Nurses
922 Quarrier Street
Suite 506, Embleton Building
Charleston, West Virginia 25301   Tel: (304) 348-3572

Wisconsin

Director
Wisconsin Bureau of Nursing
Dept. of Regulation & Licensing
1400 East Washington Avenue
P.O. Box 8936
Madison, Wisconsin 53708-8936   Tel: (608) 266-3735

Wyoming

Executive Director
Wyoming State Board of Nursing
Barrett Building, 4th Floor
2301 Central Avenue
Cheyenne, Wyoming 82002   Tel: (307) 777-7601

APPENDIX B
APPROVED NURSING DIAGNOSES, NORTH AMERICAN NURSING DIAGNOSIS ASSOCIATION, JUNE 1988

Activity intolerance
Activity intolerance, potential
Adjustment, impaired
Airway clearance, ineffective
Anxiety
Aspiration, potential for
Body temperature, altered, potential
Bowel elimination, altered: Constipation
    Colonic constipation
    Perceived constipation
Bowel elimination, altered: Diarrhea
Bowel elimination, altered: Incontinence
Breastfeeding, ineffective
Breathing pattern, ineffective
Cardiac output, altered: Decreased (specify)
Comfort, altered: Pain
Comfort, altered: Chronic pain
Communication, impaired: Verbal
Coping, family: Potential for growth
Coping, ineffective, family: Compromised
Coping, ineffective, family: Disabling
Coping, ineffective, individual
    Defensive coping
    Ineffective denial
Decisional conflict (specify)
Disuse syndrome, potential for
Diversional activity, deficit

Dysreflexia
Family process, altered
Fatigue
Fear
Fluid volume excess
Fluid volume deficit, actual
Fluid volume deficit, potential
Gas exchange, impaired
Grieving, anticipatory
Grieving, dysfunctional
Growth and development, altered
Health maintenance, altered
Health-seeking behaviors (specify)
Home maintenance, impaired
Hopelessness
Hyperthermia
Hypothermia
Incontinence, functional
Incontinence, reflex
Incontinence, stress
Incontinence, total
Incontinence, urge
Infection, potential for
Injury, potential for (specify): suffocation, poisoning, trauma
Knowledge deficit (specify)
Mobility, impaired physical
Noncompliance (specify)
Nutrition, altered: Less than body requirements
Nutrition, altered: More than body requirements
Nutrition, altered: Potential for more than body requirements
Oral mucous membrane, altered
Parental role conflict
Parenting, altered: Actual
Parenting, altered: Potential
Post trauma response
Powerlessness
Rape trauma syndrome
Role performance, altered
Self-care deficit: Feeding, bathing/hygiene, dressing/grooming, toileting
Self-concept, disturbance in body image, self-esteem, role performance,
    personal identity
Self-esteem disturbance
    Chronic low self-esteem
    Situational low self-esteem
Sensory/perceptual alteration: Visual, auditory, kinesthetic, gustatory, tac-
    tile, olfactory

Sexual dysfunction
Sexuality patterns, altered
Skin integrity, impaired: Actual
Skin integrity, impaired: Potential
Sleep pattern disturbance
Social interaction, impaired
Social isolation
Spiritual distress (distress of the human spirit)
Swallowing, impaired
Thermoregulation, ineffective
Thought processes, altered
Tissue integrity, impaired
Tissue perfusion, altered: Cerebral, cardiopulmonary, renal, gastrointestinal, peripheral
Unilateral neglect
Urinary elimination, altered patterns
Urinary retention
Violence, potential for: Self-directed or directed at others

INDEX

Page numbers in italics denote figures; page numbers followed by *t* denote tables.